A Primer of

WATER, ELECTROLYTE AND
ACID-BASE SYNDROMES

A PRIMER OF
WATER, ELECTROLYTE AND
ACID-BASE SYNDROMES

EMANUEL GOLDBERGER, M.D., F.A.C.P.

Clinical Associate Professor of Medicine, New York Medical College,
Valhalla, New York; Attending Physician (Cardiology), Montefiore
Hospital and Medical Center, New York, New York

With Contributions By

Jeffrey M. Brensilver, M.D., D-IM (Nephrology)

Assistant Professor of Clinical Medicine, Columbia University
College of Physicians and Surgeons, New York, New York

SEVENTH EDITION

 Lea & Febiger   *Philadelphia*   *1986*

Lea & Febiger
600 Washington Square
Philadelphia, PA 19106-4198
U.S.A.
(215) 922-1330

First Edition, 1959
Second Edition, 1962
Third Edition, 1965
Fourth Edition, 1970
Fifth Edition, 1975
Sixth Edition, 1980
Seventh, Edition, 1986

Translated into
Greek
Italian
Japanese
Portuguese
Spanish
Turkish

Library of Congress Cataloging in Publication Data

Goldberger, Emanuel, 1913–
   A primer of water, electrolyte, and acid-base
syndromes.
   Includes bibliographies and index.
   1. Water-electrolyte imbalances. 2. Acid-base im-
balances. 3. Fluid therapy. I. Brensilver, Jeffrey M.
II. Title. III. Title: Water, electrolyte, and acid-base
syndromes.
RC630.G6   1986   616.3'9   85-19909
ISBN 0-8121-1015-3

Pharm.
RC
630
G6
1986

Printed in the United States of America

Print number: 4   3   2   1

To my grandson

Zachary David Goldberger

Preface

In preparing this seventh edition I have added much new material, including anion gap, treatment of heat disorders, treatment of SIADH, use of oral electrolyte solutions to treat severe diarrheas and cholera, new fluid resuscitation formulas for burns, serum osmolality, use of low-dose IV and IM insulin in diabetic acidosis, use of IV HCl in metabolic alkalosis, primary aldosteronism, familial hypercalciuric hypercalcemia, dextran, mannitol, hetastarch, urea, fat emulsions, amino acids for peripheral parenteral nutrition. I have included an improved diagram to illustrate the various metabolic and respiratory acid-base disorders. The bibliographies at the end of each chapter have been brought up-to-date.

Nephrology has become a full-fledged specialty since the first edition of this book and there are now many monographs on that subject. Therefore I have been able to shorten the book by deleting the chapter on peritoneal dialysis. And I have also condensed the chapters on renal disorders. Similarly there are now many monographs on total parenteral nutrition and I have eliminated this as well as material on enteral nutrition.

As in previous editions, I have correlated electrolyte and acid-base disturbances with the clinical pictures of patients, and have continued to emphasize that "at the end of a needle there is a patient."

I want to thank Dr. Jeffrey M. Brensilver, Attending Nephrologist, St. Luke's Hospital, New York, for his help in revising the sections on renal physiology and renal disorders. I also want to thank my son, Dr. Ary Louis Goldberger, for many helpful suggestions. Last but not least, I want to express my deep appreciation to my wife for her ever-present patience, interest, and encouragement.

New York, New York   Emanuel Goldberger

Contents

PART 1

THE EXTRACELLULAR WATER

CHAPTER 1

THE BODY WATER

About a billion years ago, life began—in the sea. The sea possessed unique properties for the maintenance of life. For example, the water of the sea is a solvent for the electrolytes and the oxygen that are necessary for life. The sea is also a solvent for the carbon dioxide which accumulates during life's processes. Since the carbon dioxide is volatile, it can be easily dissipated from the surface of the sea. In addition, the volume of the sea is so great that it can absorb large amounts of heat, or lose large amounts of heat, with only relatively small changes in temperature. The volume of the sea is also so great that significant changes in its composition occur only over a period of hundreds of thousands of years. Finally, its dielectric constant, its surface tension, and other physical properties are all important in maintaining and protecting life.

As a result, the water that surrounds the cells of vertebrates and of man, namely, the extracellular water, still has an electrolyte composition similar to that which the sea had in prerecorded times, in spite of all the countless changes in evolution that have occurred. Over the eons, the rivers of the world have eroded land and have washed elements into the sea. This has caused the electrolytes of the sea to become more concentrated. In spite of this, there is still a remarkable similarity between the proportional composition of electrolytes in sea water and in extracellular water. This is shown in Figure 1–1.

TOTAL BODY WATER

The total amount of water in the body can be determined by introducing into the body a known quantity of a substance that diffuses evenly throughout the extracellular water and the cells, and then determining its concentration. Antipyrine, urea, thiourea, and more recently "heavy water" (deuterium oxide, or tritium oxide) have been used for this purpose.

Fig. 1–1.   The electrolyte concentrations of sea water compared to extracellular water. (After Gamble.)

THE EXTRACELLULAR WATER

The body water is usually divided into two main compartments: the *extracellular water* (extracellular fluid) and the *intracellular water* (intracellular fluid). The extracellular water includes the plasma water and the *interstitial water* (the fluid in the tissue spaces, lying between the cells). Gastrointestinal secretions, urine, sweat, exudates, and transudates can also be considered as specialized portions of the extracellular water, because when these are lost a severe loss of extracellular water occurs.

The relations of the body water to the body weight are as follows:

Water Compartment	Percentage of Body Weight	Volume in Liters (man, 70 kg)
Plasma water (plus)	4	2.8
Interstitial water	16	11.2
Total extracellular water (plus)	= 20	= 14.
Intracellular water	40	28.
Total average body water in a man	= 60	= 42.
Total average body water in a 70 kg woman	50	35.

These figures represent average values which I shall use in calculating water and electrolyte requirements in this book.

The total body water varies. It is related principally to the fat content of the body, and to sex. Fat has relatively little water associated with it. Therefore, a fat person will have relatively less water than a thin person. In addition, a woman has a lower content of body water than a man. The water content of the body also decreases with age.

The average water content of a man is approximately 60%. The average water content of a woman is approximately 50%.

Body water is also composed of inaccessible bone water and transcellular fluids.

Transcellular fluids include the fluids of organs such as the kidneys, liver, pancreas, and so on, the skin and mucous membranes of the gastrointestinal and respiratory tracts, cerebrospinal fluid, the intraluminal fluid of the gastrointestinal tract, and so on. It is difficult to measure the volume of the fluid in these compartments.

Body water, including percentage of fat and of lean body tissue can now be measured using a bioelectrical impedance analyzer.

The Electrolytes in the Extracellular Water

Chemists are able to determine the nature and the concentration of the electrolytes in both the extracellular water and in the cells. However, the determination of electrolyte concentration in the cells requires special research technics. Therefore, physicians must rely on the changes in electrolyte concentration in the extracellular water, particularly in the plasma or serum, in treating patients.

The relative concentration of electrolytes in the extracellular water and in the cells is shown in Figure 1–2. Notice that sodium (Na) and chloride (Cl) are the principal electrolytes in the extracellular water.

Fig. 1–2.   The relations between extracellular and intracellular water. (After Gamble.)

However, potassium (K) and phosphates (PO$_4$) are the principal electrolytes in the cells.

The extracellular preponderance of sodium and the intracellular preponderance of potassium are not due to the impermeability of the cell membrane to sodium, because recent studies with isotopic sodium have shown that the sodium passes rapidly across cell membranes. In other words, some mechanism exists by which sodium is actively extruded from the cells. The extracellular preponderance of sodium ions and the intracellular preponderance of potassium ions are maintained by an energy (ATP) dependent cell membrane "pump" that exchanges sodium and potassium ions.

Figure 1–1 shows that the electrolyte concentration of the plasma (or serum) is slightly different from the electrolyte concentration in the interstitial portion of the extracellular water. The major difference is that the protein concentration of the plasma is greater than that of the interstitial portion of the extracellular water. This is due to the fact that

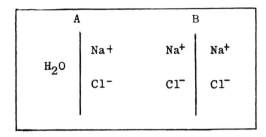

Fig. 1–3. The Donnan equilibrium. See text.

the capillary walls prevent the outward movement of most of the protein from the plasma. As a result, the sodium concentration in plasma is slightly greater than the sodium concentration in the interstitial water. Conversely, the chloride concentration in the plasma is slightly less than the chloride concentration in the interstitial water. These differences can be explained by the Donnan equilibrium.

The Donnan Equilibrium. Let us place water on one side of a membrane, and a solution of sodium chloride (NaCl) on the other (Fig. 1–3A). If the membrane is permeable to sodium and chloride ions, the sodium and chloride will pass through the membrane until their concentrations on both sides are equal (Fig. 1–3B).

Now, let us place a sodium chloride solution, NaCl, on one side of the membrane, and a sodium salt of a protein, NaR, on the other side (the symbol R represents the protein ion) (Fig. 1–4A). Let us further suppose that the membrane is impermeable to the protein ion, R, but is permeable to all other ions.

The British physicist Donnan showed that, even in such a case, the sodium chloride on the right side of the membrane will diffuse across the membrane into the left side of the solution (Fig. 1–4B). Furthermore, at equilibrium, the product of the concentrations of the sodium ions and of the chloride ions on one side of the membrane will be the same as the product of the concentrations of the same ions on the other side of the membrane. In other words,

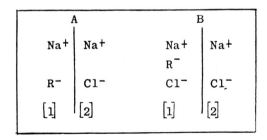

Fig. 1–4. The Donnan equilibrium. See text.

Fig. 1–5.   The cation and anion concentrations of extracellular water. (After Gamble.)

$Na_1 \times Cl_1 = Na_2 \times Cl_2$ (Fig. 1–4B).

In compartment (1), the concentration of sodium must be equal to the sum of the other ions, namely, R plus Cl. In compartment (2), on the other side of the membrane, the concentration of sodium (Na) must be the same as that of chloride (Cl). Since the products of sodium times chloride on both sides of the membrane are equal, it follows that the concentration of sodium ions in compartment (1) must be greater than in compartment (2), on the right. The reverse must be true for the chloride ions.

The Concentration of Electrolytes in the Extracellular Water

Figure 1–5 gives the values of the cations and the anions of the extracellular water. An *ion* is an atom or group of atoms with an electrical charge. When it has a positive electrical charge, it is called a *cation*. When it has a negative electrical charge, it is called an *anion*.

The terms "cation" and "anion" can be remembered by the following mnemonic device. A cation has a positive charge. It also has the letter T in it; the T resembles the (+) symbol for a positive charge.

The electrolyte concentrations are given in terms of milliequivalents per liter of serum or plasma (mEq/L).

Milliequivalents. Over 200 years ago, when modern chemistry began, it was noted that the weights of two given elements that could combine chemically with each other always had a fixed ratio or set of ratios. For example, 1 g of hydrogen would combine with 7.937 g of oxygen to form water, or with 35.5 g of chlorine to form hydrochloric acid. Chemists later determined that actually two *atoms* of hydrogen combined with one *atom* of oxygen. In other words, oxygen had a valence of 2, compared to hydrogen. In addition, weights of the hydrogen and oxygen atoms had a ratio of 1:(2 × 7.937), or 1:15.873.

For convenience, chemists later decided to set the atomic weight of oxygen arbitrarily at 16. The combining or equivalent weight of oxygen therefore became $\frac{16}{2}$ or 8; and hydrogen had both an atomic and a combining or equivalent weight of $\frac{1}{15.873}$ × 16, or 1.008.

This concept of combining or *equivalent weights* is useful. It enables the chemist to predict that 1 g of hydrogen (at.wt. 1, valence 1) will combine with 35.5 g of chlorine (at.wt. 35.5, valence 1), and that 2 g of hydrogen will combine with 16 g of oxygen (at.wt. 16, valence 2). Similarly 23 g of sodium (at.wt. 23, valence 1) or 39 g of potassium (at.wt. 39, valence 1) will combine with 35.5 g of chlorine.

An equivalent weight or *equivalent* can therefore be described as the atomic weight of an atom (or a group of atoms, such as NH_4, which reacts chemically as a unit, or of a molecule) divided by its valence. Just as a millimeter is $\frac{1}{1000}$ of a meter, a milliequivalent weight or *milliequivalent* is $\frac{1}{1000}$ of an equivalent.

The electrolytes of the body are in solution, mostly in the form of ions. Their concentration can be described in terms of weight, such as milligrams (mg) per deciliter (dl) of blood (mg/dl; a deciliter, or one-tenth of a liter, is the same as 100 ml). Since the concentrations of the various electrolytes are small, they are expressed as milliequivalents per liter, mEq/L.

These values are shown in Figure 1–5. Notice that the concentration of the cations is the same as the concentration of the anions in blood serum or plasma when expressed in terms of milliequivalents. In other words, each liter of blood has 155 mEq of cations (Na, K, Ca, Mg) and 155 mEq of anions (bicarbonate, chloride, sulfate, phosphate, organic acid anions and protein anions). However, if the concentration of these electrolytes in the blood is expressed in terms of mg/100 ml (mg/dl), no balance or relationship between the cations and anions would be evident. This is shown in Figure 1–6.

The Relationship Between Milliequivalents and Milligrams. The re-

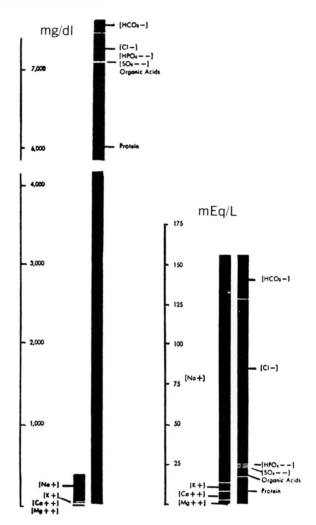

Fig. 1–6.   The value of calculations in terms of mEq/L, rather than in terms of milligrams per deciliter (mg/dl). See text.

lationship between milliequivalents and milligrams can be expressed as follows: The weight of a salt in milligrams can be converted into milliequivalents by dividing its weight in milligrams by its molecular weight, and multiplying by the valence.

Example:
1 g (1000 mg) NaCl = 17.1 mEq
proof:
Na (at.wt. 23; valence, 1) Cl (at.wt. 35.5; valence, 1) Na + Cl = 58.5
$$\frac{1000}{58.5} = 17.1 \text{ mEq}$$

Since the electrolyte concentrations in blood serum are usually expressed in mEq/L, the following formulas can be used to convert mg/dl into mEq/L, or vice versa:

$$mEq/L = \frac{mg/dl \times 10 \times valence}{atomic\ weight}$$

$$mg/dl = \frac{mEq/L \times atomic\ weight}{10 \times valence}$$

Table 1–1 gives conversion factors that enable these values to be obtained more easily.

Moles and Millimoles. There is another way of expressing the weight of chemical substances. A *mole* of a substance is the molecular weight of that substance in grams. For example, the chemical formula of the glucose molecule is $C_6H_{12}O_6$. Since carbon has an atomic weight of 12, hydrogen, 1, and oxygen, 16, the molecular weight of glucose is 12 × 6 (carbon) plus 1 × 12 (hydrogen) plus 16 × 6 (oxygen) or 180. Therefore, 1 mole of glucose = 180 g.

A *millimole* (mM) is $\frac{1}{1000}$ of a mole. Therefore, 1 millimole of glucose is $\frac{1}{1000}$ of 180 g, or 180 mg.

Similarly, the molecular weight of NaCl is: sodium (at.wt. 23) plus chlorine (at.wt. 35.5), or 58.5 g. Therefore, 1 mole NaCl = 58.5 g, and 1 millimole (mM) = 58.5 mg.

The weight of a salt in milligrams can be converted into moles or millimoles by dividing the weight in milligrams by the molecular weight, in a way similar to that used to convert milligrams into equivalents and milliequivalents.

Example:
1 g (1000 mg) NaCl = 17.1 millimoles.
1000 divided by the molecular weight of NaCl, which is 58.5 = 17.1.

The concept of moles and millimoles can also be applied to ions, such as Na, K, HCO_3, and so forth. A mole of any ion is its atomic weight (or the sum of the atomic weights of its elements) expressed in grams.

Example:
1 mole Na (at.wt. 23) = 23 g
1 mM Na = 23 mg
1 mole HCO_3 (sum of the atomic weights, H, C, and 3 – 0 = 61) = 61 g

The concentration of gases can also be expressed in terms of milliequivalents. One mole of an ideal gas at a standard temperature of 0°C, and 760 mm Hg pressure, occupies 22.4 liters. Therefore, 1 millimole occupies 22.4 ml. However, 1 mole of CO_2 occupies a slightly smaller volume of 22.26 liters, and a millimole of CO_2 occupies 22.26 ml.

The concentration of a gas dissolved in a fluid such as water can be

Table 1–1. Table for Converting Serum or Plasma Electrolyte Concentrations in mEq/L, or mg/100 ml (After Weisberg, and Others.)

Electrolyte	Calculated as:	Atomic weight	Valence	Equivalent weight	Conversion factors mEq/L from mg/dl—DIVIDE; mg/dl from mEq/L—MULTIPLY	Normal ranges (serum or plasma) mg/dl	Normal ranges (serum or plasma) mEq/L
CATIONS							
Sodium	Sodium	23	1	23	2.3	310–335	136–145
Potassium	Potassium	39	1	39	3.9	13.7–19.5	3.5–5.0
Calcium	Total calcium	40	2	20	2.	9.0–11	4.5–5.5
Magnesium	Magnesium	24	2	12	1.2	1.8–3.0	1.5–2.5
ANIONS							
Bicarbonate	CO_2 content			22.26	2.2	53–75 (avg. 62) vol. %	24–33 (avg. 28)
Chloride	Chloride	35.5	1	35.5	3.5	350–375	98–106
	Sodium chloride	58.5	1	58.5	5.8	570–620	98–106
Phosphate	Phosphorus	31	1.8	17.2	1.7	2–4.5	1.2–3.0
Sulfate	Sulfur	32	2	16.	1.6	0.5–2.5	0.3–1.5
Protein	Protein				.41	6–8 g	14.6–19.4

The phosphate is calculated as phosphorus, with a valence of 1.8. The reason for this is that at the normal pH of the extracellular water, 20% of the phosphate ions are in a form with one sodium equivalent (NaH_2PO_4), and 80% are in a form with two sodium equivalents (Na_2HPO_4). The total valence is therefore $(0.2 \times 1) + (0.8 \times 2) = 1.8$.

expressed in terms of the ml of the gas dissolved in 100 ml of the fluid, or in terms of millimoles per liter.

The following formulas can be used to convert volumes % of CO_2 (or bicarbonate) to millimoles per liter, (or milliequivalents per liter) and vice versa.

$$\text{mM } CO_2/L = \frac{\text{Vol \%}^* CO_2}{22.2} \times 10$$

$$\text{vol \% } CO_2 = \frac{\text{mM } CO_2/L^*}{10} \times 22.2$$

* at 0°C and 760 mm Hg

The Relationship Between Milliequivalents and Millimoles. A *mole* is the atomic weight of a substance in grams. An *equivalent* is the atomic weight in grams, divided by the valence. Therefore, if an ion is univalent, an equivalent or a milliequivalent is the same as a mole or a millimole. However, if an ion is bivalent, such as calcium or sulfate, 1 mole equals 2 equivalents, and 1 millimole equals 2 milliequivalents. The reason for this is that 1 millimole of calcium (2 mEq) will react with 2 millimoles of chlorine (2 mEq) to form $CaCl_2$, for example.

THE ACTIVITY CONSTANT OF IONS

Measurement of the concentration of an ion or electrolyte in the blood does not necessarily indicate that this quantity is completely available for chemical reactions, because a portion may be bound to proteins, water, or other ions. A familiar example is the serum calcium concentration, which is partly bound to serum albumin, and is partly ionized. A similar situation exists with other ions, such as sodium and particularly chloride ions, as Dahms and others have shown. The ionized and nonionized percentages of these ions in the blood can both be measured. However, the clinical importance of this information is still not known.

Cation-Anion Balance

Figure 1–5 shows that the sum of the cations in serum or plasma equals 155 mEq/L and the sum of the anions also equals 155 mEq/L.

This electrical equivalence of cations and anions in serum or plasma is maintained regardless of whether the sum of the cations (and anions) is greater or less than 155 mEq/L. It may be greater, for example, when water loss occurs. It is often less than 155 mEq/L when electrolytes are lost from the body, as in vomiting or diarrhea.

All the cations can be determined clinically, although it is usual to determine only sodium, potassium, and calcium routinely. Chloride is the only anion that is routinely determined in studying electrolyte disturbances. The bicarbonate concentration can be calculated from the CO_2 content. Under ordinary conditions it is usually between 0.6 and 1.8 mEq/L less than the CO_2 content. However, for purposes of simplicity, one can calculate all the bicarbonate concentrations by subtracting 1 mEq/L from the CO_2 content.

Astrup has described a method of calculating the bicarbonate concentration from the pH of the blood, which is measured under two different carbon dioxide tensions. This method is described in detail in Chapter 15.

The sum of phosphates, sulfates, organic acid anions and proteins is described by the symbol R, which is calculated as follows:

The Significance of Anions Labeled R. In previous editions of the book, the term R (residual ions) was used to describe unmeasured ions, such as plasma proteins and inorganic and organic acid anions in the plasma, which may be present normally or may accumulate in some patients with metabolic acidosis.

R is calculated as follows:

R = Na + K + 8 (the sum of Ca and Mg) − (HCO_3 + Cl). Normally, the value of R is 25 mEq/L or less.

However, measurement of the anion gap (see below) is a simpler way of describing an accumulation of abnormal anions.

The Anion Gap. The *anion* gap (or *delta*) also describes the residual or unmeasured anions.

Since the concentration of anions such as phosphates, sulfates, and organic acid and protein anions is not ordinarily measured, the sum of the *measured cations* (Na, K, Ca) will be greater than the sum of the *measured anions* (HCO_3 and Cl). This difference is known as the *anion gap* (or *delta*).

The following simple formula can be used to determine if an abnormal gap is present:

Anion gap = (Na + K) − (HCO_3 + Cl).

Normally, the anion gap is 16 mEq/L or less. (An anion gap of less than 9 mEq/L is extremely unlikely, and is probably due to a laboratory error.)

An alternate formula for measuring the anion gap is:

Na − (HCO_3 + Cl)

When this formula is used, the average normal value for the anion gap is 12 mEq/L, with a range of 8 to 16 mEq/L.

Example:
Na 142   K 4 HCO_3 27   Cl 103 mEq/L
Anion Gap = (Na + K) − (HCO_3 + Cl).

$$(142 + 4) - (27 + 103).$$
$$146 - 130 = 16 \text{ mEq/L}$$

This is normal.

When metabolic acidosis is present with an *abnormal* anion gap, the value of the anion gap is usually more than 22 mEq/L.

Increased Anion Gap. This can occur in the following ways:

1. Increased unmeasured anions, such as the accumulation of lactic acid in lactic acidosis; aceto-acetic acid, in diabetic ketoacidosis; organic or keto acids due to the ingestion of salicylates, paraldehyde, ethylene glycol, organic acids in hyperosmolal hyperglycemic nonketoacidotic diabetic coma; phosphoric, sulfuric and organic acids in azotemia; formic acid in methanol (methyl alcohol) poisoning; ketoglutaric acid in hepatic failure; other anions, including high doses of (sodium) penicillin, and (sodium) carbenicillin.

2. Decreased unmeasured cations, for example, potassium, in hypokalemia (if the alternate formula above is used); calcium in hypocalcemia; magnesium in hypomagnesemia.

3. Water loss.

If water loss occurs in the patient described above and the serum concentrations rise 10%, the following concentrations would be present:

Na 156.2   K 4.4 HCO_3 29.7   Cl 113.3 mEq/L

$$\text{Anion Gap} = (Na + K) - (HCO_3 + Cl)$$
$$= (156.2 + 4.4) - (29.7 + 113.3)$$
$$= 160.6 - 143.0$$
$$= 17.6 \text{ mEq/L. This is 10\% greater than the original ion gap.}$$

4. Metabolic alkalosis. The plasma proteins give up H ions and increase their net negative charge. As a result, the measured anion concentration of the plasma is apparently low. In addition, alkalosis is associated with a decreased extracellular volume (water loss—see above).

(The total anion value must equal the total cation value of the plasma. When alkalosis develops, the anion value of the proteins increases. However, the anion value of the proteins is not measured. Therefore, there is a spurious decrease of the measured anions, and an apparent increase in the anion gap.)

5. Increased unmeasured anions, such as increased phosphate, or sulfate ions, or due to treatment with intravenous solutions containing lactate, citrate or acetate ions.

6. Laboratory errors, with falsely high serum Na or falsely low serum Cl or HCO_3 values.

The Significance of an Increased Anion Gap in Metabolic Acidosis. When a metabolic acidosis is present with an increased anion gap, the value of the anion gap is usually more than 22 mEq/L. Clinically, the anion gap is important, because, when a metabolic acidosis occurs, it may or may not be associated with an accumulation of abnormal unmeasured anions (and with an increased anion gap). For example, the anion gap is increased in metabolic acidosis patients described under category #1 above. However, other patients with metabolic acidosis do not have an accumulation of unmeasured anions and do not show an increased anion gap. Instead, they show an increased concentration of chloride ions (hyperchloremic metabolic acidosis). The separation of patients with a hyperchloremic metabolic acidosis from those with an increased anion gap is clinically useful and is described in Chapter 17.

Decreased Anion Gap. This can occur in the following ways:

1. Decreased unmeasured anions, as in hypoalbuminemia. This is probably the most common cause of a decreased anion gap. A normal value of 4 g per dl of serum albumin provides 11 mEq/L of anions. Therefore, when the serum albumin content decreases from 4 to 3 g per dl, for example, the anion gap should decrease by 2.75 mEq/L.

2. Increased unmeasured cations, for example: increased serum calcium in hypercalcemia; increased serum magnesium in hypermagnesemia; or increased serum potassium in hyperkalemia (if the alternate formula above has been used). Other abnormal cations include IgG globulin in multiple myeloma or other paraproteinemias, tromethamine (TRIS buffer), polymyxin B, lithium, or bromine. Bromide intoxication may give falsely low serum chloride levels, unless the Cl is measured by means of a potentiometer technic.

3. Water Excess.

If water excess occurs and the serum electrolyte concentrations decrease by 10% in the patient described above, the following concentrations would be present:

Na 127.8   K 3.6 HCO_3 24.3   Cl 92.7 mEq/L

$$\text{Anion Gap} = (Na + K) - (HCO_3 + Cl)$$
$$= (127.8 + 3.6) - (24.3 + 92.7)$$
$$= 131.4 - 117.0$$
$$= 14.4 \text{ mEq/L. This is 10\% less than the original anion gap of}$$
16 mEq/L.

4. Laboratory errors giving a falsely low serum Na or a falsely high serum Cl or HCO_3. A falsely low serum Na may also occur if the serum is viscous. As a result, the blood sample has a smaller volume than usual.

A simultaneous increase in both the anion gap and the gap between calculated and measured osmolality (see Chap 11) suggests diabetic acidosis, alcoholic acidosis or methanol or ethylene glycol poisoning. Methanol and ethylene glycol are metabolized to organic acids which cause a metabolic acidosis with an elevated anion gap. They also cause an osmolal gap (see Chapter 11).

The Relation of Serum Sodium to Bicarbonate and Chloride Concentrations

There is another relation between the cations and anions that can be used, namely, the relation between serum sodium concentration and the sum of the serum bicarbonate and chloride ions. In Figure 1–5, it will be noted that the most important cation is sodium, and that the most important anions are bicarbonate and chloride. In most cases, the following relations between these three ions exist:

$$Na = HCO_3 + Cl + 12 \text{ mEq/L}$$

Example:
Na 142 HCO$_3$ 27 Cl 103 mEq/L
142 = 27 + 103 + 12.

In other words, if the bicarbonate and chloride ion concentrations in serum or plasma are known, the concentration of sodium can be determined from these values, using the above rule.

The major exceptions to this rule occur in patients with a metabolic acidosis who show an abnormal anion gap, because the abnormal anions are not ordinarily measured (see above). This increased anion concentration in the plasma causes the bicarbonate concentration to be reduced without necessarily affecting the sodium or chloride concentrations. The reason for this is discussed in the chapters on metabolic acidosis.

The calculated serum sodium concentration may also be incorrectly high if hyperchloremia is present.

The calculated serum sodium concentration may also be incorrectly low if the bicarbonate concentration is high due to a respiratory acidosis.

REFERENCES

Blume, R.S., MacLowry, J.D., and Wolff, S.M.: Limitations of chloride determination in the diagnosis of bromism. N Engl J Med, *279*:593, 1968.

Brozek, J.: Body composition. Ann New York Acad Sci, *110*:425, 1963.

Dahms, H., Rock, R., and Seligson, D.: Ionic activities of sodium, potassium, and chloride in human serum. Clin Chem, *14*:859, 1968.

Edelman, I.S., and Leibman, J.: Anatomy of body water and electrolytes, Am J Med, *27*:256, 1959.

Gamble, J.L.: *Chemical Anatomy, Physiology and Pathology of Extracellular Fluid,* 6th ed. Cambridge, Harvard University Press, 1954.

Hald, P.M., Heinsen, A.J., and Peters, J.P.: Estimation of serum sodium from bicarbonate plus chloride. J Clin Invest, *26*:983, 1947.

Hays, R.M.: Dynamics of body water and electrolytes. In *Clinical Disorders of Fluid and Electrolyte Metabolism,* 3rd ed., edited by Maxwell, M.H. and Kleeman C.R. New York, McGraw-Hill Book Co., 1980.

Henderson, L.J.: *The Fitness of the Environment.* New York, Macmillan, 1913.

Leaf, A., and Newburgh, L.H.: *Significance of Body Fluids in Clinical Medicine,* 2nd ed. Springfield, Charles C Thomas, 1955.

Maccallum, A.B.: The paleochemistry of the body fluids and tissues. Physiol Rev, *6*:316, 1926.

Moore, F.D., Haley, H.B., Bering, E.A., Brooks, L., and Edelman, I.S.: Further observations on total body water. Surg Gynec Obstet, *95*:155, 1952.

Moore, F.D., Olesen, K.H., McMurrey, J.D., Parker, H.V., Ball, M.R., and Boyden, C.M.:

The Body Cell Mass and Its Supporting Environment. Philadelphia, W.B. Saunders, 1963.

Olmstead, E.G.: *Mammalian Cell Water. Physiologic and Clinical Aspects.* Philadelphia, Lea & Febiger, 1966.

Robin, E.D., and Bromberg, P.A.: Claude Bernard's milieu interieur extended: Intracellular acid-base relationships. Am J Med, *27*:689, 1959.

Ross, E.J., Editor: *Clinical Effects of Electrolyte Disturbances.* Philadelphia, J.B. Lippincott, 1959.

Snively, W.D., Jr.: An example of atavistic physiology? JAMA, *204*:392, 1968.

Steele, J.M., et al.: Total body water in man. Am J Physiol, *162*:313, 1950.

Strauss, M.B.: *Body Water in Man.* Boston, Little, Brown & Co., 1957.

Ussing, H.H.: Ion transport across biological membranes. In *Ion Transport Across Membranes* (Clarke, H.T., Ed.). New York, Academic Press, 1954.

Williams, R.J.P., and Wacker, W.E.C.: Cation balance in biological systems. JAMA, *201*:18, 1967.

Anion Gaps

Askenazi, J., et al.: Spurious increases in the anion gap due to exposure of serum to air. Letter. N Engl J Med, *307*:190, 1982.

Cole, D.E.C., and Scriver, C.R.: Unexplained serum anion gap. Letter. N Engl J Med, *304*:542, 1981.

de Troyer, A., et al.: Value of anion gap determination in multiple myeloma. N Engl J Med, *296*:858, 1977.

Emmett, M., and Narins, R.G.: Clinical use of the anion gap. Medicine (Baltimore), *56*:38, 1977.

Gabow, P.A., and Kaehny, W.D.: The anion gap. Its meaning and clinical utility. The Kidney, *12*:(2), March 1979.

Graber, M.L., et al.: Spurious hyperchloremia and decreased anion gap in hyperlipidemia. Ann Intern Med, *98*:607, 1983.

Gabow, P.A., et al.: Diagnostic importance of an increased serum anion gap. N Engl J Med, *303*:854, 1980.

Goldstein, R.J., et al.: The myth of the low anion gap. JAMA, *253*:1737, 1980.

Jacobsen, D., et al.: Anion and osmolal gaps in the diagnosis of methanol and ethylene glycol poisoning. Acta Med Scandinav, *212*:17, 1982.

Keshgegian, A.A.: Hypoalbuminemia and decreased anion gap. Letter. JAMA, *247*:1697, 1982.

Madrias, N.E., Ayus, C.J., and Adrogue, H.J.: Increased anion gap in metabolic alkalosis. The role of plasma-protein equivalency. N Engl J Med, *300*:1421, 1979.

Oh, M.S., and Carroll, H.J.: Current Concepts. The anion gap. N Engl J Med, *297*:814, 1977.

Smithline, N., and Gardner, K.D., Jr.: Gaps—anionic and osmolal. JAMA, *236*:1594, 1976.

Weisberg, H.: Water, Electrolyte and Acid-Base Balance, Baltimore, Williams & Wilkins, 1953.

CHAPTER 2

THE OSMOTIC PRESSURE
AND THE VOLUME OF
THE EXTRACELLULAR WATER

OSMOTIC PRESSURE

A *solute* is a substance, such as sodium chloride, potassium phosphate, glucose, or protein, which can dissolve in a *solvent,* such as water, to make a *solution.*

If we take a solution of sodium chloride in water, for example, and place it on one side of a membrane that is permeable to both the sodium and chloride ions and to the water molecules, and if we place water on the other side of the membrane, the sodium and chloride ions and the water molecules will pass freely through both sides of the membrane until the concentration of sodium and chloride on both sides is equal.

However, we can prepare a membrane that will allow a solvent such as water to pass freely, but that will not allow a substance such as sodium chloride or glucose or protein to pass. If we place such a sodium chloride solution in a funnel, the mouth of which is sealed by such a semipermeable membrane, and then place the mouth of the funnel in a container of water, the sodium and the chloride ions will not be able to pass through the membrane. However, the water molecules will be able to pass through in either direction and they will enter the funnel and the level of the solution in the funnel will rise (Fig. 2–1). The rise continues until the hydrostatic pressure exerted by the column of fluid in the funnel is equal to the pressure exerted by the water molecules as they pass through the membrane into the funnel. When this occurs, the hydrostatic pressure prevents any further increase of volume in the salt solution. The height of the fluid in the funnel tube is therefore a measure of the osmotic pressure of the salt solution, and is dependent upon the number of particles or ions of the salt in a given volume of solution. In other words, a more concentrated salt solution would have

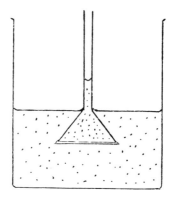

Fig. 2–1.   Diagram showing the effect of osmotic pressure. See text.

a greater osmotic pressure, and a less concentrated salt solution would have a lesser osmotic pressure.

Osmotic pressure is measured in terms of osmoles (Osm) or *milliosmoles* (mOsm). An osmole (or a milliosmole) of a substance such as glucose which does not dissociate into ions is the same as a mole (or a millimole). However, a mole of a salt such as sodium chloride which dissociates almost completely into sodium and chloride ions equals 2 osmoles.

A mole of a salt such as sodium bicarbonate, which dissociates into sodium, Na, and bicarbonate, HCO_3, ions, also equals 2 osmoles. A mole of a more complex salt such as Na_2HPO_4, which dissociates into 2-Na and 1-HPO_4 ions, equals 3 osmoles. The total osmotic pressure of a solution therefore is calculated from the sum of all the ions in solution.

We can now perform another experiment. For example, in Figure 2–2 a sodium chloride solution and a potassium phosphate solution are separated by a membrane that is impermeable to all these ions, but that is freely permeable to the water in which the ions are dissolved.

Let us assume that the concentration of sodium chloride is 310 milliosmoles per liter, and that the potassium phosphate solution has equal osmolal concentration. Since the osmotic *pressure* is the same on both sides of the membrane, there will not be any movement of water, regardless of the volume on either side of the membrane (Fig. 2–2).

However, if we place a solution of sodium chloride with a lower osmotic concentration, for example, 290 mOsm/L, on one side of the membrane, and a solution of potassium phosphate with a higher os-

NaCl	K_2HPO_4
14 liters	28 liters
310 mOsm/L	310 mOsm/L
4340 mOsm	8680 mOsm

Fig. 2–2.   Diagram showing osmotic equilibrium. See text.

before osmotic equilibrium

14 liters 290 mOsm/L 4060 mOsm NaCl	28 liters 310 mOsm/L 8680 mOsm K₂HPO₄	A.

after osmotic equilibrium

13.4 liters 303 mOsm/L 4060 mOsm NaCl	38.6 liters 303 mOsm/L 8680 mOsm K₂HPO₄	B.

Fig. 2–3.   Diagram showing the shift of water due to a disturbance in osmotic equilibrium. See text.

motic concentration of 310 mOsm/L on the other side, the osmotic pressure of the sodium chloride solution will be less than that of the potassium phosphate solution. Because of this, water will flow from the sodium chloride solution to the potassium phosphate solution in order to equalize the osmotic pressures. As a result of this, the volume of the sodium chloride solution will decrease, and the concentration of the sodium chloride will rise toward normal (Fig. 2–3). (The method of calculating the shift in water is described in Appendix 1.)

These experiments demonstrate a fundamental rule of osmotic pressure, namely: *water will flow from a region of low to a region of higher osmotic pressure.*

In the human and in animals, it is assumed that the osmotic pressures of the extracellular water and of the cells are the same. However, there are observations that this may not be correct. The osmotic pressure of the cells may be higher than that of the extracellular water and a constant gradient may normally be maintained between them by a constant active extrusion of water by the cells. However, even if this is so, it does not invalidate the concept that the osmotic pressures of the extracellular water and of the cells are in equilibrium, and that a change in the osmotic pressure of either the extracellular water or the cells will cause a flow of water either into or out of the cells.

In the human, the osmotic pressure of the extracellular water and of the cells is 310 mOsm/L. The significance of this is the following: In the plasma (or serum) and in the extracellular water, the sodium concentration is 142 mEq/L and the total cation concentration is 155 mEq/L. Practically all the osmotic pressure of the extracellular water is due to monovalent salts, which ionize into two ions each. Therefore, the osmotic pressure of the extracellular water is twice the cation (or anion) concentration, or $2 \times 155 = 310$ mOsm/L. We can therefore make the following assumption: Sodium is the chief cation of the extracellular water. Therefore, the osmotic pressure of the extracellular water should vary proportionately with the sodium concentration of the serum or plasma. In other words, we should be able to use the serum sodium concentration as a measure of the osmotic pressure of the extracellular water. Unfortunately, this relationship is valid only in normal subjects. This is discussed further in Chapter 11.

THE DIFFERENCE BETWEEN OSMOTIC PRESSURE AND ONCOTIC PRESSURE

The term "osmotic pressure" should be differentiated from the term "oncotic pressure," or "colloid osmotic pressure." The osmotic pressure of a solution varies with the number of molecules in a solution, as was pointed out above. When the molecular weight of a substance is low, there will be more molecules of the substance per unit weight, and the osmotic pressure will be greater. For example, a substance such as mannitol which has a low molecular weight will increase the osmotic pressure when given intravenously. However, a substance such as human albumin, or dextran, which has a high molecular weight around 80,000, will not increase the osmotic pressure greatly. However, such a substance exerts an oncotic pressure (colloid osmotic pressure) because it is confined by a membrane (the vascular system) to which it is relatively impermeable. Therefore, an infusion of albumin or dextran will greatly increase the oncotic pressure of the blood and will prevent the loss of excessive fluid from the capillaries. However, it will have an almost negligible effect on the osmotic pressure of the blood. Oncotic pressure is measured in terms of pressure units (mm Hg).

FACTORS REGULATING THE OSMOTIC PRESSURE AND THE VOLUME OF THE EXTRACELLULAR WATER

I have just pointed out that a primary change of osmotic pressure, either in the extracellular water or in the cells, is associated with a shift of water into or out of the extracellular water, and consequently is associated with a change in the volume of the extracellular water.

In the maintenance of life, the body has homeostatic or regulatory mechanisms that help to maintain the osmotic pressure and the volume of the extracellular water within physiological limits. The osmotic pressure of the extracellular water is controlled by the posterior pituitary antidiuretic hormone, ADH. The volume of the extracellular water is controlled partly by the adrenal cortical hormone aldosterone. We can now consider the action of these two hormones.

ADH, the Antidiuretic Hormone of the Posterior Pituitary Gland

Some authors use the symbol, AVP (arginine vasopressin), the chemical name of the antidiuretic hormone, instead of the symbol, ADH. However, the symbol, ADH, is so well known that I shall continue to use it.

ADH, the antidiuretic hormone of the posterior pituitary gland, is an octapeptide (arginine vasopressin). It is produced by neurons of the supraoptic nuclei of the hypothalamus, and is stored in axon endplates that terminate in the posterior pituitary gland.

The site of action of ADH is probably the distal tubules and collecting ducts of the kidneys. ADH increases the permeability of these structures to water. When this occurs, an increased amount of water is reabsorbed, the volume of urine decreases, and the osmolality of the urine increases.

ADH secretion can be stimulated in three ways:

1. Osmotic stimulation of ADH secretion—hyperosmolality. The most important action of ADH is to maintain the osmotic pressure of the extracellular water in relation to the osmotic pressure of the cells. The stimulus for the secretion of ADH is the *relative* osmotic pressure of the neurons (cells) of the supraoptic nuclei of the hypothalamus, that is, the osmotic pressure of these neurons in relation to the osmotic pressure of the extracellular water. When the osmotic pressure of the extracellular water becomes relatively greater than the osmotic pressure of these neurons, ADH secretion increases.

For example, if a large amount of glucose is infused into the body, it will raise the osmotic pressure of the extracellular water. Therefore the osmotic pressure of the extracellular water will rise above that of the neurons. As a result, ADH secretion will occur and water excretion by the kidneys will decrease.

2. Nonosmotic stimulation of ADH secretion. ADH secretion can also be stimulated by way of central neural pathways, from the midbrain reticular formation to the supraoptic area. These neural receptors respond to emotional stress, fever, trauma, infections, major operations, most anesthetics and most analgesics, anticholinergic drugs, barbiturates, morphine, meperidine (Demerol), cytoxan, carbamazine, vincristine, and others.

3. ADH secretion is also partly controlled by changes in blood volume. There are volume receptors in the left atrial wall that are stimulated when the left atrial pressure falls. Therefore, procedures that promote pooling of blood in peripheral vessels such as warm ambient temperature or quiet standing tend to decrease left atrial filling and stimulate ADH secretion. Similarly, intermittent or continuous positive pressure respiration also decreases left atrial filling pressure and stimulates ADH secretion. A decreased arterial blood pressure due to contraction of the vascular or extracellular volume or to a decreased cardiac output also stimulates ADH secretion.

Inhibition of ADH secretion can also occur from osmotic or nonosmotic causes.

1. Osmotic inhibition of ADH secretion—hypoosmolality. When the osmotic pressure of the neurons of the supraoptic nuclei of the hypothalamus show an increased osmotic pressure *relative* to the osmotic pressure of the extracellular water, ADH secretion is inhibited. For example, if a person drinks plain water, the immediate effect of the imbibed water is to dilute the extracellular water. This causes the osmotic pressure of the extracellular water to become lower (at least temporarily) than the osmotic pressure of the neurons. As a result, ADH secretion decreases or stops and a water diuresis occurs.

2. Nonosmotic inhibition of ADH secretion. Increased arterial blood pressure, increased tension in the left atrial wall and great pulmonary veins secondary to expansion of the vascular or extracellular volume with a rise in cardiac output, quiet resting in a supine position, exposure to cool ambient temperature, negative-pressure breathing will increase left atrial filling and decrease ADH secretion. Drugs such as alcohol, phenytoin and others will also inhibit ADH secretion.

The usual stimulus for the secretion of ADH is water loss. This causes the osmotic pressure of the extracellular water to become greater than that of the cells. ADH secretion occurs in an attempt to decrease water loss through the kidneys. In addition, ADH secretion often occurs as a result of other factors, as mentioned above.

The regulation of osmotic pressure is more important than the regulation of blood and extracellular water volume. Therefore, when the osmotic pressure of the blood and extracellular water (in relation to the osmotic pressure of the cells) decreases, and the blood and extracellular volume also decrease, *the osmotic pressure should be corrected first.*

(If the volume deficit is corrected with a solution of 5% dextrose in water, for example, which does not significantly raise the plasma osmolality, the blood and extracellular water will be further diluted, their osmotic pressures will decrease further, and more water will pass into the cells, again decreasing the blood volume, after the initial temporary increase in blood volume due to the dextrose and water infusion. However, if a solution of isotonic saline (sodium chloride solution), or dextrose in isotonic saline, or plasma, or dextran, etc., which has a significant osmolality, is infused, the increased osmolality will draw water from the cells into the extracellular water and blood, thereby increasing the blood volume as well as restoring plasma osmolality.)

Haberich and others have shown that the liver also acts as an osmoreceptor to regulate the intake of water from the gastrointestinal tract. When water is imbibed, it is absorbed into the splanchnic circulation and is brought to the liver by way of the portal vein. This causes the osmolality of the portal vein to decrease rapidly. This stimulates the liver, and afferent stimuli are sent to the hypothalamus by way of the vagus nerve. The hypothalamus then stimulates the kidneys to excrete water.

Aldosterone and the Volume of the Extracellular Water

Aldosterone is secreted by the cells of the glomerulosa zone of the adrenal cortex. Its secretion can be stimulated in several ways:

1. It responds to factors (sodium depletion, hemorrhage, or diuretic therapy, and so on) that decrease the effective circulating blood volume and reduce renal perfusion.

   Apparently, the renal afferent arterioles acts as volume receptors, which respond to decreased renal arterial pressure and decreased renal blood flow by increasing the release of renin from the juxtaglomerular cells. Renin causes the formation of angiotensin II in the blood. This directly stimulates aldosterone secretion. As a result, sodium ions (and water) are retained and the circulating blood volume rises. When this occurs, the juxtaglomerular cell secretion of renin is inhibited and aldosterone secretion stops.

2. Aldosterone secretion is also influenced by serum potassium concentration. Any factor that raises the serum potassium concentration stimulates aldosterone secretion. As a result, a diuresis of potassium ions occurs. Conversely, hypokalemia is associated with a reduced aldosterone secretion and a retention of potassium ions.

3. ACTH can also cause a transient increase in aldosterone secretion.

A deficiency of aldosterone secretion occurs usually in Addison's disease, although it may be present as an isolated abnormality (hypoaldosteronism). It is associated with a loss of sodium ions (and water), hypotension or shock, and hyperkalemia.

Patients with increased aldosterone secretion may show various syndromes. Patients with primary aldosteronism show hypokalemia but usually no edema. Patients with secondary aldosteronism due to congestive heart failure, cirrhosis of the liver, the nephrotic syndrome, or malignant hypertension may show extensive edema.

Natriuretic Hormone

It has been known for many years that dogs respond to saline infusions with a prompt increase both in sodium excretion and in glomerular filtration rate. Originally, this increased excretion of sodium was attributed to the increased filtration of sodium through the glomeruli. Studies by deWardener and many others have indicated that the increased excretion of sodium is related to a *decreased* tubular reabsorption of sodium from the proximal tubules of the kidneys. A similar loss or "escape" of sodium from the kidneys occurs when salt-retaining hormones, such as aldosterone and 11-desoxycorticosterone, are administered over a prolonged period of time to normal human subjects. This is an explanation for the observation that patients with primary hyperaldosteronism do not develop marked edema.

It is believed that the tubular excretion of sodium is controlled by a "third factor," which may be a hormone (natriuretic hormone). Its site of origin and its chemical structure are both unknown.

SIMULTANEOUS CHANGES IS OSMOTIC PRESSURE AND IN THE VOLUME OF EXTRACELLULAR WATER

Isolated changes in osmotic pressure and in the volume of extracellular water can occur. Under most conditions, there are simultaneous changes in osmotic pressure and volume. It is preferable to consider these changes from the broad clinical point of view of the patient rather than from a limited physiological point of view. Therefore, in the chapters that follow, these disturbances in volume and osmotic pressure are described in terms of the clinical syndromes with which they are associated.

REFERENCES

Barron, W.M., et al.: Transient vasopressin—resistant diabetes insipidus of pregnancy. N Engl J Med, *310*:442, 1984.

Burg, M.B., and Orloff, J.: Control of fluid absorption in the renal proximal tubules. J Clin Invest, *47*:2016, 1968.

deWardener, H.E., and Clarkson, E.M.: The natriuretic hormone. Recent developments. Clin Sci, *63*:415, 1982.

Davis, J.O.: Aldosterone and angiotensin. Interrelationship in normal and diseased states. JAMA, *188*:1062, 1964.

Davis, J.O., Urquhart, J., and Higgins, J.T., Jr.: Effects of alterations of plasma sodium and potassium concentration on aldosterone secretion. J Clin Invest, *42*:597, 1963.

Galambos, J.T., Herndon, E.G., Jr., and Reynolds, G.H.: Specific-gravity determination. Fact or fancy? N Engl J Med, *270*:506, 1964.

Gann, D.S., Delea, C.S., Gill, J.R., Jr. Thomas, J.P., and Bartter, F.C.: Control of aldosterone secretion by change in body potassium in normal man. Am J Physiol, *207*:104, 1964.

Gauer, O.H.: Osmocontrol versus volume control. Fed Proc, *27*:1132, 1968.

Gross, F.: The regulation of aldosterone secretion by the renin-angiotensin system under various conditions. Acta Endocr, Suppl, *124*, 41, 1967.

Haberich, F.J.: Osmoreception in the portal circulation. Fed Proc, *27*:1137, 1968.

Hays, R.M.: Antidiuretic hormone. N Engl J Med, *295*:659, 1976.

Jacobson, M.H., Levy, S.E., Kaufman, R.M., Gallinek, W.E., and Donnelly, O.W.: Urine osmolality. Arch Intern Med, *110*:121, 1962.

Johnston, C.I., et al.: Cross-circulation experiments on the mechanism of the natriuresis during saline loading in the dog. Circ Res, *20*:1, 1967.

Laragh, J.H.: Potassium, angiotensin and the dual control of aldosterone secretion. N Engl J Med, *289*:745, 1973.

Levensky, N.G.: Nonaldosterone influences on renal sodium transport. Ann New York Acad Sci, *139*:295, 1966.

Lichardus, B., and Pearce, J.W.: Evidence for a humoral natriuretic factor released by blood volume expansion. Nature, *209*:407, 1966.

Maffly, L.H., and Leaf, A.: The intracellular osmolality of the mammalian tissues. J Clin Invest, *37*:916, 1958.

Mills, I.H.; Atrial natriuretic factor. A new hormone? Editorial Brit M J, *289*:210, 1984.

Rector, F.C., et al.: Demonstration of a hormonal inhibitor of proximal tubular reabsorption during expansion of extracellular volume with isotonic saline. J Clin Invest, *47*:761, 1968.

Robinson, J.R.: Osmoregulation in surviving slices from the kidneys of adult rats. Proc Roy Soc London, Series B, *137*:378, 1950.

Share, L.: Effects of carotid occlusion and left atrial distention on plasma vasopressin titer. Am J Physiol, *208*:219, 1965.

Sonnenberg, H., et al.: A humoral component of the natriuretic mechanism in sustained blood volume expansion. J Clin Invest, *51*:2631, 1972.

Verney, E.B.: Absorption and excretion of water: The antidiuretic hormone. Lancet, *2*:739, 781, 1946. Also Surg Gynecol Obstet, *106*:441, 1958.

Zehr, J.E., Johnson, J.A., and Moore, W.E.: Left atrial pressure, plasma osmolality and ADH levels in the unanesthetized ewe. Am J Physiol, *217*:1672, 1969.

Zerbe, R.L., and Robertson, G.L.: A comparison of plasma vasopressin measurements with a standard indirect test in the differential diagnosis of polyuria. N Engl J Med, *305*:1540, 1981.

PART 2

SYNDROMES ASSOCIATED WITH WATER DISTURBANCES

CHAPTER 3

WATER LOSS SYNDROMES

Desiccation occurs as a result of a loss of water from the body, which can be due either to a decreased intake of water or to excessive loss of water through the lungs, skin, kidneys, or gastrointestinal tract. In most patients, it is due to a decreased intake of water.

Synonyms: Pure dehydration, dehydration hypertonicity, water deficit, water deficiency, pure water depletion.

The term "dehydration" has been used to describe not only the syndromes associated with a loss of water, but also the completely different syndromes associated with a loss of salt (sodium ions), with or without a concomitant loss of water. Therefore, I shall not use it in this book.

ETIOLOGY

Water loss can occur in the following ways:

1. Water loss secondary to inadequate water intake. This can occur in several ways:
    a. In shipwrecked sailors, people lost in the desert, or those who have been injured and are immobilized. Water loss will occur more rapidly if a castaway tries to drink sea water, because the kidneys have to excrete the extra salt with a large amount of water. Similarly, those stranded on land will become desiccated more quickly if they are directly exposed to the sun.
    b. When swallowing is difficult or impossible. This occurs in debilitated patients, comatose patients, or in patients with dysphagia.
    c. When the sense of thirst is impaired, as in elderly patients with cerebral atherosclerosis, patients with cerebral tumors, poliomyelitis of the bulbar type, meningitis, or cerebral injury. (Cerebral injury can also cause diabetes insipidus and water loss in this way.)
2. Water loss secondary to loss through the kidneys. This can occur in patients with normal or with impaired renal function.
    a. Water loss in patients with normal kidneys can occur with:
        i. Central (neurogenic, vasopressin-sensitive) diabetes insipidus. Here, the kidneys are unable to concentrate water normally, because of a lack of the posterior pituitary antidiuretic hormone ADH. Alcoholics may lose water in a similar way, because the alcohol inhibits the secretion of ADH.
        ii. Excessive water intake (psychogenic polydipsia). It has been shown that if a normal subject ingests 20 to 200 ml of water

31

every 10 minutes for 3 to 7 hours, the total urinary output of water may exceed the water intake by as much as 8%. In addition if one includes an additional 50 ml loss of water per hour, due to insensible perspiration, a severe negative water balance can develop. (Sodium and other electrolytes are also lost this way.)

    iii. Solute excess (Chap 4) or hyperosmolality (Chap 5).

   b. Water loss in patients with impaired kidney function can occur when the kidneys show a decreased ability to conserve water due to renal tubular dysfunction (*nephrogenic diabetes insipidus*). As a result, the kidneys do not respond normally to ADH.

This can occur in chronic pyelonephritis, glomerulonephritis, polycystic kidneys, during the diuretic phase of acute renal failure, partial urinary tract obstruction, or when severe prostatic obstruction is relieved too rapidly (postobstructive water loss usually improves spontaneously within several days, but some patients may not regain the capacity of the kidneys to conserve water for several weeks to months), hypokalemia, hypercalcemia, primary aldosteronism, amyloid disease, gout, multiple myeloma, Sjögren's syndrome, sickle-cell anemia affecting the kidneys, after transplantation of a kidney, as a result of high dose lithium carbonate intake, demeclocycline (declomycin), ethanol, opium antagonists, or as a toxic effect of penthrane (methoxyflurane) anesthesia. It can also occur as a congenital anomaly.

3. Water loss due to other causes, for example;

   a. Excessive loss of water from the lungs. Prolonged exposure to the sun's heat without water intake, hyperventilation and fever can cause a large loss in water volume this way. A tracheotomy accelerates the pulmonary water loss, because it reduces the dead air fraction of the tidal volume. A cerebral injury may cause hyperventilation and an increased water loss.

   b. Excessive loss of water through the skin. This occurs in burns, especially with open treatment.

PATHOPHYSIOLOGY

Water loss causes physiological changes in the following ways:

1. Changes due to osmolality. We know that the osmotic pressure of the extracellular water tends to remain equal to the osmotic pressure of the cells at all times. Following a loss of water, the osmotic pressure of the extracellular water becomes higher than that of the cells. Since water passes from a region of lower to a region of higher osmolality according to the osmotic rule, water will flow out of the cells into the extracellular water. This tends to lower the osmotic pressure of the extracellular water toward normal, and to increase its volume toward normal.

2. Changes due to hormonal effects. Because of the loss of water, the extracellular water becomes more concentrated, and the osmotic pressure of the cells becomes relatively less than that of the extracellular water. This causes the posterior pituitary gland to secrete ADH. This in turn causes the kidney tubules to reabsorb more water, which helps minimize the water loss. In addition, the water loss has caused a decrease in the volume of extracellular water. This causes the adrenal glands to secrete aldosterone. This in turn causes a retention of sodium which tends to raise

the osmotic pressure of the extracellular water still further and tends to negate the effect of the secretion of ADH.

3. A "dehydration reaction." When this happens the kidney tubules secrete large quantities of potassium ions in excess of sodium ions. The potassium that is excreted comes mostly from the cells, because potassium is found in greatest concentration in the cells. Therefore, when this loss of cellular potassium occurs, the osmotic pressure of the cells falls and becomes relatively less than that of the extracellular water. As a result, more cellular water will flow from the cells into the extracellular water to equalize the osmotic pressure.

4. Lowering of osmotic pressure of the cells by means of chemical changes within the cells. When this happens, potassium and other ions are bound to large molecular particles, such as the cellular proteins, in a manner which is not yet understood. Since the osmotic pressure is proportionate to the number of ions in solution, and not to their size, this reaction will lower the osmotic pressure of the cells still further, and will allow more water to flow from the cells to the extracellular water.

5. Changes in the brain cells. The brain cells respond to water loss in a different way from all other cells in the body, because the brain cells are able to synthesize new substances (solute) called *idiogenic osmoles*. In this way, the osmolality of the brain cells is increased, less water is withdrawn from the brain cells, and less injury to the brain cells occurs. The nature of these idiogenic osmoles is not known. They appear even within 1 hour when experimental water loss is produced.

Starvation, or partial starvation, has a sparing effect upon water loss, because a high protein diet increases urea output. This requires an increased excretion of water.

SYMPTOMS

Thirst is the earliest symptom of water loss. It occurs when the water loss is equal to about 2% of the body weight (about 3 lb, or 1.4 liters in a 70-kg [154-lb] patient). It is due to the fact that as extracellular water is lost and its osmotic pressure increases, water passes from the cells to the extracellular water. This causes a decreased volume of the cells. A center in the brain, probably in the hypothalamus, is sensitive to this decreased cell volume and causes the sensation of thirst. Later, the tongue sticks and there is an inability to swallow dry food. However, thirst may not be present, even with severe water loss in patients with cerebral lesions, for reasons already mentioned.

Thirst can also develop when the extracellular fluid volume decreases. This occurs in the following way: when the extracellular and the circulating blood volumes decrease, sympathetic stretch receptors in the atria, vena cavae, and pulmonary veins are stimulated and cause the juxtaglomerular cells of the kidneys to secrete renin. This in turn causes an increased secretion of angiotensin II. The angiotensin II stimulates thirst receptors in the hypothalamus. It also stimulates the posterior pituitary gland to secrete vasopressin. This in turn causes the kidneys to retain water. Angiotensin II also stimulates the secretion of aldosterone which causes the kidneys to retain sodium ions.

Thirst and polyuria have also been described in patients with chronic potassium loss, and in patients with hypercalcemia. The potassium loss causes injury to the kidney tubules. This prevents them from concentrating water, and causes a condition similar to diabetes insipidus (water-losing nephritis, nephrogenic diabetes insipidus). Persistent hypercalcemia causes similar changes in the kidney tubules.

SIGNS

The clinical signs depend on the extent of the desiccation. The patient appears weak and ill. Weight loss is proportional to the degree of desiccation. A fever may be present. The temperature may reach 105°F or more when the desiccation is marked.

Skin and Mucous Membranes

The following signs are present:

1. The skin may be flushed. Sweating is decreased. The axilla and groin are dry.
2. There is little saliva or tears.
3. The tongue is dry and fissured, and may be red and swollen. Phonation may be difficult and words may be poorly pronounced. These signs can also occur in patients who are not desiccated, but who are mouthbreathers, or have been receiving oxygen by mask. In desiccation, examination of the mucous membranes will reveal dryness. When you place a finger in the patient's mouth, and palpate the mucous membranes where the gums and cheek meet, you will find that your finger does not glide easily, because of the dryness of the mucous membranes.
4. Skin turgor remains normal. However, the skin may have a thick, "doughy" or "rubbery" feeling. (Loss of skin turgor occurs characteristically with sodium loss [Chap 8].)

Cardiovascular System

Since water is drawn from the cells into the extracellular fluid, as a result of the water loss, the circulating blood volume and the efficiency of the cardiovascular system remain relatively unchanged and signs of shock do *not* usually appear. However, a tachycardia may develop when fever is present.

Central Nervous System

Generalized muscle weakness, muscle rigidity, or muscle tremors may develop. Epileptiform convulsions may appear (particularly if the water loss is treated too energetically with an infusion of dextrose and water). Occasionally a patient develops muscle weakness instead of muscle rigidity. Hallucinations, delirium, and manic behavior may also develop. Death usually occurs from respiratory arrest. Before this, the patient may develop hyperpnea.

The cerebrospinal fluid may become bloody or xanthochromic, and its protein content may become elevated.

These central nervous system changes may be functional. However, the water loss can also cause subdural effusions or intracranial hemorrhage.

LABORATORY FINDINGS

Blood

In the early stages of water loss, the blood findings may be within the normal range because some cellular water passes to the extracellular fluid in response to osmotic pressure changes. However, as water continues to be lost, hemoconcentration occurs, and the hematocrit, the serum sodium, and other blood values begin to rise proportionately.

A rise in the hematocrit is a good sign of either water loss or sodium loss (unless red blood cells are also being lost by way of hemorrhage or hemolysis). The normal range of the hematocrit is 47% ± 5% for men, and 42% ± 5% for women.

The hematocrit is usually above 50%, and the serum sodium is above 150 mEq/L. This differentiates water loss from sodium loss where the hematocrit may be high, because when sodium loss occurs with a high hematocrit the serum sodium concentration is lower than normal.

A hematocrit of 55% in a patient with water loss is a much more serious sign than a hematocrit of 55% in a patient with sodium loss. The reason is that, in water loss, the extracellular fluid is diluted with water from the cells as a result of osmotic pressure changes. This tends to lower the hematocrit. Therefore, the water loss is actually greater than the rise in hematocrit would indicate.

However, when sodium loss occurs, as in vomiting, diarrhea, burns, and other conditions, water flows from the extracellular fluid into the cells because of osmotic pressure differences. This also causes the hematocrit to rise. Here, however, the water loss is actually less than the hematocrit would indicate, because it represents (in part) a shift of water into the cells rather than a true loss of water from the body. (This is described in detail in Chap 9. [It should also be pointed out that a high hematocrit can also occur with overtransfusion.])

Other serum electrolyte and protein values are also elevated, due to the water loss. An elevated blood urea nitrogen may be present. This may indicate inadequate kidney function, due to a decreased renal blood flow. The plasma osmolality is high, because of the water loss.

If the patient has abnormal quantities of nonelectrolyte substances in the blood, such as glucose in a diabetic patient, or nonprotein nitrogen products in a patient with renal disease, the serum sodium concentration may rise only slightly, or may be low, even though the water loss is marked. However, the plasma osmolality will be high in such patients (Chap 11). (The effects of an increased blood sugar concentration on the serum sodium concentration are described in Appendix IV.)

Cation-Anion Balance

The normal values of the serum electrolytes and of the anion gap are given on pages 12 and 14. The anion gap normally has a value of 16 mEq/L or less. When water loss occurs, the serum electrolytes become more concentrated and the value of the anion gap becomes proportionately higher than 16 mEq/L (Chap 1).

Other serum electrolyte disturbances may also develop because the water loss may cause renal tubular acidosis.

Urine

Because the renal blood flow is decreased, the urinary volume is small. However, it cannot fall below a minimum of 250 to 350 ml a day (unless the patient develops shock and renal shutdown). The specific gravity of the urine increases as the desiccation becomes aggravated and may exceed 1.040. However, if the patient previously was unable to concentrate urine normally, the specific gravity may not rise greatly even if severe water loss is present. Red blood cells, albumin, casts, and even acetone may be present. An important urinary finding is the continued presence of sodium and chloride. However, with severe water loss, sodium and chloride may virtually disappear from the urine.

(In diabetes insipidus, the urine specific gravity remains below 1.010 and usually below 1.005. The urine osmolality is below 280 mOsm/kg and may decrease to 40 mOsm/kg when the polyuria is extreme. Also see page 41.)

Hypernatremia (a serum sodium concentration greater than 145 mEq/L) almost always indicates that there is too little water for the amount of sodium ions and other solutes in the body. Clinically, it is important to determine whether this relative water deficit has occurred in spite of normal kidney tubular function to conserve water, or because the kidney tubules have lost their ability to conserve the excretion of water.

If hypernatremia is present with a small amount of maximally concentrated urine (that is, with a high osmolality or specific gravity), this indicates that there is adequate ADH (the antidiuretic hormone of the posterior pituitary gland) and that the kidney tubules are functioning normally. Therefore, there is an external cause for the water loss, or the patient has "essential hypernatremia."

In *essential hypernatremia,* a rare syndrome, the serum sodium concentration is continually higher than normal, but the patient does not show any apparent loss of water. Many of these patients have no symptoms. However, there may be attacks of muscle weakness or muscle paralysis, possibly related to a reduced total body potassium content, although the serum potassium concentration in these patients may be normal. Alford and Scoggins have treated a symptomatic patient with a low-sodium, high-potassium diet.

If hypernatremia is present with a dilute urine, this indicates that there is either a lack of ADH or the kidney tubules are not responsive to ADH and nephrogenic diabetes insipidus (see above) is present.

Mild hypernatremia also occurs in primary aldosteronism and in Cushing's syndrome. It can also occur as a result of drug therapy, as with methyldopa (Aldomet) or massive doses of sodium penicillin, or with large doses of sodium-retaining corticosteroids.

DIAGNOSIS

Water loss should also be differentiated from three other clinical syndromes associated with exposure to high environmental temperatures:

HEAT CRAMPS

Years ago, miners and steel factory workers who worked day after day in a hot environment developed heat cramps (miner's cramps, stoker's cramps) due to a loss of sodium and other electrolytes. However, the heat cramps that occur in athletes during hot weather, particularly early in the season, are due to a loss of water. The cramps usually affect the gastrocnemius muscles or thigh muscles, but can affect other muscles. Spasm of the abdominal muscles may simulate an acute abdomen.

Treatment consists of removal from direct sunlight, rest, ice packs to the affected muscles, and replacement of water orally.

Prevention includes adequate water during strenuous exercises or sports.

Athletes should not use so-called athletic drinks and sport beverages to replace losses of sweat. These beverages contain electrolytes and large concentrations of sweeteners to mask the bitter taste of the electrolytes. This makes the beverges hypertonic. Because they are hypertonic, they leave the stomach slowly. This produces a sensation of satiety that discourages the athlete from ingesting much-needed water (Smith).

HEAT EXHAUSTION (HEAT PROSTRATION, HEAT SYNCOPE)

This is due to a loss of water which results in reduced extracellular fluid and blood volume. As a result circulation to the brain decreases. Symptoms include weakness, visual disturbances, vertigo, pounding headache, and syncope. The skin is warm and moist. The pulse is weak and rapid, the blood pressure is decreased. The body temperature may be normal or slightly elevated.

Treatment includes removal from direct sunlight, rest, oral fluids (1 to 2 L in 2 to 4 hours). If the patient is unconscious, it may be necessary to give fluids IV. It is rarely necessary to give sodium chloride IV.

Prevention is the same as that used to prevent heat cramps (see above).

HEAT STROKE (HEAT PYREXIA)

Heat stroke can occur in two ways: 1. Induced by excessive physical exertion, in a hot environment, when it is not possible to dissipate the heat produced. This usually occurs in young healthy persons. Obesity, inadequate acclimatization to physical exertion, or potassium or salt depletion are contributing factors; 2. Not induced by excessive physical exertion. This occurs in older persons, particularly with congestive heart failure, malnutrition, or alcoholism, who are exposed to a high environmental temperature and are also deprived of an adequate amount of salt and water. It can also occur in patients who have dysfunction of the sweat glands, as in scleroderma or cystic fibrosis.

The following factors can aggravate or precipitate either type of heat stroke: drugs that *decrease thirst,* such as haloperidol; drugs that *decrease sweating,* such as anticholinergics, antihistamines, antiparkinsonism drugs, propranolol; drugs that *increase heat production,* such as amphetamines, tricyclic antidepressants, MAO inhibitors, LSD (lysergic acid diethylamide), thyroid extract.

The patient may at first complain of weakness, headache, dizziness, mental confusion, muscle cramps, a feeling of impending doom, or conversely, euphoria, as sweating decreases markedly or stops. In other patients, coma may occur abruptly. Delirium, generalized convulsions, abnormal Babinski reflexes, cerebellar disturbances, or hemoplegia may also develop.

The rectal temperature rises rapidly to 41°C (106°F) or higher and may reach 43° to 45°C (110° to 113°F). The skin is hot and dry and may show a pink or ashen color. Tachycardia is present and the heart rate may exceed 200 per minute. Respirations are rapid. The electrocardiogram may show nonspecific ST and T changes.

Complications of heat stroke include acute renal failure, particularly in the exertional type; rhabdomyolysis (skeletal muscle necrosis), only in the exertional type; disseminated intravascular coagulation; necrosis of liver cells with abnormal liver function test values and an elevated blood bilirubin (and jaundice); necrosis of heart muscle cells; electrolyte and acid-base disturbances, including hypernatremia, hypo- and hyperkalemia, hypocalcemia, hyperphosphatemia, hyperuricemia, respiratory alkalosis (in the nonexertional type) or lactic acidosis (in the exertional type of heat stroke).

Death usually occurs in the first 3 days, particularly with coma lasting more than 8 hours, shock, or a rectal temperature higher than 42°C (108°F). A patient who survives may develop delirium or aggressive behavior (which may last for several days after consciousness returns) and may require restraints. Abnormal neurological findings may persist indefinitely.

The usual recommended treatment when the rectal temperature is 41.1°C (106°F) or higher is to place the patient in an ice water tub bath, until the temperature falls to 38.8°C (102°F). An equally effective treatment is to place the patient on a bed with a large, high-powered fan blowing over him, and give vigorous massage with ice (Knochel). The rectal temperature should be taken every 10 minutes, because once it falls below 39.4°C (103°F) it may drop precipitously and shock may develop. Therefore, active cooling should be stopped when the temperature reaches 38.8°C (102°F).

The use of IV fluids or electrolytes will be determined by serum sodium and other electrolyte determinations.

When the temperature has fallen, the patient should be kept in a cool ventilated room, with an electric fan facing the bed. If the temperature rises again, active cooling with ice should be resumed. The patient should be kept in bed for at least several days until the temperature control becomes stable again.

If shock occurs, IV full-strength saline or lactated Ringer's solution may be of value. The patient may need 1200 to 1400 ml or more IV during the first 4 hours. The saline solution should not be used until the temperature has been lowered. (During the hyperpyrexia, particularly when the temperature is 39.4°C [103°F] or higher, there is marked vasodilatation. Vasoconstriction occurs as the temperature falls. If the saline solution had been given when the patient showed vasodilatation, the circulating blood volume may become excessive when vasoconstriction occurs.)

IV isoproterenol or dobutamine may be helpful if shock occurs. An alpha-adrenergic vasoconstrictor should not be infused when the temperature is still high, because it decreases the dissipation of heat.

Auxiliary treatment with chlorpromazine (Thorazine) in a dose of 50 mg intravenously at 4- to 6-hour intervals has also been used, as the temperature is being lowered. It prevents shivering or convulsions, which would cause the temperature to rise. It probably also lowers body temperature by means of a direct action on the central nervous system.

Acute renal failure is an indication for early hemodialysis, and a severe acidosis may require intravenous sodium bicarbonate (Barcenas, Hoeffler and Lie).

Prevention of heat stroke is the same as for heat exhaustion or heat cramps.

THE DIFFERENTIAL DIAGNOSIS OF CENTRAL DIABETES INSIPIDUS

The polyuria of central neurogenic (vasopressin-sensitive) diabetes insipidus should be differentiated from that caused by diabetes mellitus, chronic renal disease (nephrogenic diabetes insipidus), and by compulsive water drinking. The diagnosis of diabetes mellitus or chronic renal disease is usually simple. However, the patient with compulsive water drinking may develop impaired secretion of ADH, as does the patient with diabetes insipidus.

In diabetes insipidus, the initial disturbance is water loss due to polyuria. The excessive drinking is an attempt to overcome the loss of water. In compulsive water drinking, the initial disturbance is water excess, due to the excessive water drinking. The polyuria is an attempt to overcome the water excess. Therefore, the serum sodium concentration tends to be higher than normal in diabetes insipidus patients, and lower than normal in compulsive water drinkers.

Diabetes insipidus occurs equally in both sexes and may occur at any age. In approximately one-half the patients, no etiological factor is found. In other patients, it occurs after hypophysectomy, from basilar skull fractures, primary or metastatic brain tumors (particularly after breast carcinoma), or with cerebral histiocytosis (eosinophilic granuloma, Hand-Schüller-Christian disease), granulomatous infections (tuberculosis or sarcoidosis), other infections, or cerebral vascular insufficiency.

Patients who have had intracranial surgery may develop acute diabetes insipidus for a few days after surgery. This may then be followed by a period of severe water retention for 2 to 6 days. Then the patient may develop normal water metabolism, or permanent diabetes insipidus.

Compulsive water drinking (psychogenic polydipsia) occurs most commonly in women over 40 years. The patient with diabetes insipidus shows a rather constant intake of water from day to day. The compulsive water drinker shows a marked fluctuation in the daily volume of water imbibed, depending on the emotional state. Nocturia is common in diabetes insipidus, rare in compulsive water drinking.

A simple test for the diagnosis of diabetes insipidus is the water deprivation test. Water is withheld for 6 to 8 hours. Plasma and urine osmolality are measured at the beginning and end of the test. Normal persons will show little or no change in plasma osmolality, which remains below 300 mOsm/kg even at the end of the test. The urine osmolality is usually higher than the serum osmolality at the beginning of the test. Its osmolality becomes even higher at the end of the test so that urine/plasma osmolality ratio will always exceed 1, and even 2.

If diabetes insipidus is present, the plasma osmolality at the beginning of the test is usually higher than normal, and will rise above 300 mOsm/kg at the end of the test. The urine osmolality will be less than the plasma osmolality at the beginning of the test and will not change significantly. Therefore, the urine/plasma osmolality ratio will either remain unchanged or may even fall.

In a compulsive water drinker, the initial plasma osmolality is usually low (due to water dilution). The initial urine osmolality is also low. Both the plasma and urine osmolalities rise at the end of the test, so that the urine-plasma osmolality ratio is approximately 1. However, the plasma osmolality remains below 300 mOsm/kg.

In doing the water deprivation test, it is necessary to monitor the patient's weight carefully because a patient with severe diabetes insipidus may lose as much as 0.5 kg of body water per hour. The test should be stopped if the patient loses 3% or more of body weight.

Further discussion of diagnostic tests for diabetes insipidus, such as the infusion of hypertonic saline solution (Hickey-Hare test) or the use of nicotine or vasopressin, is beyond the scope of this book.

COURSE AND PROGNOSIS

This depends on the extent of the water loss, on the presence of associated losses of sodium and other electrolytes, on the physical condition of the patient, on the presence of central nervous system injury, and on the rapidity with which water is replaced.

When 12% of the body weight is lost, the patient loses the ability to swallow. Death usually occurs when 15 to 25% of the body weight is lost.

PROPHYLAXIS

Water loss can be avoided if one remembers the daily water requirements. For example, Table 3–1 shows the average daily water balance in an adult.

When a patient is not eating, because of starvation, a surgical oper-

Table 3–1. Daily Water Balance

Water intake		Water excretion	
In fluids	1500 ml approx.	Urine	1500 ml
In solid food	800 ml	Insensible perspiration	600 ml
In a mixed		Vaporization from lungs	400 ml
2500 calorie diet (from		In feces	100 ml
oxidation of hydrogen)	300 ml approx.		
in 100 g protein	41 ml	Total	2600 ml
in 110 g fat	118 ml		
in 244 g carbohydrate	135 ml		
	294 ml		
Total	2600 ml approx.		

ation, or any other cause, water is formed in the body as a result of three other mechanisms, namely, the lysis of muscle (lean) tissue,* the oxidation of muscle protein, and the oxidation of body fat.

The oxidation of body fat is the most important source of calories in a patient who is not eating, because each gram of fat provides 9 calories. Approximately 250 g or more of fat and 250 g of muscle tissue are catabolized daily under these circumstances.

The oxidation of 250 g of fat produces about 250 ml of water of oxidation (1 g fat produces 1.07 ml water). The lysis of 250 g of muscle tissue and the oxidation of the protein which is present in this tissue produce another 210 ml of water daily under these circumstances.

The minimal volume of water needed by the kidneys to excrete waste materials is dependent on the presence or absence of kidney disease (Fig. 3–1).

Approximately 12 ml water per kg body weight is lost by way of insensible perspiration and vaporization from the lungs daily. However, high ambient temperature, humidity, fever, and active sweating can greatly increase this loss. For example, a patient with a temperature of 104°F, breathing at a rate of 30 to 40 respirations per minute, can lose as much as 2500 ml water through the lungs daily.

As a general rule, an average adult requires approximately 1500 to 2000 ml pure water a day. If the patient has a high fever, an additional 500 to 1500 ml water daily is necessary. If the patient is sweating moderately, an additional 500 ml water daily is also needed, and if there is profuse perspiration, 100 ml water will be needed to compensate for the loss of water in the sweat. If renal disease is present, the

---

*Muscle tissue consists of approximately 73% water and 27% protein. Therefore, when 1 g of muscle tissue is lysed, 0.73 ml water is released from the cells. This is known as *preformed water, bound water, water of solution.* In addition, the oxidation of the 0.27 g of protein produces 0.11 ml water. (1 g protein produces 0.41 ml water of oxidation.) The total amount of water made available by the lysis and oxidation of 250 g of muscle tissue is therefore 250 × (0.73 ml + 0.11 ml) = 210 ml water.

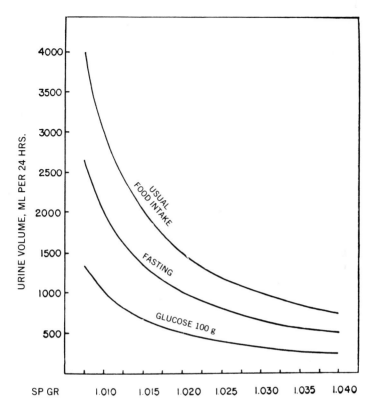

Fig. 3–1. Approximate relations of urinary volume to the ability of the kidneys to form concentrated urine. (After Gamble and after Statland.) The urinary solutes consist largely of urea and electrolytes. When kidney function is normal, 50 g of solute can be excreted in about 800 ml of urine. When renal disease is present and the kidneys are able to concentrate urine only to 1.010, for example, it would require approximately 3500 ml of urine to excrete 50 g of urinary solutes. Glucose (dextrose) has a protein-sparing effect and requires a smaller urinary volume if ingested.

Urinary specific gravity also varies with the relative amounts of urea and electrolytes. Therefore, if the patient is on a high-protein or low-sodium diet, the above diagram will not apply.

patient may require 3000 ml of water a day (Fig. 3–1).

TREATMENT

In water loss and desiccation, water, and water alone, is needed. However, the patient may have lost sodium and other ions as well as water. In such a case, these ions must be replaced. The loss of sodium in addition to water can be suspected if the patient has had a high fever and has sweated profusely, or if there has been vomiting, diarrhea, gastrointestinal drainage, and other findings. (The subject of sodium loss is discussed in detail in Chap 8.)

Type of Fluid Needed

Pure water is needed. Water alone can be given orally or rectally. However, pure water cannot be infused because it causes the red blood cells to swell and hemolyze. It must be given in an isotonic (isosmotic) solution. An isotonic solution is one which will cause neither an increase nor a decrease in the size of the red blood cells when given intravenously. A 5% dextrose (glucose) solution in water is approximately isotonic. However, 10% dextrose or 10% fructose, or invert sugar (which is half dextrose, half fructose), solutions, or even 25% and 50% dextrose solutions, can also be given intravenously without causing hemolysis of the red blood cells. The reason for this is that adequate mixing of the sugar with the blood occurs.

Volume of Fluid Needed

There are several methods of calculating the volume of water needed to treat water loss. However, one should remember that, regardless of the method of calculating water loss, additional water must be given to supply the daily water needs. For example, suppose that you calculate that a water loss of 4000 ml is present. The patient needs not only the 4000 ml, but an additional 1500 ml or more water daily to cover the daily water losses due to insensible perspiration, urinary output, and other causes.

Method 1. A simple way to calculate the water deficit is the following:

a. If thirst is present, but other clinical signs are minimal, one can assume that the water deficit is about 2% of the body weight. Thus, in a 70-kg (154-lb) patient, the water deficit would be approximately 1400 ml.
b. If the patient has gone 3 to 4 days without water, and if there is marked thirst, a dry mouth and oliguria, the water deficit is approximately 6% of the body weight. In a 70-kg patient, the water deficit would be approximately 4200 ml.
c. The above signs are present. In addition, if there are marked physical weakness and severe mental changes, such as confusion or delirium, the water deficit is 7 to 14% of the body weight. In a 70-kg patient, this would be approximately 5 to 10 liters.

Method 2. If the patient has been weighed daily, and it is known, for example, that he has lost 4 kg weight during an *acute* period of desiccation, the water deficit is approximately 4000 ml, or 4 liters.

Method 3. This method is based on the fact that the plasma sodium concentration varies inversely with the volume of extracellular water.

It assumes, however, that only water has been lost and that the sodium content of the body has remained unchanged.

The following formula is used:

$$Na_2 \times BW_2 = Na_1 \times BW_1.$$

Na_2 represents the present serum sodium concentration. BW_2 represents the present body water volume. Na_1 represents the original, or normal, serum sodium concentration of 142 mEq/L. BW_1 represents the original volume of body water. This is 60% of the body weight of a man (50% in a woman).

The loss of body water therefore equals $BW_1 - BW_2$.

Example:
Man, weighing approximately 70 kg. Present serum sodium concentration, 162 mEq/L.

$$Na_2 \times BW_2 = Na_1 \times BW_1$$
$$162 \times X = 142 \times 42$$
$$X = \frac{142 \times 42}{162} = 37 \text{ liters.}$$

The water loss is therefore $42 - 37 = 5$ liters.

Route of Fluid Administration

If the patient can drink water, the water should be given orally, unless vomiting is present. Water can also be given by means of an intranasal gastric tube, or rectally by means of a Murphy drip. However, if oral administration is impossible, it is best to use an intravenous solution of dextrose in water.

Rate of Administration

Ordinarily the water loss can be corrected in a period of 2 days. One-half the necessary volume of water is given the first day. This can be done either orally or by means of an infusion of 5% dextrose in water. A rate of administration of 120 to 1000 ml per hour can be used. (The relation between the number of drops per minute and the total volume per hour is described on page 352.)

(Water must never be given by nasogastric tube to a comatose patient unless a cuffed endotracheal tube is in place.)

If severe water loss is present and water is infused too rapidly, it may cause transient water intoxication and convulsions, because the brain cells have a higher osmolality than the other cells of the body, because idiogenic osmoles have been synthesized (see above). If water is given too rapidly, the brain cells will swell excessively. This can be avoided by giving the infusion slowly and by determining the serum sodium concentration after one-half the calculated volume of dextrose in water has been infused.

Patients with neurogenic diabetes insipidus usually respond to IM vasopressin tannate in oil (Pitressin), to aqueous Pitressin, or to a nasal spray of synthetic lysine-8-vasopressin (lypressin, Dyapid-Sandoz). Desmopressin (DDAVP-Ferring), a synthetic analog of argenine vasopressin, the natural human antidiuretic hormone (ADH), is now available for intranasal use.

Patients also respond to the thiazides and to the antidiabetic chlorpropamide. The thiazides probably act by decreasing the amount of sodium ions that reach the distal tubules of the kidneys. This is secondary to the sodium deficit induced by the thiazides. The thiazides are particularly effective in patients with nephrogenic diabetes insipidus.

Chlorpropamide and other sulfonylureas probably potentiate the action of ADH on the kidney tubules. (They can also cause hypoglycemia as a side efect, particularly if the patient fasts.)

The thiazides and chlorpropamide have additive effects and can be used simultaneously. Small doses, such as 125 to 375 mg chlorpropamide and 50 mg hydrochlorothiazide daily, are effective.

Clofibrate has also been used when central diabetes insipidus is not complete.

REFERENCES

Alford, F.P., and Scoggins, B.A.: Symptomatic normovolemic essential hypernatremia. Am J Med, *54*:359, 1973.

Arieff, A.I., Guisado, R., and Lazarowitz, V.C.: Pathophysiology of hyperosmolar states. I. *Disturbances in Body Fluids*. Edited by T.E. Andreoli, J.J. Grantham, S.C. Rector, Jr., American Physiology Society, Bethesda, Maryland, 1977.

Barlow, E.D., and deWardner, H.E.: Compulsive water drinking. Quart J Med, *28*:235, 1959.

Barcenas, C., Hoeffler, H.P., and Lie, J.T.: Obesity, football, dog days and siriasis. A deadly combination. Am Heart J, *92*:237, 1976.

Barron, W.M., et al.: Transient vasopressin-resistant diabetes insipidus of pregnancy. N Engl J Med, *310*:442, 1984.

Baxter, C.R., and Teschan, P.E.: Atypical heat stroke with hypernatremia, acute renal failure, and fulminating potassium intoxication. Arch Intern Med, *101*:1040, 1958.

Belding, H.S.: Hazards to health. Work in hot weather. N Engl J Med, *266*:1052, 1962.

Beyer, C.B.: Heat stress and the young athlete. Recognizing and reducing the risks. Postgrad Med, *76*:109, 1984.

Black, D.A.K., McCance, R.A., and Young, W.F.: A study of dehydration by means of balance experiments. J Physiol, *102*:406, 1944.

Boyd, A.E., and Beller, G.A.: Heat exhaustion and respiratory alkalosis, letter. Ann Intern Med, *83*:835, 1975.

Bricker, N.S., and Klahr, S.: Obstructive uropathy. In *Diseases of the Kidney*, 2nd ed. (Strauss, M.B., and Welt, L.G., Eds.). Boston, Little, Brown & Co., 1971.

Brunner, F.P., et al.: Hypokalemia, metabolic alkalosis, and hypernatremia due to "massive" sodium penicillin therapy. Br Med J, *4*:550, 1968.

Costrini, A.M., et al.: Cardiovascular and metabolic manifestations of heat stroke and severe heat exhaustion. Am J Med, *66*:296, 1979.

Clowes, G.H.A., and O'Donnell, T.F., Jr.: Heat stroke. N Engl J Med, *291*:564, 1974.

Coburn, J.W., and Reba, R.C.: Potassium depletion in heatstroke. Milit Med, *131*:678, 1966.

Cushard, W.G., Jr., et al.: Oral therapy of diabetes insipidus with chlorpropamide. Calif Med, *115*:1, 1971.

Dashe, A.M., Cramm, R.E., Crist, C.A., Habener, J.F., and Solomon, D.H.: A water deprivation test for the differential diagnosis of polyuria. JAMA, *185*:699, 1963.

DeRubertis, F.R., Michelis, M.F., and Davis, B.B.: "Essential" hypernatremia. Arch Intern Med, *134*:889, 1974.

Dies, F., Rangel, S., and Rivera, A.: Differential diagnosis between diabetes insipidus and compulsive polydipsia. Ann Intern Med, *54*:710, 1961.

Elkinton, J.R., and Taffel, M.: Prolonged water deprivation in the dog. J Clin Invest, *21*:787, 1942.

England, A.C., et al.: Preventing severe heat injury in runners. Ann Intern Med, *97*:196, 1982.

Feig, P.U., and McCurdy, D.K.: The hypertonic state. N Engl J Med, *297*:1444, 1977.

Fine, J.: Disseminated intravascular coagulation in heat stroke, letter. JAMA, *233*:1164, 1975.

Fitzsimons, J.T.: The physiological basis of thirst. Kidney Int, *10*:3, 1976.

Fourman, P., and Leeson, P.M.: Thirst and polyuria, with a note on the effects of potassium deficiency and calcium excess. Lancet, *1*:268, 1959.

Gamble, J.L.: *Chemical Anatomy, Physiology and Pathology of Extracellular Fluid,* 6th ed. Cambridge, Harvard University Press, 1954.

Gold, J.: Development of heat pyrexia. JAMA, *173*:1175, 1960.

Gordon, G.L., and Goldner, F.: Hypernatremia, azotemia and acidosis after cerebral injury. Am J Med, *23*:543, 1957.

Hariprasad, M.K., et al.: Hyponatremia in psychogenic polydipsia. Arch Intern Med, *140*:1639, 1980.

Hayek, A., and Ramirez, J.: Demeclocycline-induced diabetes insipidus. JAMA, *229*:676, 1974.

Hays, R.M.: Antidiuretic hormone. N Engl J Med, *295*:659, 1976.

Hoagland, R.J., and Bishop, R.J., Jr.: A physiologic treatment of heat stroke. Am J Med Sci, *241*:415, 1961.

Hockaday, T.D.R.: Diabetes insipidus. Br Med J, *1*:210, 1972.

Kaplan, S.A., Yuceoglu, A.M., and Strauss, J.: Vasopressin-resistant diabetes insipidus. J Dis Child, *97*:308, 1959.

Knochel, J.P.: Environmental heat illness. Arch Intern Med, *133*:841, 1974.

Knochel, J.P.: Dog days and siriasis. How to kill a football player. JAMA, *233*:513, 1975.

Knochel, J.P.: Clinical physiology of heat exposure. In *Clinical Disorders of Fluid and Electrolyte Metabolism,* 3rd ed., Maxwell, M.H., and Kleeman, C.R., editors. New York, McGraw-Hill Book Co., 1980.

Knochel, J.P., and Caskey, J.H.: The mechanism of hypophosphatemia in acute heat stroke. JAMA, *238*:425, 1977.

Leaf, A.: The clinical and physiologic significance of the serum sodium concentration. N Engl J Med, *267*:24, 1962.

Leaf, A.: Dehydration in the elderly, Editorial. N Engl J Med, *311*:791, 1984.

Marriott, H.L.: Water and salt depletion. Br Med J, *245*:285, 328, 1947.

Massry, S.G., and Coburn, J.W.: Clinical physiology of heat exposure. In *Clinical Disorders of Fluid and Electrolyte Metabolism.* 2nd ed. (Maxwell, M.H., and Kleeman, C.R., Eds.). New York, McGraw Hill Book Co., 1972.

Mellinger, R.C., and Zafar, S.: Primary polydipsia syndrome of inappropriate thirst. Arch Intern Med, *143*:1249, 1983.

Middleton, D.B.: Treatment of hypernatremic dehydration. N Engl J Med, *291*:683, 1974.

Moore, F.D.: Common patterns of water and electrolyte change in injury, surgery and disease. N Engl J Med, *258*:277, 325, 377, 427, 1958.

Morris-Jones, P.H., and Houston, I.B.: Prognosis of the neurological complications of acute hypernatremia. Lancet, *2*:1385, 1967.

Murphy, R.J.: Heat illness in the athlete. Am J Sports Med, *12*:258, 1984.

Nelson, D.C., et al.: Hypernatremia and lactulose therapy. JAMA, *249*:1295, 1983.

O'Donnell, T.F., and Clowes, G.H.A.: The circulatory abnormalities of heat stroke. N Engl J Med, *287*:734, 1972.

Phillips, P.A., et al.: Reduced thirst after water deprivation in healthy elderly men. N Engl J Med, *311*:753, 1984.

Price, J.D.E., and Lauerner, R.W.: Serum and urine osmolalities in the differential diagnosis of polyuric states. J Clin Endocr, *26*:143, 1966.

Raff, S.B., and Gershberg, H.: Night sweats. A dominant symptom in diabetes insipidus. JAMA, *234*:1252, 1975.

Roberts, K.E.: Mechanism of dehydration following alcohol ingestion. Arch Intern Med, *112*:52, 1963.

Robinson, A.G.: DDAVP in the treatment of central diabetes insipidus. N Engl J Med, *294*:507, 1976.

Sandifer, M.: Hyponatremia due to psychotropic drugs. J Clin Psychiatry, *44*:301, 1983.

Sawyer, R.B., et al.: Hypernatremia with pharmacological doses of steroids. Am J Surg, *114*:691, 1967.

Shibolet, S., et al.: Heatstroke. Its clinical picture and mechanism in 36 cases. Quart J Med, *36*:525, 1967.

Simon, N.M., Garber, E., and Arieff, A.J.: Persistent nephrogenic diabetes insipidus after lithium carbonate. Ann Intern Med, *86*:446, 1977.

Smith, N.J.: The prevention of heat disorders in sports. Am J Dis Child, *138*:786, 1984.

Sohar, E., Michaeli, D., and Shibolet, S.: Heatstroke caused by dehydration and physical effort. Arch Intern Med, *122*:159, 1958.

Statland, H.: *Fluid and Electrolytes in Practice,* 3rd ed. Philadelphia, J.B. Lippincott Co., 1963.

Sturtz, G.S., and Burke, E.C.: Obstructive water losing uropathy. JAMA, *166*:45, 1958.

The Medical Letter: Demopressin for diabetes insipidus, 20: no. 5, March 10, 1978.

Weitzman, R., and Kleeman, C.R.: Water metabolism and the neurohypophyseal hormones. In *Clinical Disorders of Fluid and Electrolyte Metabolism,* 3rd ed., Maxwell, M.H., and Kleeman, C.R., editors. New York, McGraw-Hill Book Co., 1980.

Welt, L.G.: Water balance in health and disease. In *Diseases of Metabolism* (Duncan, G.G., Ed.). Philadelphia, W.B. Saunders Co., 1964.

Welt, L.G.: Hypo- and hypernatremia. Ann Intern Med, *56*:161, 1962.

Zelman, S., and Guillan, R.: Heat stroke in phenothiazine-treated patients. A report of three fatalities. Am J Psychiatr, *126*:1787, 1970.

CHAPTER 4

WATER LOSS SYNDROMES
(Continued)
WATER LOSS DUE TO SOLUTE EXCESS

This type of water loss is caused by the urinary excretion of an excessive amount of solutes such as sodium, chloride, potassium, and other anions and cations, or nonionic solutes such as dextrose, fructose, or other sugars, or urea, amino acids, or other nitrogenous products, which act as osmotic diuretics and cause an obligatory loss of water.

Synonym: Solute loading hypertonicity.

ETIOLOGY

Water loss due to solute excess can occur:

1. When an unconscious patient is given nasogastric feedings that supply a large amount of solutes, such as salt, dextrose, proteins and other substances, with an inadequate volume of water. When a patient is given nasogastric feeding with a high protein mixture, particularly if the daily protein intake is more than 150 g, much of the protein is not utilized and is converted to urea, which is excreted in the urine along with water.
2. When a patient with a bleeding peptic ulcer is given frequent feedings of milk and cream without water. Here, the absorption of partially digested blood, as well as the milk and cream, causes a great increase in the solute concentration of the blood.
3. When a patient convalescing from a severe burn is given a high carbohydrate diet, particularly more than 300 g of carbohydrate a day. The patient may not be able to metabolize such a large amount of carbohydrate and the excessive glucose is excreted in the urine along with water (burn stress pseudodiabetes).
4. With many conditions associated with hyperosmolality (Chap 5).

PATHOPHYSIOLOGY

Substances such as dextrose, amino acids, and others that are used for nasogastric feedings act as osmotic diuretics. In other words, when they reach the kidneys in excessive concentrations, they are automatically excreted along with a large amount of water. This can cause a large water loss. The kidneys may also excrete sodium with the water. This may cause a sodium loss in addition to a water loss.

When the water loss occurs, the compensatory mechanisms described in Chapter 3 occur.

SYMPTOMS, SIGNS, AND LABORATORY FINDINGS

These are similar to those which occur in ordinary water loss due to a decreased water intake or the inability of the kidney tubules to conserve water. However, the following differences are present:

1. In water loss due to solute excess, the patient may gain weight, instead of losing, as the syndrome develops.
2. In water loss due to solute excess, the patient passes large amounts of urine as the water loss develops, whereas in water loss due to decreased water intake or defective renal tubular function, the patient becomes oliguric as the water loss develops.
3. In water loss due to solute excess, the plasma osmolality can rise to very high levels, due to the excessive amounts of solutes in the blood, but the hematocrit remains essentially normal. For example, a plasma osmolality of 340 mOsm/kg can be present with a hematocrit of 45%. In ordinary water loss, the plasma osmolality and the hematocrit will rise proportionately. For example, a plasma osmolality of 340 mOsm/kg with a hematocrit of 55 or 66% or higher is not uncommon.
4. The polyuria associated with solute excess can be differentiated from the polyuria due to water excess, as occurs in diabetes insipidus for example, in the following ways: When solute excess is present, the urine specific gravity tends to be higher (1.009 to 1.035 or higher) than when the polyuria is due to water diuresis (1.001 to 1.005). Similarly, when solute excess is present, the urine osmolality is higher (250 to 320 mOsm/kg) than when the polyuria is due to water diuresis (50 to 150 mOsm/kg) (Berman).

DIAGNOSIS

Water loss due to solute excess should be suspected in patients who are receiving nasogastric tube feedings, or in diabetic or other patients who are receiving large amounts of saline but who show clinical signs of desiccation. A serum sodium concentration of 150 mEq/L or more indicates the presence of water loss (unless the patient has been receiving large volumes of saline solution intravenously).

When water loss is present with hyperglycemia, the serum sodium concentration in relation to the glucose concentration may be of value in differential diagnosis. In water loss due to solute excess, the increased serum sodium occurs when the blood sugar falls, as in a patient with diabetic acidosis who is being treated with insulin and saline solution. In water loss caused by a brain injury or cerebral disease, an increased serum sodium may be present in association with an elevated blood glucose.

COURSE AND PROGNOSIS

Water loss due to solute excess is even more serious than water loss due to decreased water intake, because nasogastric tube feedings are usually used for seriously ill patients. Death will occur unless the condition is recognized early.

PROPHYLAXIS

When a patient is being given nasogastric tube feedings, particularly if the daily protein intake is 150 g or more, he or she should be observed carefully for clinical signs of desiccation. If such signs develop, the concentration of the tube feedings should be decreased, and more water should be given.

TREATMENT

The treatment is the same as that for water loss due to a decreased water intake. The volume of water lost can be calculated from the increased serum sodium concentration, and the water can be given orally or intravenously. In addition, if the patient has been receiving nasogastric tube feedings these should be stopped temporarily. During treatment with water, the patient will continue to pass large volumes of urine.

REFERENCES

Berman, L.B.: An abundance of urine. JAMA, 229:203, 1974.

Engel, F.L., and Jaeger, C.: Dehydration with hypernatremia, hyperchloremia and azotemia complicating nasogastric tube feeding. Am J Med, 17:196, 1954.

Fonkalsrud, E.W., and Keen, J.: Hypernatremic dehydration from hypertonic enemas in congenital megacolon. JAMA, 199:584, 1967.

Gault, M.H., et al.: Hypernatremia, azotemia, and dehydration due to high-protein tube feeding. Ann Intern Med, 68:778, 1968.

Moore, F.D.: Metabolic Care of the Surgical Patient. Philadelphia, W.B. Saunders Co., 1959.

Wilson, W.S., and Meinert, J.K.: Extracellular hyperosmolarity secondary to high-protein nasogastric tube feeding. Ann Intern Med, 47:585, 1957.

CHAPTER 5

WATER LOSS SYNDROMES (Continued)

WATER LOSS DUE TO HYPEROSMOLALITY

Water loss due to hyperosmolality can occur whenever the extracellular water becomes hyperosmolal for any reason. The hyperosmolality due to the administration of food in excess of water has been described in Chapter 4. In this chapter, hyperosmolality which may occur in diabetic patients (hyperosmolal, hyperglycemia, nonketoacidotic diabetic coma) and the hyperosmolality associated with the parenteral or rectal administration of substances that increase the osmolality of the blood will be described.

HYPEROSMOLAL, HYPERGLYCEMIC, NONKETOACIDOTIC DIABETIC COMA

Hyperosmolal, hyperglycemic, nonketoacidotic diabetic coma may occur in middle-aged or elderly diabetic patients whose diabetes is not severe. Most of the patients are over sixty years. Rarely, the condition occurs in young patients.

Precipitating factors include treatment with corticosteroids, chlorpromazine, antimetabolites, or phenytoin (Dilantin), thiazide diuretics, furosemide or ethacrynic acid, propranolol, cimetidine, diazoxide, mannitol, mafenide burn ointment, glycerol therapy for cerebral edema. peritoneal dialysis with a high glucose solution, or diseases such as pancreatitis or carcinoma of the pancreas, acute pyelonephritis, acute myocardial infarction, subdural hematoma, hemorrhage from the gastrointestinal tract, burns, systemic lupus erythematosus, pemphigus, and hypothermia.

Pathophysiology

The precipitating factor is reduced insulin activity. This may be due to a decreased insulin reserve or to increased endogenous insulin antagonists. The decreased insulin activity is adequate to control the acidosis, but is not adequate to control the hyperglycemia.

The condition slowly develops over many days. The hyperglycemia increases and the osmotic pressure of the extracellular water rises much higher than that of the cells. As a result, water flows from the cells to the extracellular water. This decreases the water content of the cells and temporarily increases the water content of the extracellular water. However, the large amount of glucose that is brought to the kidneys acts as an osmotic diuretic. When the glucose is filtered through the glomeruli and enters the kidney tubules, it has to be excreted with water. The large amount of glucose excreted produces a large water loss. The increased serum sodium concentration that results from the water loss also contributes to the hyperosmolality.

Cerebral symptoms and signs occur because of the blood-brain barrier. The glucose level and the osmolality of the *blood* are much higher than the glucose level and osmolality of the *cerebrospinal fluid*. As a result, water passes from the cerebrospinal fluid into the blood to equalize the different osmotic pressures (Chap 2). This produces severe dehydration of the brain cells. Intracerebral or subarachnoid hemorrhages may also develop.

Renal tubular dysfunction may also be present and may be one of the factors that cause a loss of water (Chap 3).

Symptoms and Signs

During this time, the patient continues to eat, but becomes thirsty from the water loss. He or she often drinks a large amount of juice which contains carbohydrate to slake the unquenchable thirst. This aggravates the condition. (Many patients are not aware that they are diabetic.)

When the water loss becomes excessive, the patient becomes less aware that he or she is thirsty and drinks less. Therefore, the hyperglycemia and the hyperosmolality increase.

At this time, abnormal neurological signs may develop. These include stiffness of the neck, extensor plantar responses, focal or generalized convulsive seizures, and coma. In addition, the patient shows the characteristic physical signs of water loss (Chap 3) and may show signs of shock, arterial or venous thrombosis, or acute renal failure. A high fever may develop because of the water loss.

(Coma due to overdosage with oxazepam [Serax] may simulate non-ketoacidotic diabetic coma because the oxazepam gives a false-positive reaction for glucose.)

Laboratory Findings

The serum glucose concentration is usually above 1000 mg/dl. The serum osmolality is greatly increased. The serum sodium concentration may or may not be increased (see Appendix IV). The serum potassium concentration may be normal or decreased. The plasma shows no acetone or only a trace. The pH is within normal or may show a slight acidosis. The BUN concentration is elevated because of decreased renal blood flow. Therefore, the serum creatinine concentration remains essentially normal and the BUN:creatinine ratio becomes much higher than the normal 10:1 ratio (Chap 21).

The urine characteristically shows a 4 plus glucose reaction, but no ketonuria. (Occasionally, the urine may show a small or moderate amount of ketones.)

The white blood count may rise even to 50,000/cu ml.

The patient continues to have a seemingly adequate urine output. This may be misleading because the physician may misinterpret this as a sign of adequate water intake.

Treatment

Relatively small amounts of regular insulin are needed. Twenty units of regular insulin can be given intramuscularly initially. This can be followed by 5 units of regular insulin intramuscularly every hour until the blood glucose level falls to 300 mg/dl. When this occurs, the insulin can be stopped. (Some patients may show insulin resistance.)

The insulin therapy can result in severe hypokalemia, particularly if the serum potassium level was low before treatment. In such cases, potassium chloride, in a dose of 20 to 40 mEq, can be added to each liter of intravenous fluid. However, no parenteral potassium chloride should be given until the patient shows an adequate urinary output.

If the patient is able to drink, water should be given orally. Water can also be given by way of a nasogastric tube.

There are differences of opinion about the best fluid to give intravenously. Most physicians prefer to start with a hypotonic saline solution (half-strength), and agree that dextrose solutions should *not* be used at the beginning of treatment. Dextrose solutions can be given when the blood glucose concentration has fallen to 250 mg/dl.

A variable amount of intravenous fluid is needed. It has been calculated that as much as 6 to 16 liters of fluid may be needed the first 24 hours. If hypotonic solutions are continually used, there is a danger that water excess will develop. Therefore, isotonic saline can be used when the serum sodium concentration (corrected for the hyperglycemia [Appendix IV]) begins to fall. Replacement of potassium ions may also be necessary.

Prognosis

In spite of treatment, the mortality of hyperosmolal, hyperglycemic, nonketoacidotic diabetic coma patients is almost 50%.

HYPEROSMOLALITY DUE TO OTHER CONDITIONS

Water loss due to hyperosmolality can also occur in diabetic patients who do not have nonketoacidotic diabetic coma, for example:

In untreated diabetic acidosis, a large amount of glucose is excreted by the kidneys. This is associated with polyuria and water loss.

A similar clinical picture of water loss due to hyperosmolality can occur in another way when diabetic acidosis is present. When the blood glucose concentration is high, the osmotic pressure of the extracellular water becomes greater than that of the cells, and water will flow from the cells into the extracellular water, diluting it. When the serum sodium concentration is measured in such a patient, it may be low. However, this is more apparent than real, since it is produced by the dilution of the extracellular water (Appendix IV).

When the patient is given insulin, the blood glucose concentration falls, the osmotic pressure of the extracellular water also falls and becomes lower than that of the cells. Water therefore flows from the extracellular water into the cells, and the concentration of the extracellular electrolytes, including the serum sodium concentration, becomes elevated. If a large amount of sodium chloride and other sodium salts, such as bicarbonate or lactate, and other substances have been used in the treatment of the diabetic acidosis, the total electrolyte concentration may rise steeply and a serious water loss due to the excretion of these substances may develop, even though the diabetic acidosis is controlled.

Hyperosmolality can also occur after repeated angiocardiography with contrast material, after the intravenous use of sodium sulfate for hypercalcemia, after repeated hypertonic enemas for congenital megacolon. It can occur as a complication of therapeutic abortion, when hypertonic sodium chloride solution is inadvertently injected intraperitoneally or intravascularly instead of into the amniotic cavity.

Hyperosmolality is also often present in patients with chronic renal disease, due to the marked increase in nitrogenous substances in the extracellular water and blood. In many of these patients, the hyperosmolality may be overlooked because the serum sodium concentration is low (for reasons discussed in Appendix IV). However, the serum osmolality is high.

A similar syndrome may occur in patients convalescing from severe burns. These patients may be unable to metabolize diets high in carbohydrate, particularly over 300 g of carbohydrate a day. This syndrome can be prevented by avoiding a high carbohydrate intake.

REFERENCES

Arieff, A.I., and Carroll, H.J.: Nonketotic hyperosmolar coma with hyperglycemia. Medicine, 51:73, 1972.

Arieff, A.I., et al.: Pathophysiology of hyperosmolar states, in T.E. Andreoli, J.J. Grantham, and F.C. Rector, Jr., (eds.) *Disturbances in Body Fluid Osmolality,* Chap. 11, Bethesda, Maryland, American Physiology Society, 1977.

Boyer, J., Gill, G.N., and Epstein, F.H.: Hyperglycemia and hyperosmolality complicating peritoneal dialysis. Ann Intern Med, *67*:568, 1967.

Boyer, M.H.: Hyperosmolar anacidotic coma in association with glucocorticoid therapy. JAMA, *202*:1007, 1967.

Fulop, M., Tannenbaum, H., and Dreyer, N.: Ketotic hyperosmolar coma. Lancet, *2*:635, 1973.

Gerich, J.E., Martin, M.M., and Recant, L.: Clinical and metabolic characteristics of hyperosmolar nonketotic coma. Diabetes, *20*:228, 1971.

Giammona, S.T., Lurie, P.R., and Segar, W.E.: Hypertonicity following selective angiocardiography. Circulation, *28*:1096, 1963.

Lindsey, C.A., et al.: Plasma glucagon in nonketotic hyperosmolar coma. JAMA, *229*:1771, 1974.

McCurdy, D.K.: Hyperosmolar hyperglycemic nonketotic diabetic coma. Med Clin N Am, *54*:683, 1970.

Perry, T.L.: et al.: Nonketotic hyperglycemia. N Engl J Med, *292*:1269, 1975.

Podolsky, S.: Nonketotic diabetic coma in the cardiac patient. Cardiovasc Reviews & Reports, *4*:201, 1983.

Questions and Answers: Hypernatremia from intravascular saline infusion during therapeutic abortion. JAMA, *220*:1749, 1972.

Rosenberg, S.A., et al.: The syndrome of dehydration, coma, and severe hyperglycemia without ketosis in patients convalescing from burns. N Engl J Med, *272*:931, 1965.

Ross, E.J., and Christie, S.B.M.: Hypernatremia. Medicine, *48*:441, 1969.

Sament, S.: Hyperosmolar coma in diabetes. Lancet, *1*:1153, 1966. Also N Engl J Med, *276*:1385, 1967.

Sherwood, L.M.: Hypernatremia during sodium sulfate therapy. N Engl J Med, *277*:314, 1967.

Whelton, M.J., Walde, D., and Havard, C.W.H.: Hyperosmolar non-ketotic diabetic coma, with particular reference to vascular complications. Br Med J, *1*:85, 1971.

Woods, J.E., et al.: Hyperosmolar non-ketotic diabetic coma, with particular reference to vascular complications. Br Med J, *1*:85, 1971.

Woods, J.E., et al.: Hyperosmolar nonketotic syndrome and steroid diabetes. Occurrence after renal transplantation. JAMA, *232*:1261, 1975.

Zileli, M.S., et al.: Oxazepam intoxication simulating non-ketoacidotic coma. JAMA, *215*:1986, 1971.

CHAPTER 6

WATER EXCESS SYNDROMES

Water excess occurs when a patient receives more water than the kidneys can excrete.

Synonyms: Water intoxication, overhydration, dilution syndrome.

ETIOLOGY

When the posterior pituitary gland, the kidneys, and the adrenal glands are normal, it is almost impossible for a person to take enough water by mouth to produce water excess (except in the case of a psychotic patient). However, water excess can be experimentally produced by infusing water at a rate faster than the kidneys can excrete it (about 13 ml per minute).

Water excess is likely to occur when the following groups of patients are given excessive water or hypotonic (hyposmotic) solutions either orally, subcutaneously, intravenously, or rectally:

1. When ADH secretion is excessive. This can occur as a result of fear, pain, analgesics or anesthetics, an acute infection such as pneumonia, an acute medical stressful situation such as an acute myocardial infarction, an acute surgical stressful situation, such as trauma or a major operation, or even being hospitalized. Excessive ADH secretion can also occur in many other clinical conditions (see Chap 7).
2. When the renal blood flow is low and the kidneys are not able to excrete water normally. This is seen in:
   a. Addison's disease, and other conditions of adrenocortical insufficiency.

   Water excess can also occur and produce stupor and coma in patients with hypopituitarism (pituitary coma). This occurs especially if a water tolerance test is being performed. The excessive water retention that these patients show is due to the fact that they lack ACTH. As a result, there is a deficient secretion of adrenal cortical steroids which normally enable the kidneys to excrete water when necessary. The situation is similar to that which occurs in Addison's disease.

   b. Acute renal insufficiency. Water excess occurs when the physician attempts to increase the urinary volume by giving large infusions of dextrose in water.
   c. Severe congestive heart failure, or cirrhosis of the liver with low renal blood flows.

3. In a patient with normal kidneys and posterior pituitary gland who is given large volumes of water rectally. This occurs, for example, in children with congenital megacolon who are treated too vigorously with enemas. A barium enema may also cause water excess. The barium spreads throughout the colon and the water comes into contact with a large absorbing surface. This can be aggravated if water is subsequently used to help evacuate the barium.

4. When a continual intravenous infusion (usually of 5% dextrose in water) is administered to a hospitalized patient to keep a vein open (KVO). If a microdrip bulb is not attached to the IV tubing, and if the rate of flow is not kept minimal, as much as a liter or more of fluid will be infused in each 24-hour period.

5. In hospitalized patients as a result of fluids taken with medication, little sips of water, or mouth washing. It has been calculated that as much as 500 to 1000 ml water can be imbibed daily in this way. In addition, chronically or seriously ill patients are usually anorexic and prefer liquids to solids. If they imbibe sodium-free liquids, such as ginger ale, water, or fruit juices, rather than eating solid food, this can also result in water excess.

6. From absorption of the irrigating fluid during transurethral electroresection of the prostate.

7. Sodium loss from any reason (vomiting, diuretics, low-sodium intake, and so on). The reason for this is that when sodium loss occurs, the osmotic pressure of the blood and the extracellular water is lower than that of the cells. Therefore, water flows from the blood and extracellular water into the cells, which swell. Water excess aggravates this condition.

For example, water excess is rare in compulsive water drinkers (who usually show symptoms suggestive of diabetes insipidus unless another factor, such as the use of diuretics, is also present). Habitual excessive beer drinking (exceeding 4 liters daily) may also cause water excess with severe neurological signs. Here again, other factors, such as sodium loss, are probably also present.

PATHOPHYSIOLOGY

When a normal person is given an excess of water, the water will dilute the extracellular water, and its osmotic pressure will become less than that of the cells. As a result, water will flow into the cells. This will cause the posterior pituitary gland to stop secreting ADH, and a water diuresis will occur. However, if the patient is in an antidiuretic state due to excessive secretion of ADH, the water will be retained. This causes a further decrease in the osmotic pressure of the extracellular water, and a further flow of water into the cells.

The retention of water causes an increased volume of the extracellular water. Normally, when the volume of the extracellular water rises, aldosterone secretion stops and the kidneys stop retaining sodium, which is then excreted along with water (Chap 2). Here, the increased volume of the extracellular water also causes aldosterone secretion to stop. Therefore, the kidneys excrete sodium, but a free water diuresis does not occur because of the excessive ADH which is present. This loss of sodium ions by the kidneys merely aggravates the water excess, because it causes the osmotic pressure of the extracellular fluid to fall still further. Thus, a vicious cycle is created. A patient with latent epilepsy may develop a convulsive seizure when only minimal water excess is present.

The mechanism causing convulsions is not known. One explanation is that the convulsions are due to the entrance of water into the cells of the central nervous system. However, Helwig studied the histological changes in the brains of laboratory animals and one human being who died of water excess and did not find any actual neuronal swelling.

SYMPTOMS

Wynn has pointed out that in acute water excess the symptoms start dramatically and suddenly. The patient develops strange behavior, loss of attention, confusion, staring, aphasia, incoordination, sleepiness interposed with periods of violent behavior, shouting, delirium, and extreme muscle weakness. This may be followed by convulsive seizures, coma and overbreathing.

If the water excess occurs slowly, the patient may complain of weakness, apathy, sleepiness, and may have anorexia, nausea and vomiting. Headache and muscle cramps are rare. Later, personality changes occur, with disorientation or psychotic behavior, convulsive seizures, or coma.

Salivation and lacrimation may be marked, and a watery diarrhea may occur because of the water excess. However, there is no unusual sweating. The patient may complain of thirst, though it is difficult to explain this symptom. When water excess develops slowly, the patient may have minimal symptoms.

SIGNS

There is a history of an acute gain of weight.

Skin

The skin is warm, moist and may be flushed. It may become edematous and show "fingerprinting," which is elicited in the following way: If you roll your finger over a bony prominence such as the patient's sternum or tibia, your fingerprint will become visible on the patient's skin.

Central Nervous System

There is gross muscle weakness, and isolated muscle twitching may occur. The tendon reflexes are usually diminished or absent. However, when convulsions or coma occur, a positive Babinski reflex may appear. The patient may also develop a hemiplegia. Papilledema may occur in association with an increased pressure of the cerebrospinal fluid.

The electroencephalogram may show abnormalities such as theta and delta waves.

Cardiovascular System

The cardiovascular system remains normal. Subcutaneous edema or pulmonary edema may occur, or become aggravated, particularly if the patient has congestive heart failure.

LABORATORY FINDINGS

Blood

Hemoglobin and mean corpuscular hemoglobin concentration (MCHC) are decreased because of the water dilution. The mean corpuscular volume (MCV) of the red blood cells is increased because the osmotic pressure of the plasma (and the extracellular water) is lower than that of the cells. This causes water to enter the cells, including the red blood cells, making them swell. The hematocrit remains relatively unchanged because the swelling of the red cells is proportional to the increased plasma volume.

Serum Electrolyte Concentrations

The serum sodium and other electrolyte concentrations may be low as a result of the water dilution. The blood urea nitrogen is normal or low, unless it was previously high. Potassium is either normal or low.

The serum sodium concentration is below 130 mEq/L. It may fall to 115 mEq/L, or even lower. However, the rate of lowering is more important than the absolute concentration reached, and convulsions may occur when the serum sodium concentration falls rapidly, even to 120 mEq/L.

A marked lowering of the bicarbonate may occur in acute water excess. This is due to overbreathing and the development of an acute respiratory alkalosis.

Urine

The urinary volume may be low or high. The specific gravity is usually low, especially if the urinary volume is high. Sodium and chloride may be present in the urine, in spite of the low sodium and chloride concentrations in the serum. In some patients, however, the urinary sodium and chloride content becomes low.

DIAGNOSIS

Water excess should be suspected when a postoperative patient develops strange behavior, a convulsive seizure or hemiplegia, or becomes comatose. A sudden lowering of the serum sodium concentration is also a good sign of water excess, unless sodium has been lost by some extrarenal route, such as vomiting, diarrhea, or paracentesis.

The presence of a low serum sodium concentration by itself is not pathognomonic of water excess. It can occur also in patients with a true sodium loss, or in diabetic or uremic patients when the serum glucose or BUN concentration is high (see Appendix IV). However, in water excess, the serum osmolality is characteristically low, whereas, in diabetic patients with low serum sodium concentrations, the serum osmolality may be high or normal, and will be low only when water excess is also present.

A low serum sodium concentration can also occur in the syndrome of inappropriate secretion of ADH (the antidiuretic hormone) (Chap 7).

Chronic Cellular Hypoosmolality

In early editions of this book, there was a chapter on chronic cellular hypoosmolality (*synonyms:* internal dilution hyponatremia, asymptomatic hyponatremia, new steady state, sodium paradox), due to a primary decrease in the osmotic pressure of the cells. When this occurs, there is a shift of water from the cells to the extracellular water, to equalize the intra- and extracellular osmotic pressures. As a result, the serum sodium concentration becomes low.

Theoretically, chronic cellular hypoosmolality can occur. However, it is not possible to measure the osmotic pressure of cells. In addition, I believe that most, if not all, patients, such as the chronically ill or malnourished, or those with various forms of tuberculosis, who have been described as showing chronic cellular hypoosmolality can be described more simply in terms of simple water excess or as having an inappropriate secretion of ADH (Chap 7).

COURSE AND PROGNOSIS

If moderate water excess is present and no further water is given, the patient will usually recover spontaneously. However, if the patient has developed a convulsive seizure, or has become comatose, or has developed a hemiplegia, death may occur even when the patient is treated vigorously.

The water excess syndrome which occurs after trauma and postoperatively is usually self-limited. However, if it occurs in a severe form, the serum potassium concentration may rise to very high levels. This may be dangerous to life, particularly since the toxic effects of potassium ions on the heart are aggravated by hyponatremia, which is present, and by hypocalcemia, which may also be present.

The exact cause of the marked increase in serum potassium concentration which may occur is not known. The elevated serum potassium and the low serum sodium concentrations resemble the electrolyte patterns of acute adrenal cortical insufficiency. However, it has been shown that the concentration of free blood corticosteroids is high (40 to 80 mg/dl) in these patients after extensive surgery. This indicates that the adrenal cortex is functioning normally.

PROPHYLAXIS

There is a tendency to give postoperative patients and patients with acute renal shutdown too much water. Methods of avoiding this are described in Chapters 33 and 34. Similarly, the physician should remember that water excess can occur if too much water is given, regardless of the route of administration.

TREATMENT

Type of Fluid Needed

Water excess is treated in two ways:

1. Fluids should be withheld for 24 hours. In this way at least 1000 ml will be lost through the skin and lungs, and a large volume will be excreted in the urine. This alone will correct a moderate water excess.
2. If convulsions or hemiplegia have occurred, or if the patient is comatose, fluids must be withheld. In addition, hypertonic sodium chloride solution (3 to 5%) should be given.

    If the patient is acidotic, and chloride ions are contraindicated, a one-third or one-half molar lactate solution can be used instead of the hypertonic sodium chloride solution.

Volume of Fluid Needed

It is not necessary to calculate the exact volume of water excess which is present in order to determine the volume of 5% sodium chloride solution needed. The reason for this is that the body is not a closed system, and a relatively small volume of hypertonic sodium chloride solution will prevent death and enable the kidneys to respond by the excretion of large volumes of water.

A simple rule to use is to give the patient 6 ml hypertonic (5%) sodium chloride solution per kg of body weight.

Example: Patient weighing 70 kg.
6 × 70 = 420 ml. 5% sodium chloride solution needed.
This will raise the serum sodium concentration approximately 10 mEq/L.

The derivation of this rule is given in Appendix III.

If there is doubt whether water excess is present, one-fourth to one-half of the calculated hypertonic sodium chloride solution can be given and the patient can be checked by noting signs of clinical improvement, or a rise in serum sodium concentration.

Route of Fluid Administration

Hypertonic sodium chloride solution can be given only intravenously.

Rate of Fluid Administration

The hypertonic sodium chloride solution should be given at a rate of 100 ml per hour. One hundred ml should be infused. Then the patient should be observed for a half hour. At this time, another 100 ml can be infused. Not more than 400 ml 5% sodium chloride solution should be infused in 1 day.

Other Treatment

D'Angelo and his associates have suggested that the excessive secretion of ADH which occurs postoperatively in mitral commissurotomy patients can be suppressed by giving absolute alcohol in a dose of 20 to 50 ml daily on the second, third, or fourth postoperative day. The alcohol may be given in fruit juice by mouth or, if the patient is nauseated, as a 5% intravenous solution in 5% dextrose in water. The alcohol acts as a diuretic and may cause a marked increase in urinary output.

REFERENCES

Baskin, J.L., Keith, H.M., and Scribner, B.H.: Water metabolism in water intoxication: review of basic concepts. Am J Dis Child, *83*:618, 1952.

Beresford, H.R.: Polydipsia, hydrochlorothiazide, and water intoxication. JAMA, *214*:879, 1970.

Bewley, T.H.: Acute water intoxication from compulsive water drinking. Br Med J, *2*:861, 1964.

D'Angelo, G.J., Murdaugh, H.V., Jr., and Sealy, W.C.: The nature and treatment of the postcommissurotomy hyponatremic syndrome. Surg Gynecol Obstet, 106:87, 1958.

Demanet, J.C., et al.: Coma due to water intoxication in beer drinkers. Lancet, 2:1115, 1971.

Desmond, J.: Serum osmolality and plasma electrolytes in patients who develop dilutional hyponatremia during transurethral resection. Canad J Surg, 13:116, 1970.

Editorial: The hazard of water enemas. Lancet, 1:559, 1959.

Gupta, D.R., and Cohen, N.H.: Oxytocin, "salting out" and water intoxication. JAMA, 220:681, 1972.

Holmes, J.H., Sitprija, W., et al.: Fluid intake with medication. Arch Intern Med, 116:813, 1965.

Lipsmeyer, E., and Ackerman, G.L.: Irreversible brain damage after water intoxication. JAMA, 196:286, 1966.

Marx, G.F.: Koenig, J.W., and Orkin, L.R.: Dilutional hypervolemia during transurethral resection of the prostate. JAMA, 174:1834, 1960.

Richards, M.R., and Hiatt, R.B.: Untoward effects of enemata in congenital megacolon. Pediatrics, 12:253, 1953.

Shalhoub, R.J., and Antoniou, L.D.: The mechanism of hyponatremia in pulmonary tuberculosis. Ann Intern Med, 70:943, 1969.

Swanson, A.G., and Iseri, O.A.: Acute encephalopathy due to water intoxication. N Engl J Med, 258:831, 1958.

White, J.C.: The risks of excessive water drinking in epileptic patients, letter. N Engl J Med, 312:246, 1985.

Wynn, V., and Rob, C.G.: Water intoxication: differential diagnosis of hypotonic syndromes. Lancet, 1:587, 1954. Also Metabolism, 5:490, 1956.

Zimmerman, B., and Wangensteen, O.H.: Observations on water intoxication in surgical patients. Surgery, 31:654, 1954.

CHAPTER 7

WATER EXCESS SYNDROMES (Continued)

INAPPROPRIATE ADH SECRETION SYNDROMES (SIADH)

The syndrome of inappropriate ADH (antidiuretic hormone) secretion (SIADH) is a form of dilutional hyponatremia and low serum osmolality due to the retention of water, produced by an inappropriate or an excessive secretion of ADH. In addition, there is failure to excrete a dilute urine in the presence of the low serum osmolality, and excessive loss of sodium ions in the urine in the absence of renal or adrenal disease. The syndrome is not caused by excessive water intake.

In 1953, Leaf and associates showed that when long-acting pitressin was given to humans, water retention, hyponatremia, a decreased serum osmolality, and an increased urine osmolality due to increased sodium excretion (*renal sodium wasting*) developed.

In 1957, Schwartz and associates described 2 patients with bronchogenic carcinoma who showed similar signs. They postulated that the syndrome was due to an "inappropriate" secretion of ADH. (Ordinarily, when hyponatremia and a decreased serum osmolality occur, urine with a low sodium concentration and a low osmolality is formed because of an increased urinary excretion of free water, in an attempt to restore the serum osmolality to normal.) Since then, the syndrome has been described in many other groups of patients.

PATHOPHYSIOLOGY

The physiological mechanisms for the secretion of ADH have been described in Chapter 2.

The basic physiological disturbance in this syndrome is an inappropriate or an excessive secretion of ADH. The secretion of ADH results in water retention and an expansion of the blood and extracellular volume. This causes a suppression of aldosterone secretion. As a result, sodium ions are lost through the kidneys into the urine. The serum osmolality falls because of the increased retention of water and the loss of sodium ions. The urine osmolality rises because of the decreased urinary excretion of water and the continued excretion of sodium ions. As a result, the osmolality of the urine becomes higher than the osmolality of the plasma.

The inappropriate ADH secretion can be due to many factors:

1. ADH secretion due to cerebral stimulation, as in:
   a. Central nervous system diseases (*cerebral salt wasting*), such as brain abscess, hypopituitarism, encephalitis, Guillain-Barré syndrome, head injuries, meningitis, subarachnoid hemorrhage, concussion, electroconvulsive therapy.
   b. Stress reactions, including fear, pain, trauma, or major operations. The period of postoperative ADH secretion is usually 12 to 36 hours, but may last longer.
   c. Endocrine disturbances, such as myxedema, Addison's disease, hypopituitarism.
   d. Drugs, including: hypoglycemic drugs, such as chlorpropamide (Diabenese), tolbutamide (Orinase); thiazide diuretics, and spironolactone; antineoplastic drugs, such as cyclophosphamide, vincristine; tricyclic drugs acting on the central nervous system, such as amitriptyline (Elavil), barbiturates, carbamazepine (Tegretol), fluphenazine (Permitil, Proloxin), haloperidol (Haldol), thioridazine (Mellaril), thiothixene (Navane), miscellaneous drugs, including acetaminophen (Tylenol), tranylcypromine (Parnate), clofibrate (Atromid S), isoproterenol, morphine, meperidine (Demerol), oxytocin, and most anesthetics.

   Chlorpropamide probably produces the SIADH by potentiating the action of ADH on the kidneys, although it may also stimulate ADH secretion centrally.
2. Secretion of ADH-like peptides by tumor or inflammatory tissue, for example, tumors of the lung (particularly oat cell bronchogenic carcinoma), pancreas, thymus, duodenum, or other organs, Ewing's sarcoma, or inflammatory lung diseases such as pneumonia, tuberculosis, chronic pulmonary infections, status asthmaticus, and pulmonary aspergillosis with cavitation.
3. Hypovolemia due to diuretics, positive-pressure respirators, loss of gastrointestinal fluids, and so on. When excessive doses of a diuretic are given, the blood and extracellular volume may decrease and in this way may stimulate excessive ADH secretion. This is potentiated if the diuretic also causes hypokalemia.
4. Excessive ADH secretion due to unknown factors, such as acute intermittent porphyria.

SYMPTOMS AND SIGNS

Symptoms and signs are related to the rapidity with which the water excess has developed, and to the extent of the lowering of the serum sodium concentration.

The water excess usually develops slowly so that symptoms and signs are rarely present when the serum sodium concentration is more than 125 mEq/L. However, when the serum sodium concentration falls to 115 mEq/L or less, serious neurological disturbances, including mental depression, convulsive seizures, or coma, commonly develop. In addition, symptoms and signs will be aggravated by any coincidental condition that produces water excess and/or sodium loss.

Many nonspecific symptoms may also be present, related to the underlying disease rather than to the water excess.

LABORATORY FINDINGS

Blood

The serum sodium concentration and the serum osmolality are low.

The serum chloride concentration is also low. The serum potassium concentration may be normal or low. It is low, in association with a high serum bicarbonate concentration (metabolic alkalosis), when the syndrome has been produced by excessive diuretic therapy. Hypokalemia may also occur when the patient has a chronic wasting disease and does not eat adequately.

The BUN concentration is normal.

Bioassay of ADH in the plasma will show elevated levels.

Urine

The excretion of sodium ions in the urine continues despite the low serum sodium concentration. The sodium excretion will be equal to or greater than the sodium intake. (The sodium concentration in the urine is usually more than 20 mEq/L. However, if the patient is on a low-sodium diet, sodium excretion in the urine may be less than this.)

The urine is usually hypertonic to plasma because the plasma is diluted with water, and the urine contains an appreciable amount of sodium ions. Therefore, the urine osmolality is usually higher than the plasma osmolality.

Bioassay for ADH in the urine (measured by radioimmunoassay) will usually reveal an increased ADH excretion.

Normal amounts of adrenocortical hormones are excreted in the urine.

DIAGNOSIS

An inappropriate ADH secretion syndrome can be suspected if the following conditions are present:

1. Hyponatremia and decreased osmolality of the serum.
2. Urine osmolality usually higher than serum osmolality.

3. Continued urinary excretion of sodium in spite of hyponatremia (unless the patient is on a low-sodium diet).
4. Normal renal function tests (BUN, serum creatinine, creatinine clearance).
5. Normal aldosterone blood levels and normal urinary excretion of aldosterone.
6. Absence of hypotension or dehydration.
7. Absence of clinical edema.
8. Improvement in the clinical condition by fluid restriction.

Example: Oat cell carcinoma of the lung
Na 121   K 3.7 HCO_3 29   Cl 85
Serum osmolality: 240 mOsm/kg
Urine osmolality: 590 mOsm/kg
BUN 15 mg/dl
Serum creatinine 0.9 mg/dl

TREATMENT

There is no specific treatment. If convulsions or other serious neurological symptoms of water excess develop, hypertonic sodium chloride solution may be needed intravenously (Chap 6). If lesser symptoms are present, the intake of water should be restricted, even to 500 ml a day, for several days, and the amount of salt in the diet can be increased. Patients with bronchogenic carcinoma may improve when the tumor is removed surgically, or when nitrogen mustard therapy is used. Phenytoin (Dilantin) has also been used to inhibit the excessive ADH secretion.

If the syndrome is due to excessive diuretic therapy, the diuretic should be stopped and potassium chloride should be given to correct the hypokalemia. Sodium chloride may also be helpful, although it is contraindicated when the syndrome is due to other causes.

When severe neurological signs such as coma develop, a 5° headdown position may cause a water diuresis and produce an increased serum sodium concentration (Segar and Moore).

Intravenous furosemide (Lasix) has been used to correct the neurological signs of water excess rapidly, in association with intramuscular DOCA (desoxycorticosterone acetate). The furosemide achieves a renal loss of water. The DOCA increases sodium reabsorption in the distal renal tubules. This is followed by 3% sodium chloride intravenously when the urinary sodium concentration begins to fall (Greenberg and Yudis). Similarly, intravenous furosemide has been used in association with 3% sodium chloride and with potassium chloride intravenously (Hantman *et al.*).

Demeclocycline (Declomycin), a broad spectrum antibiotic, has recently been used to treat the SIADH because it can interfere with the action of ADH on the kidneys and therefore can produce a diabetes insipidus-like effect (Cherrill *et al.*). A dose of 300 mg can be given 3 times a day. It may take several days before its effects are noted. Transient azotemia may occur as a side effect.

Lithium carbonate has also been recommended for the SIADH syndrome, because it interferes with the action of ADH on the distal tubules of the kidneys. However, it may cause toxicity, and it may interfere with the action of aldosterone, so that a loss of sodium ions may occur. It can also cause a nephrogenic type of diabetes insipidus.

Intravenous or oral urea has also been used (see Urea in Part 5).

The underlying condition producing the SIADH should be treated, if possible.

PROPHYLAXIS

The inappropriate ADH secretion syndrome is aggravated by any condition associated with a loss of sodium ions or an excess of water in the extracellular spaces. Therefore, diuretics should not be used unless necessary, and when used should be given in minimal doses. Similarly, intravenous fluids must be given very cautiously, to avoid water excess. Oral water intake should also be limited, depending on the serum sodium concentration.

REFERENCES

Ajilouni, K., et al.: Thiothixene-induced hyponatremia. Arch Intern Med, *134*:1103, 1974.

Baker, J.W., et al.: Elevated plasma antidiuretic hormone levels in status asthmaticus. Mayo Clin Proc, *51*:31, 1976.

Baylis, P.H., et al.: Water disturbances in patients treated with oral lithium carbonate. Ann Intern Med, *88*:607, 1978.

Beresford, H.R.: Polydipsia, hydrochlorothiazide, and water intoxication. JAMA, *214*:879, 1970.

Cherrill, D.A., Stote, R.M., Birge, J.R., and Singer, I.: Demeclocycline treatment in the syndrome of inappropriate antidiuretic hormone secretion. Ann Intern Med, *83*:654, 1975.

Decaux, G., et al.: Hyponatremia in the syndrome of inappropriate secretion of antidiuretic hormone. Rapid correction with urea sodium chloride and water restriction therapy. JAMA, *247*:471, 1982.

Decaux, G., et al.: Treatment of the syndrome of inappropriate secretion of antidiuretic hormone with furosemide. N Engl J Med, *304*:329, 1981.

Decaux, G., et al.: Hyponatremia in the syndrome of inappropriate secretion of antidiuretic hormone. Rapid correction with urea, sodium chloride, and water restriction therapy. JAMA, *247*:471, 1982.

DeFronzo, R.A., et al.: Water intoxication in man after cyclophosphamide therapy. Ann Intern Med, *78*:861, 1973.

Dempster, W.J.: Syndrome of inappropriate secretion of antidiuretic hormone. Lancet, *1*:970, 1971.

DeRubertis, F.R., et al.: Complications of diuretic therapy. Severe alkalosis and syndrome resembling inappropriate secretion of antidiuretic hormone. Metabolism, *19*:709, 1970.

Dingman, J.F.: What is an 'inappropriate' ADH syndrome? Mod Med, May, 36, 1973.

Fine, D., and Shedrovilzky, H.: Hyponatremia due to chlorpropamide. A syndrome resembling inappropriate secretion of antidiuretic hormone. Ann Intern Med, 72:83, 1970.

Fishman, M.P., Kleeman, C.R., and Bethune, J.E.: Inhibition of antidiuretic hormone secretion by diphenylhydantoin. Arch Neurol, 22:45, 1970.

Fishman, M.P., et al.: Diuretic-induced hyponatremia. Ann Intern Med, 75:853, 1971.

Goldstein, C.S., et al.: Idiopathic syndrome in inappropriate antidiuretic hormone secretion possibly related to advanced age. Ann Intern Med, 99:185, 1983.

Greenberg, S.R., and Yudis, M.: Rapid reversal of inappropriate antidiuretic-hormone syndrome. Lancet, 1:547, 1971.

Gupta, D.R., and Cohen, N.K.: Oxytocin, "salting out," and water intoxication. JAMA, 220:681, 1972.

Hamburger, S., et al.: Thiazide-induced syndrome of inappropriate secretion of antidiuretic hormone. JAMA, 246:1235, 1981.

Hantman, D., et al.: Rapid correction of hyponatremia in the syndrome of inappropriate secretion of antidiuretic hormone. An alternative to hypertonic saline. Ann Intern Med, 78:870, 1973.

Hendler, N., et al.: Problems with lithium as treatment of inappropriate ADH secretion, letter. N Engl J Med, 294:446, 1976.

Kaplowitz, L.G., and Robertson, G.L.: Hyponatremia in rocky mountain spotted fever. Role of antidiuretic hormone. Ann Intern Med, 98:334, 1983.

Khokhar, N.: Inappropriate secretion of antidiuretic hormone. Postgrad Med, 62:73, 1977.

Lauersen, N.H., and Birnbaum, S.J.: Water intoxication associated with oxytocin administration during saline-induced abortion. Am J Obstet Gynecol, 121:2, 1975.

Marcaron, C., and Olufunsho, F.: Hyponatremia of hypothyroidism. Arch Intern Med, 138:820, 1978.

Miller, M., and Moses, A.M.: Urinary antidiuretic hormone in polyuric disorders and in inappropriate ADH syndrome. Ann Intern Med, 77:715, 1972.

Novick, R.K.: Drug-induced dilutional hyponatremia. N Engl J Med, 292:810, 1975.

Raskind, M.A., et al.: Acute psychosis, increased water ingestion and inappropriate antidiuretic hormone secretion. Am J Psychiat, 132:407, 1975.

Rosenow, E.C., II, Segar, W.E., and Zehr, J.E.: Inappropriate antidiuretic hormone secretion in pneumonia. Mayo Clin Proc, 47:169, 1972.

Sandifer, M.: Hyponatremia due to psychotropic drugs. J Clin Psychiatry, 44:301, 1983.

Schwartz, W.B., Bennet, W., Curelop, S., and Bartter, F.C.: A syndrome of renal sodium loss and hyponatremia probably resulting from inappropriate secretion of antidiuretic hormone. Am J Med, 23:529, 1957.

Sexton, D.J., and Clapp, J.: Inappropriate and antidiuretic hormone secretion. Occurrence in a patient with Rocky Mountain Spotted Fever. Arch Intern Med, 137:362, 1977.

Sladen, A., Laver, M.B., and Pontoppidan, H.: Pulmonary complications and water retention in prolonged mechanical ventilation. N Engl J Med, 279:448, 1968.

Tanay, A., et al.: Long-term treatment of the syndrome of inappropriate antidiuretic hormone secretion with phenytoin. Ann Intern Med, 90:50, 1979.

Weissman, P.N., Shenkman, L., and Gregerman, R.I.: Chlorpropamide hyponatremia. Drug-induced inappropriate antidiuretic-hormone activity. N Engl J Med, 284:65, 1971.

White, M.G., and Fetner, C.D.: Treatment of the syndrome of inappopriate secretion of antidiuretic hormone with lithium carbonate. N Engl J Med, 292:390, 1975.

PART 3

SYNDROMES ASSOCIATED WITH SODIUM DISTURBANCES

CHAPTER 8

SODIUM LOSS SYNDROMES

The sodium loss syndrome is due to a loss or depletion of sodium from the extracellular water. There may be no accompanying water loss; if water loss is present, it is proportionately less than the loss of sodium ions.

Synonyms: Sodium depletion, pure salt depletion, desalting water loss, sodium deficiency, low sodium syndrome, dehydration.

PATHOPHYSIOLOGY

The sodium loss which occurs in the sodium loss syndrome is not related to a decrease in total exchangeable body sodium. The sodium loss which causes the physiological disturbances, symptoms and signs is localized to the extracellular water. The total exchangeable body sodium may be low or normal, and may often be high. As a matter of fact, an internal shift of sodium and water to a localized area, such as in severe burns, or in peritonitis, or in an accumulation of pleural or ascitic fluid, can cause a severe and fatal sodium loss syndrome without any sodium having been lost from the body. In addition, a severe and even fatal sodium loss syndrome can occur in a patient with congestive heart failure who shows marked edema (which indicates that there is an excess of total exchangeable body sodium).

We know that the concentration in the extracellular water is relatively so great that the loss of sodium (with a loss of chloride or other anions) can cause a marked decrease in the osmotic pressure of the extracellular water. When this occurs, water will flow from the extracellular water into the cells, because of the lowered osmotic pressure of the extra- cellular water. As a result, the volume of the extracellular water, in- cluding the volume of the blood plasma, will fall and produce a de- creased circulating blood volume and shock. The shock which occurs as a result of sodium loss is characterized by the fact that it will not respond to pressor substances, such as norepinephrine (Levophed), dopamine (Intropin), and other similar drugs, but only to solutions containing isotonic, hypotonic, or concentrated sodium salts.

In addition, the loss of sodium is associated with a loss of circulating

Table 8–1.   *Water and Electrolyte Losses in Gastrointestinal Secretions,*
and in Sweat (After Lockwood, and Randall)

Fluid	Average volume (ml per 24 hr)	Electrolyte concentrations (mEq/liter)			
		Na$^+$	K$^+$	Cl$^-$	HCO$_3^-$
Blood plasma		136–145	3.5– 5.0	98–106	23–28
Gastric juice*	2500				
achlorhydric		8–120	1–30	100	20
containing HCl		10–110	1–32	8– 55	0
Bile	700–1000	134–156	3.9– 6.3	83–110	38
Pancreatic juice	>1000	113–153	2.6– 7.4	54– 95	110
Small bowel					
(Miller-Abbott suction)	3000	72–120	3.5– 6.8	69–127	30
Ileostomy					
(a) recent	100–4000	112–142	4.5–14	93–122	30
(b) adapted	100–500	50	3	20	15–30
Cecostomy	100–3000	48–116	11.1–28.3	35– 70	15
Feces	100	<10	<10	<15	<15
Sweat	500–4000	30–70	0– 5	30– 70	0

*The electrolyte concentrations in gastric juice vary widely—the higher the acidity, the lower the sodium concentration. Thus, when normal gastric acidity is present, the average sodium concentration of gastric juice is approximately 45 mEq/L. When hypoacidity or anacidity is present (as in elderly patients or those with carcinoma of the stomach), the average sodium concentration of gastric juice is approximately 100 mEq/L.

plasma proteins, particularly albumin, from the bloodstream. This causes the osmotic pressure of the blood to become lower than that of the extravascular portion of the extracellular water. As a result, water flows out of the plasma and the circulating blood volume falls still further. The reason for the loss of plasma albumin is not clear. It may be that as the cardiac output falls there is a decreased return of the extracellular and lymphatic fluid (which is rich in albumin) to the heart.

ETIOLOGY

Sodium loss can occur in the following situations:

1. Loss of sodium in gastrointestinal secretions. The electrolyte concentrations of the various gastrointestinal secretions are shown in Table 8–1. Notice that when these secretions are lost, a marked loss of sodium as well as other electrolytes occurs. The sodium can be lost as a result of:
   a. Vomiting.
   b. Dysentery, cholera, diarrhea, ulcerative colitis, pseudomembranous colitis.
      A patient with a mucus-secreting villous adenoma of the rectum or sigmoid may excrete several liters of mucus a day, and as a result may develop shock from the loss of sodium ions and water (in the mucus). In addition, a large amount of potassium ions may also be lost in this way, and symptomatic hypokalemia may also develop.
   c. Gastric, biliary, pancreatic or intestinal lavage by means of a Levin or Abbott-Miller tube.
   d. Gastrointestinal or biliary fistulas.

    e. Cation exchange resins. These absorb sodium from food in the stomach and cause its excretion in the stool. (Cations, such as potassium and magnesium, are also lost in addition to the sodium.)

2. Loss of sodium through the skin. This can occur in

    a. Excessive sweating, particularly if a large amount of water is imbibed to quench thirst.

    b. Extensive, exudative skin lesions or burns.

    c. Fibrocystic disease of the pancreas (mucoviscidosis).

       The diagnosis of cystic fibrosis of the pancreas is based on four criteria: increase in the concentration of sodium or chloride in sweat; absence of the pancreatic enzyme, trypsin, obtained by duodenal drainage; signs of chronic pulmonary involvement (obstructive emphysema and history of bilateral bronchopneumonia); and a family history of this disorder. All these criteria need not be present.

3. Loss of sodium in bronchial secretions. This is a relatively rare cause of sodium loss. It occurs, for example, in patients with bronchorrhea due to pulmonary adenomatosis. Some patients can expectorate 500 ml or more of bronchial secretions daily for weeks or months.

4. Sequestration of sodium within the body. This can occur in several ways:

    a. In small bowel obstruction, where large volumes of intestinal fluid can exudate into the intestinal lumen. In these patients, little or no visible loss of fluids may be noted because the patient may not vomit.

    b. A sequestration of extracellular water in the abdomen in peritonitis patients, in acute spreading cellulitis, in acute venous obstruction, such as portal vein thrombosis, and in so-called tourniquet lesion, with "release edema."

    c. In severe burns, where the edema accumulates under the burn, withdrawing salt, water, and protein from the plasma and the extracellular water. This edema continues to accumulate for 48 to 72 hours after the burn, and may be complicated by an external loss of water and salt through the burned skin.

       The external loss of extracellular water and sodium into the burn area is maximal in wet burns and scalds and reaches 1000 to 2000 ml a day. In dry, charred burns, such a loss of sodium and water is minimal. However, in dry burns treated with the open method, there may be a considerable loss of water by evaporation, particularly as sloughing begins. This can cause a severe water loss syndrome. (Burns are discussed in detail in Chap 9.)

    d. As a result of hypodermoclysis of dextrose in distilled water. When this is done, sodium, chloride and other electrolytes diffuse into the subcutaneous pool of dextrose and water. (No solution should ever be given subcutaneously unless it contains electrolytes in either isotonic or half-isotonic strength (see Chap 34).

5. Sodium loss through the kidneys. This can occur in the following ways:

    a. With intrinsic renal disease. The usual patient with chronic renal disease does not lose an excessive amount of sodium ions through the kidneys. However, many patients with renal atherosclerosis may lose a small but definite amount of sodium ions daily this way and can develop a sodium loss syndrome quickly if they are placed on a low-sodium diet, or if they lose sodium ions extrarenally in any other way. The terms *renal salt wasting* or *salt-losing nephritis* have been used to describe patients with chronic renal disease who lose so many sodium ions that they require massive amounts of sodium chloride daily to prevent a sodium loss syndrome. Transient salt wasting can occur during the polyuric phase of acute renal failure, after relief of urinary obstruction, and rarely after transplantation of a kidney.

b. In the syndrome of inappropriate secretion of antidiuretic hormone (ADH) (Chap 7). These patients show a retention of water and an increased circulating blood volume due to the continuous secretion of ADH. However, aldosterone secretion decreases or stops as a result of the increased circulating blood volume and the kidneys excrete a large amount of sodium ions. The low serum sodium concentration in these patients is therefore partly due to water excess and partly due to true sodium loss.

c. In Addison's disease and other forms of adrenocortical insufficiency, as after the withdrawal of cortisone or other corticosteroids.

d. In diabetic acidosis. Sodium loss may occur in patients with diabetic acidosis even if they have not vomited. Apparently, the diuresis of large quantities of glucose is associated with a large urinary loss of sodium. This is due to the fact that the glucose excreted by the kidneys acts as an osmotic diuretic and causes sodium and other electrolytes to be eliminated into the urine.

e. As a result of drugs:
  i. Carbonic anhydrase inhibitors, such as Diamox. These drugs inhibit the action of carbonic anhydrase in the kidney tubular cells (Chap 12). When this happens, hydrogen ions are retained, and sodium and potassium are excreted instead.
  ii. Excessive ammonium chloride administration. The ammonium ion is converted to urea by the liver. The chloride is excreted along with sodium and other cations.
  iii. Diuretics such as the thiazides, spironolactone, furosemide, and ethacrynic acid.

6. Loss of sodium from serous cavities, or the subcutaneous tissues. This can occur after abdominal paracentesis, when a large volume of ascitic fluid is removed, or after repeated thoracenteses, or with the use of Southey tubes to relieve severe edema of the lower extremities. In such cases, the fluid quickly reaccumulates, or the patient becomes thirsty and drinks a large amount of water. This further lowers the osmotic pressure of the extracellular water, and causes more water to flow into the cells, thereby further decreasing the volume of the extracellular water.

7. Loss of sodium as a result of severe hemorrhage.

In all the above patients, the sodium loss syndrome is aggravated by a low-sodium diet. In addition, just as sodium loss aggravates the water excess syndrome (Chap 6), water excess will aggravate the sodium loss syndrome.

SYMPTOMS AND SIGNS

The clinical picture depends on the rapidity of the sodium loss. When it occurs acutely, the clinical picture is that of severe shock. When it occurs slowly, the following symptoms and signs may appear.

General Symptoms

These include weakness, apathy, and lassitude. McCance, in his classic studies of experimentally induced salt loss, described how he and the other subjects all suffered from excessive fatigue and a general sense of exhaustion. They were content to sit and do nothing for hours on end. Muscle weakness was also present, and McCance found that his arm became tired while shaving and his jaws became tired when he ate.

Headache is an early signs. It is dull and becomes more marked on standing. In addition, giddiness and a feeling of faintness on standing may occur because of the decreased circulating blood volume. Muscle cramps may also occur. These can be precipitated if the patient drinks water freely, because the water aggravates the sodium loss.

When the sodium loss is marked, mental confusion, delirium, delusions, stupor or coma may develop.

Gastrointestinal symptoms such as anorexia, nausea or vomiting may occur. Thirst is characteristically absent; however, cases of sodium loss have been reported where thirst has been present. This is due to the decreased extracellular and circulating blood volume (see Chap 3).

The patient appears apathetic and acutely ill. The eyeballs may be sunken and soft on palpation. The eyes have a glassy stare. The tongue may appear softened and shrunk, and may show longitudinal wrinkling.

The Skin

Skin turgor and elasticity disappear. Normally, when the skin of the inner forearm or arm is picked up and released, it returns to its previous shape almost immediately. When sodium loss is present, the skin tends to remain folded for one-half minute or more. (This sign can occur in elderly or cachectic patients in the absence of sodium loss.)

Cardiovascular Signs

These depend on the extent to which the circulating blood volume has diminished. There may be orthostatic hypotension, tachycardia, a low blood pressure and small pulse pressure, and a collapsing pulse. The extremities may be cold and the body temperature subnormal. The peripheral pulses may be absent. In severe cases, the typical signs of shock with cold, clammy skin and sweating may be present.

The peripheral veins, such as the hand veins, may be collapsed and may fill slowly (in more than 5 seconds) when the hand is held dependent, or if an occlusive venous tourniquet is placed around the hand.

A patient with congestive heart failure who develops sodium loss may show an aggravation of the heart failure, such as increasing edema, the development of pulmonary edema, or pleural effusion. A patient with coronary artery disease may show increased coronary insufficiency, or may develop a myocardial infarct.

LABORATORY FINDINGS

Blood

Hemoconcentration is present, with an elevated hematocrit. However, the mean corpuscular volume of the red blood cells is high, due to the entrance of water into the cells. This occurs because the osmotic pressure of the extracellular water is lower than that of the cells, because of the loss of sodium. For this same reason, the mean corpuscular hemoglobin concentration is low. In spite of the hemoconcentration, the serum sodium concentration is low—135 mEq/L, or lower. This differentiates sodium loss from water loss, where a high hematocrit is associated with a high serum sodium concentration.

The concentration of chloride or bicarbonate is also low, depending on which ion has been lost in association with the sodium. The BUN concentration is high because of the decreased renal blood flow. The serum potassium concentration is often high. (There is a tendency for the serum potassium and sodium concentrations to vary in opposite directions. However, the exact mechanism by which hyponatremia causes hyperkalemia is not known.)

Urine

The specific gravity is usually normal. The urinary volume is low and anuria may occur as a result of shock. Sodium and chloride concentrations are characteristically low in the urine.

The concentration of sodium in the urine tends to be proportional to the serum sodium concentration. In the sodium loss syndrome, it is therefore low, and is characteristically below 10 mEq/L, and may even fall below 1 mEq/L. The urinary sodium concentration should be measured at a time when a sodium salt is not being given intravenously, and when the patient is not receiving a diuretic. In addition, the sodium concentration in the urine should be determined from a 24-hour collection.

When hyponatremia is associated with low urinary excretion of sodium ions, regardless of the dietary intake of salt, this is a sign either that the extracellular and blood volume is low, or that a condition, such as congestive heart failure with edema, cirrhosis of the liver, or the nephrotic syndrome, associated with an increased retention of sodium ions by the kidneys, is present. (A patient with inappropriate secretion of ADH (SIADH) (Chap 7) may also have a low urinary excretion of sodium ions, if the dietary salt intake is low.)

A urinary sodium concentration of more than 10 mEq/L can occur in the sodium loss syndrome in two different conditions:

1. When the kidneys are unable to conserve sodium ions, as in patients with renal salt wasting.
2. When the adrenal cortex is not secreting sufficient aldosterone, as in Addison's disease or transient adrenocortical insufficiency. This may occur postoperatively.

A high urinary sodium concentration also occurs in the syndrome of inappropriate secretion of ADH (SIADH) (Chap 7), when the dietary intake of salt is adequate.

DIAGNOSIS

Hyponatremia without true sodium loss may also occur when marked hyperglycemia, hyperlipidemia, azotemia, or hyperproteinemia is present (see Chap 11). This type of hyponatremia is asymptomatic and the patient does not require treatment. However, one should be certain that the hyponatremia is caused by one of these conditions, because sodium loss or water excess may also be present.

The use of serum osmolality measurements to differentiate true sodium loss or water excess from other syndromes associated with a low serum sodium concentration is described in Chapter 11.

The sodium loss syndrome is also frequently confused with another condition in which a low serum sodium concentration is found, namely, water excess syndrome.

The laboratory findings in water excess and sodium loss are similar because in both conditions the osmotic pressure of the extracellular water is lower than that of the cells, and each condition aggravates the other. However, the clinical picture of the two conditions is different. Patients with water excess will give a history of weight gain. Central nervous system disturbances, particularly convulsions, dominate the clinical picture. In sodium loss, weight loss, loss of skin turgor and shock are characteristic. Water excess is described in detail in Chapters 6 and 7.

Acute Adrenal Crisis

Adrenal crisis (acute adrenocortical insufficiency) can be suspected when a patient receiving long-term corticosteroid therapy, or one who has had bilateral adrenalectomy or hypophysectomy, for example, develops one or more of the following symptoms and signs: severe weakness or lethargy, nausea and vomiting and abdominal pain, hypotension

or shock, hyponatremia and hyperkalemia, hyperthermia and hypoglycemia.

The decreased circulating blood volume that occurs as a result of the
sodium loss is often associated with decreased renal blood flow and a
high BUN concentration. A metabolic acidosis is also present. The
plasma cortisol level will be low. Some patients may show an apparently normal plasma cortisol level, but this is really inappropriately
low in the presence of the stress situation.

PROPHYLAXIS

In the absence of sweating, a normal person requires little salt. It has
been shown that as little as 200 mg of sodium (approximately 0.5 g of
salt) or less is needed daily.

When sweating is present, the patient will require salt as well as
water. So-called *insensible* perspiration contains practically pure water.
It occurs continually in cold as well as warm weather. *Sensible* or visible
sweat, on the other hand, occurs with excessive heat production by the
body, as a result of fear, and as a result of other strong stimuli. It can
be considered as a hypotonic (hyposmotic) solution with a sodium and
chloride concentration ranging from about 30 to 70 mEq and a small
amount of potassium (Table 8–1). When sensible perspiration is excessive, the patient will require supplemental salt. This can be given
in the form of salt tablets (0.5 g). Water with one tablet per pint (0.5 g
per 500 ml) (0.1% solution) can be imbibed freely. As a general rule,
one 0.5-g (7½ grain) salt tablet and 1 pint of water for each pound of
weight lost should provide a satisfactory amount of salt and water.

A patient who is perspiring excessively and cannot take salt orally
can be given an infusion composed of 1 part of isotonic saline (sodium
chloride) solution and 2 parts dextrose in water. (This contains approximately 50 mEq sodium per liter and is similar to the composition
of sweat, Table 8–1.)

Sodium loss can be prevented if the physician is aware of the conditions in which it can occur, and is alert to recognize premonitory
symptoms and signs.

Several preventive measures can be taken. For example, if the patient
has pyloric obstruction and is vomiting greatly, or if gastric suction is
being used, a volume-for-volume replacement of the water and electrolytes (including potassium) should be done daily. The volume of
gastric fluid in the suction bottle can be measured every 4, 6 or 12
hours, and an equivalent amount of fluid infused. In addition, since
the patient is not taking fluids orally, enough water, sodium, potassium,
and protein for ordinary daily needs (Chap 34) must be given.

The type of fluid used for replacement of gastrointestinal losses depends on the type of fluid being lost.

If fluid is being lost by gastric suction, or from vomiting due to pyloric obstruction, an adequate gastric replacement solution can be prepared in the following way:

> If the gastric juice is highly acid (pH 1.5 to 2.5) replace one third of the volume lost with isotonic saline solution and two thirds with dextrose in water, and add 20 mEq potassium chloride (1.5 g) per liter.
> If the gastric juice has a low acidity (pH 5.0 to 5.5), give half strength saline solution to which 20 mEq potassium chloride (1.5 g) per liter has been added. Such solutions can be given at a rate up to 500 ml per hour.

In acute gastric dilatation, the fluid may have a high chloride concentration of 150 mEq/L. In such a patient, isotonic saline solution should be used to replace the fluid lost.

If gastrointestinal fluids are being lost from a pancreatic or small intestinal fistula, or from intestinal obstruction, the electrolyte concentration of lactated Ringer's solution (Chap 35) is similar to that of the duodenal and small intestinal secretions, and it can be used to replace duodenal or small intestinal losses. Additional KCl can be added, if necessary.

In pancreatic fistulas, the fluid may have a high sodium concentration, even 185 mEq/L. Isotonic saline solution should be used to replace fluid losses. In addition, it may be necessary to use small amounts of hypertonic 5% sodium chloride to maintain a normal sodium concentration.

Ileostomy fluid may have a high potassium concentration, even 70 mEq/L. Sufficient potassium must be added to the lactated Ringer's solution to maintain the serum potassium concentration.

A volume-by-volume replacement of the intestinal fluid losses should be made, and the patient's daily needs for water, sodium, potassium, and protein (Chap 33) should be maintained.

One should remember that patients with small bowel obstruction may lose enormous volumes of fluid, as much as 5 to 10 liters, in the distended intestine, even though vomiting is not present. Similarly, patients with duodenal or jejunal fistulas can lose 3 to 6 liters daily through the fistula alone. Patients with pancreatic fistula usually lose less than 2 liters a day through the fistula. A patient with acute gastric dilatation who is being treated with nasogastric suction can lose 8000 ml or more fluid a day, which must be replaced (also see Chap 34).

Bile secretion has a composition which is approximately similar to that of the plasma. Therefore, losses from a biliary fistula can be replaced with lactated Ringer's solution (Chap 35).

When gastrointestinal suction is being used, the tube should be irrigated with isotonic saline, or saline solution to which 1 g of potassium chloride per liter has been added, but not with water.

TREATMENT

In treating sodium loss, one should:

1. Treat shock. Large quantities of sodium chloride, water and plasma may be needed (see below). In addition, I have already mentioned the fact that severe shock due to sodium loss will not respond to pressor amines, such as dopamine (Intropin), or norepinephrine (Levophed). However, pressor amines may become effective after an infusion of sodium chloride has been started. (The pressor amines can be used immediately if they are given in a solution which contains sodium chloride. Norepinephrine should be given in a solution which contains dextrose as well as sodium chloride, in treating a patient with shock due to sodium loss. Otherwise it will oxidize and become ineffective.)
2. Stop further sodium loss from the body. This has already been discussed under Prophylaxis. In addition, if Addison's disease is present, hydrocortisone or large quantities of salt orally are indicated (also see below). If the patient is on a low-sodium diet, the sodium intake should be increased. In a patient with renal salt wasting as much as 15 to 20 g of salt orally may be needed daily.
3. Give sufficient sodium chloride, water and plasma, if necessary, to compensate for the loss of sodium. In addition, other electrolytes such as potassium, chloride or bicarbonate may have to be replaced.

Type of Solution Needed

Most patients with acute sodium loss and shock respond to isotonic 0.9% sodium chloride (saline). In addition, colloid solutions, such as whole blood, plasma, or plasma expanders such as dextran (Chap 36) may be helpful in treating the shock.

In patients with chronic sodium loss, hypertonic 5% sodium chloride solution can be given intravenously (see Chap 6).

If the patient is acidotic, one-third molar sodium lactate (Chap 35), or 3.75% sodium bicarbonate (Chap 35) can be substituted for the 5% sodium chloride.

Potassium Solutions. When gastrointestinal secretions are lost, potassium as well as sodium is lost and must be replaced. Table 8–1 gives average values for the electrolyte concentrations in the various gastrointestinal secretions. The potassium can be given as potassium chloride in the infusion bottle. As much as 80 mEq/L potassium (6 g KCl) per liter can be placed in the infusion bottle, but the potassium must be infused at a rate which does not exceed 20 mEq (rarely, 35 mEq) per hour. In addition, if the patient is oliguric, potassium should not be given until the urinary volume increases.

Even when sodium loss is not related to a loss of gastrointestinal secretions, potassium chloride orally may be helpful in raising the serum sodium concentration. It probably is effective by entering the cells and exchanging with intercellular sodium ions, which pass into the extracellular water and blood.

Volume of Solution to Be Used

There are several methods for calculating the volume of sodium chloride and colloid solution to be given. Any one of the following is satisfactory:

Method 1. If one knows the acute weight loss, the loss of sodium (in mEq) equals 142 times the loss of weight in kilograms (kg). This assumes that the normal sodium concentration of the extracellular water is 142 mEq/L and that the weight loss has been due entirely to a loss of extracellular water and its electrolytes.

Example: The patient has lost 2 kg weight in a period of one day. Therefore, the loss of sodium would be 142 × 2 = 284 mEq sodium.
1 mEq sodium = approximately 1 ml hypertonic 5% NaCl solution.
1 mEq sodium = approximately 6 ml isotonic 0.9% NaCl solution.
Therefore, the patient would receive 284 × 6 = 1704 ml, or approximately 2 liters of isotonic sodium chloride (saline) solution.

Method 2. If accurate weight loss is not available, the sodium loss can be calculated from the hematocrit. This method also assumes that only extracellular water and electrolytes have been lost, and that there has not been any hemorrhage.

Example: Woman wt. 70 kg; hematocrit 55%.
We know that the normal extracellular water volume is approximately 20% of the body weight. (The plasma volume is about 4% of the body weight, or one-fifth the volume of the extracellular water.) The average normal hematocrit is 42% ± 5% in a woman and 47% ± 7% in man.
Therefore, a rise in the hematocrit from 42 to 55% in a woman indicates that approximately 25% of the extracellular water has been lost (55 − 42 = 13%; $^{13}/_{42}$ = ¼, or 25% loss).
The extracellular water volume of this patient is 20% of 70 kg = 14 liters. The loss of sodium and water is 25% of 14 liters = 3.5 liters. Therefore, 3.5 liters of isotonic sodium chloride solution are urgently needed.

Method 3. The sodium loss can also be calculated from changes in the serum sodium concentration. Superficially, it might seem that the changes in serum sodium concentration in relation to the volume of extracellular water should be measured. However, when sodium salts are given, a similar rise must occur in the osmolality of both the extracellular water and of the cells. This is the reason that changes in the serum sodium concentration must be calculated in relation to the total body water volume (unit serum sodium deficit per mEq/L *times* volume of body water).

Example: Patient wt. 70 kg; serum sodium 122 mEq/L.
We know that the total body water volume is 60% of the weight, 0.6 × 70 = 42 liters. The unit sodium deficit equals 142 mEq/L (the normal concentration) − 122 mEq/L = 20 mEq/L.
In other words, a deficit of 20 mEq sodium is present in each liter of body water. Since the total body water volume is 42 liters, the total sodium deficit

is 20 × 42 = 840 mEq. However, it is neither necessary nor desirable to give such a large quantity of sodium chloride.

Not more than one-half this amount, or 840/2 = 420 mEq, should be given. One reason for this is that as the sodium and water are infused the circulation improves and the kidneys are able to excrete water. This increases the serum sodium concentration and helps decrease the need for further salt.

Method 4. Treatment of Sodium Loss Complicated by Water Excess. This usually occurs in patients with chronic sodium loss. It also is common in patients with congestive heart failure, who have lost sodium, and also occurs in patients with sodium loss who have been incorrectly treated with dextrose in water, or with pressor amines in dextrose and water.

These patients should be treated by withholding water and giving sodium chloride. The water intake can be kept below 1000 ml a day, and even withheld for the first 12 hours. Salt can be added to the diet. For example, if a cardiac patient who has been on a low-sodium diet complains of progressive weakness and shows other signs of sodium loss, 2 to 3 g of table salt can be added daily to the food. This can be done by using an ordinary No. 0 gelatin capsule. When the capsule is filled with salt, it holds almost 1 g (400 mg sodium). The salt is sprinkled on the food, because salt on the food tastes better than salt in the food. This can be done easily by puncturing an end of the capsule a few times with a pin, making the capsule a miniature salt shaker.

If a patient with congestive heart failure who shows sodium loss and water excess is given hypertonic sodium chloride intravenously, the heart failure may become aggravated. However, I have used hypertonic sodium chloride intravenously, even in congestive heart failure patients, if signs of acute water intoxication, such as the sudden development of delirium, are present. A small infusion of 50 to 100 ml 5% sodium chloride is usually adequate.

Patients with cardiac decompensation and a combination of sodium loss and water excess (as indicated by a low serum sodium concentration) can now be treated with "loop" diuretics, such as furosemide (Lasix) or ethacrynic acid (Edecrin). Both these diuretics are able to cause a diuresis of water in excess of sodium ions.

Rate of Administration of the Solution

When shock is present, isotonic sodium chloride can be given rapidly, at a rate of 1 to 2 liters per hour. Marriott, for example, describes the following schedule in the treatment of shock due to severe acute sodium losses:

500 ml in 10 minutes. Then,
500 ml in 15 minutes. Then,
500 ml in 10 minutes. Then,
500 ml in 30 minutes. Then,
500 ml every 2 hours until the blood pressure is normal.

Such massive doses are rarely needed, because after the first 500 ml or 1 liter has been infused, the shock can be alleviated either with plasma or dextran.

When isotonic sodium chloride is given at a rate faster than 500 ml an hour, the patient should be watched constantly by the physician for the development of signs of congestive heart failure or metabolic acidosis.

The rate of administration of hypertonic sodium chloride solution is described in Chapter 6.

Route of Administration

Intravenous administration is advisable. However, large volumes of isotonic sodium chloride solution can be given by means of a nasogastric tube, or rectally by means of a Murphy drip apparatus, or by hypodermoclysis. Salt can also be given orally. Isotonic sodium chloride solution is irritating to the gastrointestinal tract of many patients, and may be deleterious in the treatment of patients with cholera. However, Moyer has found that large amounts of a salt solution having less than 0.6% salt can be imbibed without difficulty, especially if the solution also contains sodium bicarbonate. He recommends a mixture of 3 to 4 g (1 level teaspoonful) of sodium chloride and 1.5 to 2 g (1 level teaspoonful) of sodium bicarbonate or citrate per liter of water. Salt tablets can also be given orally in mild sodium loss.

Carpenter has made extensive studies in the treatment of patients with cholera. He has shown that cholera stool is approximately isotonic and has a bicarbonate concentration of 45 to 50 mEq/L.

WHO (World Health Organization) has recommended the use of the following oral replacement solution for severe diarrhea, including cholera:

	g per Liter		mmol per Liter
Sodium chloride	3.5	Na	90.
Potassium chloride	1.5	K	20.
Sodium bicarbonate	2.5	Cl	80.
Glucose	20.	HCO_3	30.

Dextrose is used in the solution because it stimulates active transport of sodium ions and water from the intestines into the bloodstream.

The oral solution can be given on a basis of equal volumes for stool losses. If the stool volume exceeds oral intake in any 4-hour period, intravenous therapy should be given if possible.

Treatment of Renal Salt Wasting

When a patient with moderate renal salt wasting is placed on a low sodium diet, a continued excretion of sodium ions in the urine occurs, so that a sodium loss syndrome may develop, often in a few days. This can be prevented by allowing a regular diet without added salt. (This contains about 7 g of salt a day.) When renal salt wasting is severe, as in a patient with medullary cystic disease of the kidneys, as much as 10 to 40 g of salt a day may be needed to maintain sodium balance.

Treatment of Acute Adrenocortical Insufficiency (Adrenal Crisis)

Acute adrenocortical insufficiency is associated with a deficiency of both the glucocorticoid and mineralocorticoid adrenal cortical hormones.

Emergency treatment includes the following (after Himathongkam et al.):

Treatment of Glucocorticoid Lack. A solution of 100 mg hydrocortisone succinate (Solu-Cortef) dissolved in 2 to 10 ml water is given as an intravenous bolus. Then 100 mg hydrocortisone succinate is given continuously in an intravenous infusion every 8 hours, for at least 36 or 48 hours. A total dose of 300 mg hydrocortisone over 24 hours is adequate to control the stressful situation that precipitated the crisis.

After this period, 5 mg hydrocortisone, or cortisone acetate, is given orally every 6 hours. In addition, 50 mg cortisone acetate can be given intramuscularly every 12 hours, to maintain adequate cortisol blood levels until the acute crisis disappears. The glucocorticoid dosage can be decreased over a period of several days, to a maintenance dose of approximately 10 mg hydrocortisone 2 or 3 times a day.

Treatment of Mineralocorticoid Lack. While the patient is receiving large doses of hydrocortisone, it is not necessary to use any supplementary adrenal mineralocorticoid hormones. However, when the daily hydrocortisone dosage decreases below 100 mg, it may be necessary to give the patient a mineralocorticoid such as fludrocortisone acetate (Florinef), 0.1 mg every 24 hours, or desoxycorticosterone acetate (DOCA), 2.5 to 5.0 mg intramuscularly every 24 hours, to prevent a loss of sodium ions in the urine.

Treatment of Hyponatremia and Hypotension. Intravenous saline solution is necessary to raise the serum sodium concentration, increase the circulating blood volume, and counteract the hypotension. One liter of 5% dextrose in isotonic saline is given intravenously in a period of 1 to 2 hours. Most patients need additional intravenous saline, at a rate of 1 liter every 3 to 6 hours for the next 24 hours. If an excessive amount of sodium chloride solution is infused, pulmonary or cerebral edema may occur.

If the blood pressure does not respond to the intravenous hydrocortisone and saline, it may be necessary to use a pressor amine, such as phenylephrine (Neo-Synephrine) or dopamine (Intropin) intravenously.

Treatment of Hyperkalemia. The hyperkalemia responds to the intravenous glucocorticoids and saline solution. If the serum potassium concentration is higher than 6.5 mEq/L and if cardiac arrhythmias are present, 1 or 2 ampuls of 44.5 mEq sodium bicarbonate (Chap 35) can be given intravenously every 1 to 2 hours, until the serum potassium concentration falls and the arrhythmias disappear.

One should remember that high-dose glucocorticoid therapy may produce severe *hypo*kalemia by the second to the fourth day of therapy, which may require treatment with potassium chloride.

Treatment of Hypoglycemia. This usually responds to the intravenous infusion of dextrose in saline. If the patient has diabetes and is taking insulin, the blood sugar level should be checked repeatedly to prevent severe hypoglycemia.

Treatment of Hyperpyrexia. Fever usually disappears with the intravenous therapy described above. An alcohol sponge bath can be used if necessary. The fever may also be a sign of a bacterial or viral infection, which may require treatment. When adrenal crisis develops without an apparent cause, one should suspect that an infection has precipitated the crisis.

CLINICAL APPROACH TO A HYPONATREMIC PATIENT

This and the preceding two chapters have described in detail the multiple causes of hyponatremia. Because of the complexity and clinical importance of this subject, this final section is devoted to a review of the bedside and laboratory approaches to a hyponatremic patient.

First, it is important to remember that not all low serum sodium values indicate true hyponatremia. Laboratory error must always be ruled out. A useful way of checking the consistency of a laboratory report is to calculate the anion gap (Chap 1). An anion gap of less than 9 mEq/L is unlikely and suggests that the "hyponatremia" is due to a laboratory error.

Next, hyperlipidemia or hyperproteinemia must also be excluded as a cause of pseudohyponatremia (Chap 11).

A concomitant measurement of serum glucose concentration must always be obtained, because hyperglycemia will produce a misleading hyponatremia due to osmotic fluid shifts. Every elevation of the serum glucose concentration of 100 mg/dl will decrease the serum sodium concentration approximately 1.6 mEq/L (Appendix IV). Similarly, an increased BUN concentration will cause a slight decrease in serum sodium concentration.

When true hyponatremia has been ascertained, the most important step is a clinical assessment of the patient's extracellular fluid volume. Hyponatremic patients can be divided as follows:

1. Patients with decreased extracellular fluid volume, due to sodium loss (indicated by decreased skin turgor, hypotension, shock, and so on; see above).
2. Patients with increased extracellular fluid volume, due to water excess. These patients can be further subdivided into those with and those without edema.

In medical patients, the most important causes of hyponatremia with decreased extracellular fluid volume are adrenocortical insufficiency, gastrointestinal sodium loss syndromes (due to vomiting, diarrhea, and so on), excessive sweating, or excessive diuresis, with replacement of the losses with water rather than a sodium-containing solution. Salt-losing nephritis is rare and is discussed in Chapter 20. Adrenocortical insufficiency is listed first because it is important to rule out an incipient Addisonian crisis in every patient with hyponatremia and a decreased extracellular fluid volume. The combination of a low serum sodium concentration and a high serum potassium concentration, a history of recent corticosteroid use, and the physical stigmata of Addison's disease (increased pigmentation, and so on) should be carefully sought.

The treatment of a hyponatremic patient with a decreased extracellular fluid volume requires the replacement of sodium ions and fluid, as has been discussed above.

Patients who show hyponatremia and *edema* indicate an excessive total body sodium content, in spite of the low serum sodium concentration. This problem is commonly encountered in patients with congestive heart failure, cirrhosis, or the nephrotic syndrome. The low serum sodium concentration can result from numerous factors, including excessive diuretic therapy, excessive water intake, and the inability of the kidneys to excrete water normally. The primary therapy in these patients is water restriction, in contrast to the sodium and volume replacement needed in patients with hyponatremia and a decreased extracellular fluid volume.

Patients with hyponatremia, no edema, and no signs of decreased extracellular fluid volume usually have evidence of water excess produced iatrogenically, inappropriate secretion of ADH syndromes (SIADH), or compulsive water drinking. The diagnosis of SIADH is made by finding a low serum sodium concentration and a low serum osmolality, usually a high urine sodium concentration and high urine osmolality, and normal adrenal and renal functions. A work-up for a suspected SIADH patient should include chest x-ray examination and sputum culture (to detect tuberculosis or pulmonary fungal infection, or pulmonary carcinoma), careful neurological assessment, thyroid studies (to rule out myxedema), and a careful listing of all medications the patient has been taking (see Chap 7).

In the general assessment of the hyponatremic patient, urinary sodium determinations are valuable. (This can be done on a "spot" sample of urine and does not require 24-hour collection.) As mentioned above, SIADH is typically associated with an inappropriately high urine sodium concentration (usually more than 20 mEq/L), despite the hyponatremia. A high urine sodium concentration with hyponatremia can also be seen in adrenocortical insufficiency, salt-losing nephritis, and with excessive diuretic therapy.

Conversely, patients with hyponatremia and extracellular fluid loss due to gastroinestinal losses will have a low urine sodium concentration. Patients with hyponatremia and edema due to congestive heart failure, cirrhosis, and the nephrotic syndrome also typically retain sodium ions and show a low urine sodium concentration.

Finally, it is important to emphasize that hyponatremia may be due to more than one cause, or to a combination of sodium loss and water excess. For example, a patient with congestive heart failure may develop hyponatremia because of a low sodium intake, excessive water intake, excessive diuresis, vomiting, removal of a large pleural effusion, and so on.

REFERENCES

Ashraf, N., et al.: Thiazide-induced hyponatremia associated with death or neurologic damage in outpatients. Am J Med, *70*:63, 1981.

Berry, R.E.L.: The 'third kidney' phenomenon of the gastrointestinal tract. Arch Surg, *81*:193, 1960.

Cash, R.A., Nalin, D.R., Forrest, J.N., and Abrutyn, E.: Rapid correction of acidosis and dehydration of cholera with oral electrolyte and glucose solution. Lancet, *2*:549, 1970.

Carey, R.J., and Burbank, C.B.: Mucus-secreting villous adenoma of the colon presenting as circulatory collapse. N Engl J Med, *267*:609, 1962.

Carpenter, C.C.J.: Clinical studies in Asiatic cholera. Bull Johns Hopkins Hosp., *118*:165, 174, 197, 216, 243, 1966.

Carpenter, C.C.J.: Oral rehydration. Is it as good as parenteral therapy? Editorial. N Engl J Med, *306*:1103, 1982.

Cece, J.D., and Toigo, A.: Pancreatic cystic fibrosis in an adult. JAMA, *181*:31, 1962.

Cooke, R.E., and Crowley, L.G.: Replacement of gastric and intestinal fluid losses in surgery. N Engl J Med, *246*:637, 1952.

Dahl, L.K.: Salt intake and salt need. N Engl J Med, *258*:1152, 1205, 1958.

Dwek, J.H., et al.: Salt wasting bronchorrhea and its mechanisms. Arch Intern Med, *137*:791, 1977.

Elkinton, J.R., Winkler, A.W., and Danowski, T.S.: The importance of volume and of tonicity of the body fluids in salt depletion shock. J Clin Invest, *26*:1002, 1947.

Fuisz, R.E.: Hyponatremia. Medicine, *42*:149, 1963.

Gup, A.M., and Briggs, G.W.: Elevated sweat sodium and chloride in adult without cystic fibrosis. Arch Intern Med, *112*:113, 1963.

Harrington, J.T., and Cohen, J.J.: Measurement of urinary electrolytes. Indications and limitations. N Engl J Med, *293*:1241, 1975.

Himathongkam, T., et al.: Medical emergency management. Acute adrenal insufficiency. JAMA, *230*:1317, 1974. Also, Emergency Med, April 1976, page 71.

Hughes, J.M.: Salt-losing nephritis. Arch Intern Med, *114*:190, 1964.

Kassirer, J.P., and Gennari, F.J.: Salt wasting. Consequence or functional adaptation? N Engl J Med, *296*:42, 1977.

Kerpel-Fronius, E.: Uber die Beziehungen zwischen Salz- und Wasseraushalt bei exper-imentellen Wasserverlusten. Z Kinderheilk, *57*:489, 1935.

Knights, E.M., Jr., Brush, J.S., and Schroeder, J.: Simplified screening test for cystic fibrosis of the pancreas. JAMA, *169*:1279, 1959.

Krumlovsku, F.A.: Hyponatremia. Rational Drug Ther, 9:no. 5, May 1975.

Laragh, J.H.: The effect of potassium chloride on hyponatremia. J Clin Invest, *33*:807, 1954.

Leaf, A.: The clinical and physiological significance of the serum sodium concentration. N Engl J Med, *267*:24, 77, 1962.

Leshin, M.: Acute adrenal insufficiency. Recognition, management, and prevention. Uro-logic Clin N Am, *9*:229, 1982.

Lockwood, J.S., and Randall, H.T.: The place of electrolyte studies in surgical patients. Bull. New York Acad Med, *25*:228, 1949. Also Surg Clin N Amer, *32*:3, 1935.

Marriott, H.L.: Water and salt depletion. Br Med J, *1*:245, 285, 328, 1947.

McCance, R.A.: III. Experimental salt deficiency. Lancet, *1*:823, 1936.

Medical Letter on Drugs and Therapeutics: Gatorade and other oral electrolyte solutions, *2*:71, 1969.

Moore, F.D.: Common patterns of water and electrolyte change in injury, surgery and disease. N Engl J Med, *258*:277, 325, 377, 427, 1958.

Nadal, J.W., Pedersen, S., and Maddock, W.G.: Comparison between dehydration from salt loss and from water deprivation. J Clin Invest, *20*:691, 1941.

Nalin, D.R., et al.: Oral maintenance therapy for cholera in adults. Lancet, *2*:370, 1968.

Pierce, N.F., and Hirschhorn, N.: Oral fluid. A simple weapon against dehydration in diarrhoea. How it works and how to use it. WHO Chron, *31*:87, 1977.

Pierce, N.F., et al.: Replacement of water and electrolyte losses in cholera by an oral glucose-electrolyte solution. Ann Intern Med, *70*:1173, 1969.

Questions and Answers: Fluid and electrolyte replacement in sweating athletes. JAMA, *212*:1713, 1970.

Santosham, M., et al.: Oral rehydration therapy of infantile diarrhea. N Engl J Med, *306*:1070, 1982.

Schwachman, H., and Gahm, N.: A simple test for the detection of excessive chloride on the skin. N Engl J Med, *255*:999, 1956.

Sherman, R.A., and Eisenger, R.P.: The use (and misuse) of urinary sodium and chloride measurements. JAMA, *247*:3121, 1982.

Stanbury, S.W., and Mahler, R.F.: Salt-wasting renal disease. Quart J Med, *28*:425, 1959.

Taclob, L.T., and Needle, M.A.: Hyponatremic syndromes. Med Clin N Am, *57*:1425, 1973.

Toigo, A., Dietz, A.A., Crane, J.B., and Reisner, D.: Sweat electrolytes in chronic pul-monary disease. Ann Intern Med, *58*:961, 1963.

Vere, D.W., and King, C.E.: The reaction to subcutaneous drainage in anasarca. Lancet, *1*:779, 1960.

Westerman, R.L.: Oral electrolyte solutions for fluid and electrolyte replacement. Ques-tions and Answers. JAMA, *248*:370, 1982.

CHAPTER 9

SODIUM LOSS SYNDROMES
(Continued)

BURNS

Burns can be classified as follows:

1. *First degree burns.* The injury is limited to the outer layer of the epidermis. Erythema, edema, and pain occur, but vesicles are rarely seen.
2. *Second degree burns.* The injury involves both the epidermis and the dermis, but does not destroy the dermis. Vesicles, bullae and blebs occur with oozing. The skin is pink and reddened, and is painful. Second degree burns usually result from contact with hot liquids or exposure to flashes of short duration.
3. *Third degree burns.* The epidermis and the dermis are destroyed. A third degree burn is usually due to contact with a flash or flame of longer duration. The skin is pearly-white or charred, dry and anesthetic, because the nerve endings have been destroyed.

In this chapter, we shall be concerned with the physiological disturbances caused by second and third degree burns.

PATHOPHYSIOLOGY

Burns can cause the following physiological disturbances:

1. Even a first degree burn causes capillary dilatation and an increased capillary permeability. When second and third degree burns occur, massive amounts of water, plasma electrolytes and plasma proteins pour into the burned and injured areas.

   The most rapid exudation of fluid occurs in the first 6 to 8 hours after the burn. However, the exudation may continue for a total of 48 to 96 hours. This causes a severe sodium loss syndrome (Chapter 8) and may require treatment with large amounts of water, electrolytes and colloid solutions. Adults with a burn of 20% or more will almost always develop the sodium loss syndrome.
2. Extensive burns, especially third degree burns, cause destruction of red blood cells. The anemia which results may be severe.
3. Hyperkalemia may occur, due to the release of intracellular potassium ions from the burned cells. Similarly, a metabolic acidosis may result

from the accumulation of organic acids from the burned cells. A moderate azotemia (BUN concentration 30 to 60 mg/dl) may also develop. Hypocalcemia, even with tetany, can develop 12 to 24 hours after a large deep burn, probably due to saponification of burned subcutaneous tissue.
4. The urine may contain hemoglobin from destruction of red blood cells.

From a physiological point of view, burns can be classified in the following stages:

1. *Stage of sodium loss and shock.* This occurs in the first 48 to 72 hours. Adequate therapy with water, electrolytes, with or without colloid solutions usually causes the patient to gain from 8 to 10% weight during this period of time, after a severe burn.
2. *Stage of sodium and water reabsorption and diuresis.* This occurs from the third or fifth to the twelfth or fourteenth day because the edema fluid in the tissues surrounding the burn begins to be reabsorbed and excreted by the kidneys.
3. *Stage of anemia and malnutrition.* This occurs from the fifth day onward. In this stage, it is important to maintain the patient's blood count and to feed him or her adequately, in order to stop the negative nitrogen balance due to the destruction of tissue.

COURSE AND PROGNOSIS

Shock, oliguria, and fever are unfavorable signs. The prognosis of a person with a burn of less than 20% is uniformly good. However, at least one out of two patients will die when 50% or more of the body surface is burned. The cause of death is usually overwhelming infection that does not respond to antibiotic therapy.

TREATMENT

Stage of Sodium Loss and Shock

All investigators agree that burn patients at this stage require electrolytes with or without colloid solutions. However, there is no agreement about the types or volumes of the electrolyte or colloid solutions that should be used. It is interesting to note that very different treatments appear to be almost equally effective.

At the 1978 Consensus Development Conference on Supportive Therapy in Burn Care, the participants agreed on the following general principles of fluid treatment for severe burns (Schwartz):

1. In the initial 24 hour post-burn period, an isotonic balanced (Lactated Ringer's) salt solution is as adequate as colloid-containing solutions, and that no other solution (neither colloid nor 5% dextrose in water) needs to be given at this time. The calculated dose of lactated Ringer's solution should range between 2 and 4 ml/kg/% body surface burned.
2. At approximately 24 hours post-burn, colloid-containing solutions can be given to expand the plasma volume.
3. The total time required for resuscitation can be shortened by the rapid

reconstitution of plasma volume as soon as leaky capillaries are sealed, i.e. between 24 and 32 hours post-burn.

The Parkland Hospital (Baxter) formula corresponds to these recommendations.

A burned patient can be treated like other patients with sodium-loss syndrome, with merely oral or parenteral saline or similar sodium-containing solutions. The fluid and electrolyte requirements of a burned patient depend partly on the extent of the burn. This can be determined in a simple way by the following *rule of nines*:

Anterior head—4½% of the body surface.
Posterior head—4½% of the body surface.
Each upper extremity—9% of the body surface.
Each lower extremity—18% of the body surface.
Anterior thorax and abdomen—18% of the body surface.
Posterior thorax and back—18% of the body surface.

The Treatment of Limited Burns (10 to 15% of the body surface). A patient with a burn of only 10 to 15% of the body surface can usually be treated by means of a sodium-containing electrolyte solution, given orally. The solution should be iced. The container can be placed in a pan of ice at the patient's bedside, so that the solution remains chilled. (However, if repeated vomiting or diarrhea occurs, oral therapy should be stopped.)

Many oral electrolyte solutions have been described, for example:

Moyer's solution, consisting of 1 level teaspoonful (approximately 3 g) sodium chloride, and 1 level teaspoonful (approximately 1.5 g) sodium bicarbonate (baking soda), to 1 liter of iced drinking water. (It is hypotonic and provides 69 mEq sodium ions, 52 mEq chloride ions, and 17 mEq bicarbonate ions per liter.)
Markley's solution, consisting of 5.5 g sodium chloride and 4.0 g sodium bicarbonate in 1 liter iced drinking water. (It is isotonic and provides 140 mEq sodium ions, 94 mEq chloride ions, and 47 bicarbonate ions per liter.)

The oral solution can be imbibed at a rate of 50 to 100 ml per hour, as tolerated; 1 to 2.5 liters can be imbibed in 24 hours. (The volume taken in the first 24 hours should not exceed 5% of the body weight.) The patient is also allowed soft food, occasionaly broth or fruit juice, but *no* tap water.

The Treatment of Extensive Burns (20% or more of the skin surface). A patient with an extensive burn can also be treated with a sodium-containing electrolyte solution, just as a less seriously burned patient, and just as other patients with sodium-loss syndrome. However, the solution is usually given intravenously because of the large volume needed. Part (or even all) of the solution can be given orally, using one of the oral formulas described above, if the patient tolerates it.

The following discussions present widely used methods of giving fluids intravenously.

Table 9–1.   *Formulas for Estimating Adult Burn Patient Resuscitation Needs**

Formula	Electrolyte solution	Colloid solution**	5% Dextrose in water
	First 24 Hours		
Parkland Hospital (Baxter)	Lactated Ringer's 4 ml/kg/% burn		
Brooke Army Med. Center (Reiss)	Lactated Ringer's 1.5 ml/kg/% burn	0.5 ml/kg/% burn	2000 ml
Hypertonic Sodium chloride (250 mEq Na/L)	Volume to maintain urine output at 30 ml/hr		
	Second 24 Hours		
Parkland Hospital (Baxter)		20–60% of calculated plasma volume***	To maintain adequate urinary output
Brooke Army Med. Center	½ to ¾ of first 24 hr needs	½ to ¾ of first 24 hr needs	2000 ml
Hypertonic Sodium chloride (250 mEq Na/L)	⅓ isotonic saline orally up to 3500 ml limit		

*Adapted from Pruitt.
**The usual colloid solutions are blood plasma or human serum albumin.
***Calculated plasma volume is 39 ml/kg for men; 40 ml/kg for women.

The Parkland Hospital or Baxter Formula (Table 9–1). In the first 24 hours, lactated Ringer's solution, 4 ml per kg body weight per % of total body surface burned, is given.

Example: Patient, 70 kg weight, with a 50% second degree burn.
The total volume of lactated Ringer's solution needed during the first 24 hours is:
$4 \times 70 \times 0.5 = 14$ liters.

One-half of the calculated volume is given rapidly during the first 8 hours; one-quarter is given in the next 8 hours; the final one-quarter is given in the final 8 hours.

The goal of the intravenous fluid is to establish a urine flow of 50 to 70 ml an hour, a pulse rate less than 120 per minute, a normal pH and serum bicarbonate concentration, and a lucid patient with stable vital signs. (It may be difficult or impossible to measure blood pressure if the upper extremities are burned.) When a urine flow greater than 50 ml per hour has been established and the patient's clinical condition improves, the rate of flow of the infusion can be adjusted.

When most or all of the lactated Ringer's solution has been infused, 18 to 24 hours after the burn, a small amount of plasma or serum albumin (see Table 9–1) can be given intravenously if the patient does not show optimum vital signs.

After the first 24 hours, lactated Ringer's solution is not used. Instead, dextrose in water should be administered in an amount necessary to maintain a normal serum sodium concentration. Two (or more) liters of dextrose in water may be needed in this second 24-hour period.

The Brooke Army Medical Center Formula (Reiss et al.) (Table 9–1). (This is a modification of the Evans formula.)

First 24 hours:
Colloid (plasma or human serum albumin): 0.5 mg per kg body weight per % of total body surface burned.
Lactated Ringer's solution: 1.5 ml per kg body weight per % of total body surface burned.
Dextrose in water solution: 2000 ml.

Second 24 hours:
Approximately one-half the volumes of the lactated Ringer's solution and of the colloid solution.
Dextrose in water solution: 2000 ml.

One-half of this amount is given in the first 8 hours after the burn. One-quarter is given in the next 8-hour period; the final one-quarter is given in the next 8-hour period.

Whole blood should not be used at first because of the presence of hemoconcentration. However, it can be given when the hematocrit falls below normal (usually on the second to seventh day after the burn). (If the patient shows an anemia but the central venous pressure is elevated, a packed red blood cell transfusion should be given instead.)

Dextran can be used as a plasma substitute, but not more than 1 liter a day should be given (Chap 35).

(In the original Evans formula, isotonic saline solution was used instead of lactated Ringer's solution. However, a large amount of sodium chloride intravenously may cause a metabolic acidosis [Chap 17], or it may aggravate the metabolic acidosis that is usually present in a severely burned patient.)

When the extent of the burn is more than 50% of the body surface, colloid and lactated Ringer's solutions should be given in an amount calculated for only a 50% burn. In this way, the patient will not receive an excessive amount of fluid (which can cause pulmonary edema when the burn edema fluid begins to be reabsorbed into the circulation on the third day or later).

In addition, not more than 10,000 ml of total fluids should be given in 1 day, regardless of the extent of the burn and the weight of the patient, except under unusual circumstances.

If the patient is able to tolerate oral fluids, plain water or sweetened tea can be considered as part of the daily water intake.

The urinary output should be maintained between 30 and 50 ml per hour, and vital signs should be stable. (It may be difficult or impossible to take blood pressure readings if the upper extremities are burned.)

If the urinary output falls below 30 ml per hour, it is a sign that more electrolyte and colloid solutions should be given. If the urinary output exceeds 50 ml per hour, this may be a sign of excessive fluid administration.

The hematocrit should be determined every 3 to 4 hours for the first 2 or 3 days. It should be maintained at approximately 45%.

When either the Parkland or the Brooke formula, or any other formula, is used, one must remember that a formula is only a guide to the treatment of the patient, and that changes in the clinical condition of the patient or in laboratory test reports may require extensive changes in the intravenous or oral therapy.

Patients with burns caused by high-voltage electricity require larger amounts of fluid during early resuscitative therapy.

Stage of Sodium and Water Reabsorption and Diuresis

Fluid intake should be decreased when the edema fluid begins to be reabsorbed and diuresis occurs. Too much fluid given at this time may cause pulmonary edema. However, the diuresis may be so great that a water loss syndrome with desiccation may occur. This situation is similar to the water loss syndrome that occurs with an excessive solute intake (Chap 4). In addition, the patient may be losing a large amount of water from the burned skin, from fever, and from seepage into dressings.

The physician must observe the patient closely for clinical signs of water loss, such as thirst and dryness of the mucous membranes (Chap 3). If these signs are present, water must be given freely. As much as 4 to 6 liters a day may be needed.

The best method of determining water needs in this stage is the serum sodium concentration. It should be maintained at about 136 mEq/L, or the hematocrit should be maintained at about 45%.

In addition, the patient may lose a large amount of potassium in this stage. To avoid this, potassium chloride can be added to the infusions in a daily dose of approximately 80 mEq/L (6 g KCl).

After the third to the fifth day, a vigorous attempt should be made to give the patient adequate nourishment. Nasogastric tube feedings of a high protein solution are valuable (also see Chap 4). In addition, repeated transfusions may be necessary.

Diet Requirements After Severe Burns

Curreri et al. have developed a simple formula for caloric food intake to minimize weight loss during the acute burn period, namely:

Daily calories needed are equal to the sum of the patient's weight in kg multiplied by 25, plus the % of the total body surface burn multiplied by 40.

Other treatment is outside the scope of this book.

REFERENCES

Asch, M.J., White, M.G., and Pruitt, B.A.: Acid base changes associated with topical Sulfamylon therapy. Ann Surg, *172*:946, 1970.

Baxter, C.R.: Crystalloid resuscitation of burn shock. In *Contemporary Burn Management* (Polk, H.C., Jr., and Stone, H.N., Eds.). Boston, Little, Brown & Co., 1971.

Baxter, C.R.: Guidelines for fluid resuscitation. J Trauma, *21*:687, 1981.

Burke, J.F., et al.: 1981—approach to burn therapy. Surg Annual, *13*:1, 1981.

Caldwell, F.T., Jr., and Bowser, B.H.: Critical evaluation of hypertonic and hypotonic solutions to resuscitate severely burned children. A prospective study. Ann Surg, *189*:546, 1979.

Curreri, P.W., et al.: Dietary requirements of patients with major burns. J Am Diet Assoc, *65*:415, 1974.

Demling, R.H.: Fluid resuscitation after major burns. JAMA, *250*:1438, 1983.

Evans, E.I., et al.: Fluid and electrolyte requirements in severe burns. Ann Surg, *135*:804, 1952.

Hinton, P., et al.: Electrolyte changes after burn injury and effect of treatment. Lancet, *2*:218, 1973.

Hutcher, N., and Haynes, B.W.: The Evans formula revisited. J Trauma, *12*:453, 1972.

Markley, K., Bocanegra, M., Bazan, A., Temple, R., Chiappori, M., Morales, G., and Carrion, A.: Clinical evaluation of saline solution therapy in burn shock. JAMA, *170*:1633, 1959; *161*:1465, 1956.

Markley, K.: Comparison of sodium salts and plasma therapy in burned patients in Peru. Ann New York Acad Sci, *150*:845, 1968.

Monafo, W.W., et al.: Hypertonic sodium solutions in the treatment of burn shock. Am J Surg, *126*:778, 1973.

Monafo, W.W.: *The Treatment of Burns*. St. Louis, Warren H. Green, Inc., 1971.

Moyer, C.A., Margraf, H.W., and Monafo, W.W.: Burn shock and extravascular sodium deficiency. Treatment with Ringer's solution with lactate. Arch Surg, *90*:799, 1965.

Peaston, M.J.T.: Metabolic acidosis in burns. Br Med J, *1*:809, 1968.

Pruitt, B.A., Jr.: Fluid resuscitation for extensively burned patients. J Trauma, *21*:690, 1981.

Reiss, E.J.A., et al.: Fluid and electrolyte balance in burns. JAMA, *152*:1309, 1953.

Schwartz, S.I.: Consensus summary on fluid resuscitation. J Trauma, *19*:(Suppl II)876, 1979.

Shires, G.T., and Black, E.A.: Editors: Consensus development conference supportive therapy in burn care. J Trauma, *19*:Suppl. II, Nov. 1979.

Warden, G.D., et al.: Hypernatremic state in hypermetabolic burn patients. Arch Surg, *106*:420, 1973.

CHAPTER 10

SODIUM EXCESS SYNDROMES (EDEMA)

PATHOPHYSIOLOGY

In Chapter 8, it was pointed out that the serum sodium concentration and the total exchangeable body sodium do not vary proportionately. Therefore, a low serum sodium concentration may be associated with a low, normal, or high total exchangeable body sodium. Similarly, a high serum sodium concentration may be associated with a low, normal, or high total exchangeable body sodium.

An excessive total exchangeable body sodium is almost always associated with an excess of water, except possibly in certain patients with hypernatremia due to cerebral lesions. In other words, *an excess of total exchangeable body sodium is not manifested by hypernatremia, but by edema.*

Edema occurs in several ways:

Cardiac Edema

Cardiac edema occurs when the heart fails as a pump and the renal blood flow decreases as a result of this. This is followed by a retention of sodium ions and water.

The decreased renal blood flow stimulates the production of renin. This in turn stimulates the secretion of aldosterone. As a result, the distal renal tubules reabsorb an excessive amount of sodium ions (and water); therefore the plasma volume increases, the venous pressure rises, and edema occurs.

Activity of a natriuretic hormone (third factor) may be suppressed. It is believed that the excretion of sodium ions by the renal tubules is controlled by this hormone, though its site of origin and chemical structure are unknown. (The first two factors affecting excretion of sodium ions by the kidneys are the glomerular filtration rate and the effects of aldosterone.)

It has been known for many years that dogs respond to a saline infusion with a prompt increase both in glomerular filtration rate and the excretion of sodium ions. This increase is caused by a decreased tubular reabsorption of sodium ions from the proximal renal tubules. A similar loss or "escape" of sodium ions from the kidneys occurs when a salt-retaining hormone such as aldosterone or 11-desoxycorticosterone is administered over a prolonged period of time to normal subjects. This explains why patients with primary aldosteronism do not develop severe edema.

The decreased effective arterial blood volume may also stimulate the secretion of ADH (vasopressin), the antidiuretic hormone of the posterior pituitary. The ADH level in the blood may also become abnormally high when chronic passive congestion of the liver is present (caused by right-sided congestive heart failure) because the liver may not be able to normally degrade and inactivate the circulating ADH. If excessive ADH secretion occurs, water rather than sodium ions is retained and the serum sodium concentration will fall.

The relation of hormonal imbalances to the formation of edema is actually very complicated; for example, aldosterone secretion may be high only when edema formation starts. Congestive heart failure is also not usually associated with excessive ADH secretion. And, if it occurs, water rather than sodium ions is retained and the serum sodium concentration falls. In congestive heart failure there is also increased adrenocortical activity. As a result, the sodium content of sweat, saliva, and urine decreases.

Circulatory Edema

In this group of patients, the heart does not fail as a pump. However, other factors cause the continued secretion of aldosterone. This type of edema occurs, for example, in cirrhotic and nephrotic patients. The primary disturbance is a decreased circulating blood volume.

In *cirrhosis of the liver,* edema is associated with ascites, which is due essentially to obstruction of the lymphatic flow from the liver. This, in turn, is affected by any factor that interferes with the return of blood through the hepatic and portal veins. The ascites can occur as a result of the following factors:

1. Obstruction of the portal vein itself rarely causes ascites. However, obstruction of the hepatic vein is almost always associated with ascites. Conversely, if the inferior vena cava is ligated below the insertion of the hepatic veins, ascites will not develop.

   In cirrhosis, the inflammatory process in the liver obstructs both venous return through the hepatic veins and the portal venous return. Marked congestion of the lymphatics of the liver occurs. The transudation of fluid from the lymphatics on the surface of the liver is the direct cause of the ascites.

Ascites is associated with a marked increased secretion of aldosterone, which can occur in several ways: It has been shown that if the hepatic veins of a dog are ligated a marked increased aldosterone secretion occurs almost immediately, *before* ascites develops (Orloff and associates). The mechanism by which this occurs is not known. Later, when ascites has developed, the entrance of fluid into the abdominal cavity may decrease the circulating blood volume and cause a secondary aldosteronism in this way. In addition, a tense ascites may compress the inferior vena cava and decrease the venous return and cardiac output, which also stimulates aldosterone secretion.

2. When liver injury is present for a long time, the liver loses its capacity to form serum albumin. When hypoalbuminemia develops, the osmotic pressure of the blood decreases. This enhances the effect of the hydrostatic pressure of the blood and increases the ascites and the edema.

3. In addition, cirrhotic patients may show an increased amount of ADH in the blood, which causes water retention and also aggravates the ascites. The cause of the ADH secretion is not known.

4. Cardiac factors may also be present to cause the ascites and the edema, because patients with chronic cirrhosis may show microscopic signs of myocardial degeneration. (This may be due partly to malnutrition, and partly to chronic potassium loss.) Another cardiac factor which may contribute to the development of the ascites and edema is the development of abnormal vascular anastomoses in the liver and lungs, which may cause an increased venous return and high-output type of heart failure.

(Ascites can of course occur not only in cirrhosis of the liver and in severe right-sided congestive heart failure, but in constrictive pericarditis, the nephrotic syndrome, pancreatitis, malignant disease of the abdomen, in intraabdominal infections, myxedema, and so on.)

The development of edema in the *nephrotic syndrome* is apparently related primarily to the increased glomerular permeability to albumin. Long-continued loss of serum albumin decreases the oncotic pressure of the blood and causes an increased flow of water from the blood to the tissue spaces. As a result, the circulating blood volume decreases. This stimulates aldosterone secretion, which in turn causes the retention of sodium and water which leads to edema, just as in a cardiac patient.

Hormonal Edema

In Cushing's syndrome, and during ACTH or corticosteroid therapy with hydrocortisone or its derivatives, the edema which occurs may be due to increased aldosterone secretion as a result of either the disease process or the drugs.

Edema Associated with Excessive ADH Secretion

Cardiac edema is not ordinarily associated with an excessive secretion of ADH. However, under special circumstances, an excessive ADH secretion may develop, for example, postoperatively, during acute infections, and in other ways (see Chap 7). If this occurs, a patient with congestive heart failure whose diet has been too low in sodium, or who has lost an excessive amount of sodium ions by vomiting, paracentesis, as a result of excessive administration of diuretics, or in any other way, and who has been drinking water freely, or has been given an excessive amount of water parenterally, may develop edema related to the abnormal retention of water. Such a patient will show an abnormally low serum sodium concentration (see Chap 6).

Idiopathic Cyclic Edema

This consists of periodic nonpitting edema of the face, hands, and feet, and occurs in women who still have their menses. However, it is not related to premenstrual tension. Patients also complain of abdominal distention and a sense of fullness in the bladder. The edema is minimal when the patient awakens and becomes more marked during the day. This is due to fluid retention in the upright position. However, the way in which an upright position produces the fluid retention is not known. Some patients may gain as much as 12 pounds a day. The usual weight gain is 2 to 4 pounds. Many patients are emotionally disturbed. The syndrome may last for years.

Laboratory tests may show hypoalbuminemia, hyponatremia, hypokalemia, or hypomagnesemia. The loss of serum albumin may be due to abnormal transudation from the blood into the extracellular spaces as a result of abnormal capillary permeability. Hyponatremia, hypokalemia, and hypomagnesemia are usually the effects of the diuretics the patient has been given.

TREATMENT

The treatment of edema depends on the physiological mechanisms that have produced it. In cardiac patients, an attempt should be made to strengthen the force and efficiency of cardiac contractions. Digitalis is the drug of choice. In addition, a low-sodium diet tends to prevent the retention of sodium ions associated with cardiac edema.

A patient placed on a sodium-restricted diet must avoid not only salt but also processed and packaged foods, such as canned foods, delicatessen products, and most cheeses. (Further details of low-sodium diets are beyond the scope of this book.)

Diet lists describing the sodium content of foods may also be misleading. For example, the sodium content of foods can be expressed either as grams of sodium *ions,* or as grams of sodium chloride (salt). For example, 1 g of sodium ions is equivalent to 43 mEq sodium ions. However, 1 g of sodium chloride is equivalent to 17 mEq sodium ions.

Therefore, a 2-g sodium (ion) diet and a 5-g sodium chloride diet contain approximately similar amounts of sodium ions.

Medications may be an inadvertent source of sodium intake. For example, each gram of carbenicillin disodium (Geopen-Roerig) contains approximately 5.9 mEq (136 mg) sodium ions. If a patient is given a daily dose of 24 g of carbenicillin, this will contain 142 mEq (6.2 g) of sodium ions. Each 2.5 g of sulfadiazine (Parke Davis) for parenteral use, contains 9.3 mEq (215 mg) of sodium ions.

Widely used proprietary drugs that have a relatively high sodium content include Alka-Seltzer, Bisodol powder, Bromo-Seltzer, Metamucil instant mix, Sal Hepatica, sodium bicarbonate and so on. Fleet enema also has a high sodium content, although it is not totally absorbed from the rectum.

Another possible source of sodium is drinking water, because the water content may be more than 8.7 mEq (200 mg) sodium per liter in some cities. In addition, home water-softening units replace the magnesium and calcium salts that may be present in the water with sodium chloride. In Chicago, the water is moderately hard, and about 5.2 mEq (120 mg) sodium per liter is added when the water is processed.

Diuretics are also effective in treating cardiac edema. The commonly used diuretics are of two major types: (1) the *thiazides* such as chlorothiazide (Diuril), hydrochlorothiazide (HydroDIURIL, Esidrix), trichlormethiazide (Metahydrin, Naqua), and so on, and similar nonthiazide diuretics such as the sulfonamyls (Hygroton), and the quinazolines (Hydromox and Zaroxolyn), and (2) the newer *loop* diuretics such as furosemide (frusemide, Lasix), ethacrynic acid (Edecrin), and bumetanide (Bumex).

The various diuretics can cause a urinary excretion of sodium, potassium, bicarbonate, and phosphate ions, and a urinary excretion of free water, depending on the site or sites of their action in the kidneys. Figure 10–1 is a schematic diagram of a nephron, showing the major sites of actions of the commonly used diuretics. The various diuretics act in the following ways:

Carbonic Anhydrase Inhibitors (Diamox). Carbonic anhydrase inhibitors work in the following way: In the kidneys, all the bicarbonate ions that pass the glomeruli and enter the proximal tubules (glomerular filtrate) are reabsorbed. This occurs because hydrogen and bicarbonate ions are produced by the tubule cells by means of the enzyme, carbonic anhydrase. The hydrogen ions pass into the tubular urine and react with sodium bicarbonate to form carbonic acid, which is excreted. The sodium ions pass back into the tubule cells, react with bicarbonate ions and then pass back into the plasma as sodium bicarbonate. As a result, sodium ions are conserved by the kidneys.

When a carbonic anhydrase inhibitor is given, the formation of carbonic acid in the proximal tubule cells (Fig. 10–1 [1]) is inhibited, and

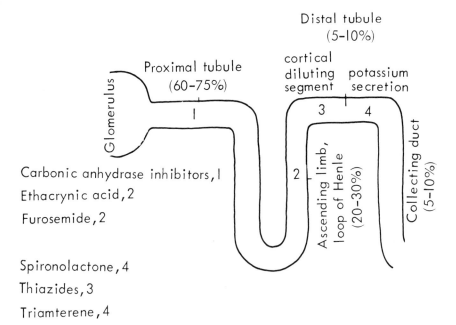

Fig. 10–1. Sites of action of diuretics in the nephron. See text. (Adapted from P.G. Gazes: *Clinical Cardiology.* Chicago, Year Book Publishers, 1975.)

a large amount of sodium bicarbonate and water is excreted in the urine. This causes a diuresis and also a rise in the hydrogen and chloride concentration in the blood and a tendency to a metabolic acidosis. The serum potassium concentration may fall because a large amount of potassium ions is also excreted in the urine. (There is an exchange mechanism for potassium and hydrogen ions in the kidney tubule cells. This causes hydrogen and potassium ions to be excreted in inverse proportional concentrations in the urine.)

A carbonic anhydrase inhibitor loses its effectiveness after 2 to 3 days. Therefore it should be used only intermittently, for example, for 2 or 3 days, then a rest period of at least 2 days before it is started again. In the intervals when it is not given, the patient can receive a thiazide, or furosemide or ethacrynic acid. A carbonic anhydrase inhibitor can be given simultaneously with a thiazide or with ethacrynic acid. There is some evidence that it can interfere with the effectiveness of chlorthalidone (Hygroton).

Ethacrynic Acid (Edecrin). Ethacrynic acid inhibits the reabsorption of sodium ions in the ascending limb of the loop of Henle (Fig. 10–1 [2]) and decreases distal tubular reabsorption of sodium and chloride ions. As a result, an increased amount of sodium and chloride ions and slightly less potassium and bicarbonate ions are excreted in the urine. Ethacrynic acid is effective when either a metabolic alkalosis or acidosis is present. However, it may aggravate either of these conditions.

Furosemide (Lasix). The actions of furosemide are similar to those of ethacrynic acid (see Ethacrynic acid above). It is particularly effective when renal insufficiency is present.

Spironolactone (Aldactone). Spironolactone inhibits the physiological effects of the adrenocortical hormone aldosterone, on the distal renal tubules (Fig. 10–1 [4]), and in this way produces an increased excretion of sodium and chloride ions. It also increases the urinary excretion of free water. It characteristically decreases the urinary excretion of potassium ions and can cause hyperkalemia. It also increases the urinary excretion of ammonium and phosphate ions.

Because most of the sodium ions are reabsorbed in the proximal renal tubules, spironolactone is relatively ineffective when given alone, and a diuretic, such as a thiazide, ethacrynic acid, or furosemide, which blocks reabsorption of sodium ions in a region of the nephron proximal to the site of action of spironolactone, should be given concomitantly.

Thiazides and Related Diuretics. The thiazides and related sulfonamide diuretics, such as chlorthalidone (Hygroton), and quinethazone (Hydromox) inhibit the reabsorption of sodium ions in the distal renal tubules (Fig. 10–1 [3]) and in this way increase the urinary excretion of sodium ions. Hyponatremia can therefore develop. There is also an increased urinary excretion of chloride ions, so that hypochloremia can also develop.

Hyponatremia and a sodium loss syndrome may develop with any of the above diuretics, particularly if the diuretic is given to a patient who is on a low sodium diet. Hyperglycemia and/or hyperuricemia may also develop when a thiazide, ethacrynic acid, or furosemide is used.

When the diuretics (with the exception of spironolactone or triamterene) are given regularly for a long time, supplementary potassium chloride is needed to prevent both hypokalemia and hypochloremia and a metabolic alkalosis. Both spironolactone and triamterene cause a retention of potassium ions so that hyperkalemia may occur as a toxic effect. Therefore, when either of these is prescribed, the patient must not take supplemental potassium chloride. Otherwise a severe and even fatal hyperkalemia can develop.

The urinary excretion of potassium ions is also increased, so that hypokalemia often occurs. Plasma renin activity is also greatly increased by the thiazides, probably as a result of the decreased plasma volume produced by the thiazides. This causes an increased secretion of aldosterone, which may contribute to the hypokalemia.

The urinary excretion of bicarbonate and magnesium ions also is increased. When given for a long time the thiazides decrease the excretion of calcium ions and can raise the serum calcium level. The thiazides also have a slight carbonic anhydrase inhibitor activity (see Carbonic anhydrase inhibitors, above). The diuretic effect of the thiazides is not affected by the acid base balance of the patient.

Triamterene (Dyrenium). Triamterene has a weak action similar to spironolactone and depresses reabsorption of sodium ions in the distal renal tubules (Fig. 10–1 [4]) (also see Spironolactone, above). It also increases the urinary excretion of chloride ions, but slightly less than the urinary excretion of sodium ions. The urinary excretion of potassium ions is characteristically decreased, so that hyperkalemia may develop. The serum sodium level is lowered.

All the diuretics have side effects, some of which can be serious. Therefore, it is important to be familiar with the indications, contraindications, side effects and toxicity, reactions with other drugs, and dosages of each of these diuretics. (This statement also applies to the use of all drugs.) For example, if a patient who is on long-term lithium therapy receives a thiazide diuretic, or any diuretic that promotes the urinary excretion of both potassium and sodium ions, the serum lithium level may rise greatly and produce lithium toxicity. Therefore, the lithium dosage must be reduced and serum lithium levels must be checked constantly. (A potassium-sparing diuretic, such as spironolactone or triamterene, is safer for such patients.)

When diuretics are given to a patient on a low-sodium diet, a severe sodium loss syndrome (Chap 8) may develop. Hyperglycemia and/or hyperuricemia may also develop when the thiazides, ethacrynic acid, or furosemide are used.

Spironolactone and triamterene are weak diuretics, as was mentioned above, and are rarely prescribed by themselves. Spironolactone is particularly effective as a diuretic when right-sided congestive heart failure (with congestion of the liver) is present.

Amiloride (Midamor) is a new potassium-sparing diuretic with actions similar to triamterene and aldactone.

When congestive heart failure and edema are severe, digitalis, the thiazides, ethacrynic acid or furosemide, and spironolactone or triamterene can be used concomitantly.

The corticosteroids, particularly prednisone, in small oral doses (15 mg a day for several days) have also been used for refractory cardiac edema, particularly in patients with coronary artery disease. The exact mechanism by which prednisone is effective is not known. It may act as a direct antagonist of aldosterone or directly cause increased renal blood flow and increased excretion of sodium ions and water. The corticosteroids inhibit ACTH. They also cause sodium ions to move from the cells into the extracellular water. This increases plasma volume and in this way also increases renal blood flow.

Peritoneal dialysis, using a 4.25% dextrose solution, can also be used when edema and severe congestive heart failure do not respond to medical therapy.

The treatment of congestive heart failure associated with a retention of water, rather than a retention of sodium ions, is described on page 62. These patients often show a metabolic alkalosis, with low serum sodium, chloride, and potassium concentrations, associated with the excessive use of thiazide diuretics or with furosemide or ethacrynic acid. The treatment is described in Chapters 26 and 27.

Patients with *cirrhosis of the liver* and ascites can be treated with a low sodium diet and with an aldosterone-antagonist, such as spironolactone (Aldactone). Or small doses of furosemide (Lasix), with or without supplemental potassium chloride, if indicated, can be used. (Excessive doses can precipitate hepatic coma or the hepato-renal syndrome.) If severe hypoproteinemia is present, infusions of salt-poor albumin may temporarily increase the colloid osmotic pressure and produce a diuresis.

Ammonium chloride or a carbonic anhydrase inhibitor (such as Diamox) should *not* be used, because it may precipitate hepatic coma.

Even when maximal diuresis is obtained, it is not possible to decrease the volume of ascitic fluid by more than 1000 ml a day. Therefore, a weight loss of 1 to 2 pounds a day is satisfactory. If excessive diuresis is produced, a low sodium syndrome, hepatic coma or progressive renal insufficiency (hepatorenal syndrome) may develop.

Discussion of use of the peritoneovenous shunt in the treatment of refractory ascites is outside the scope of this book.

Paracentesis should not be done, if possible, because it results in a loss of serum proteins, it decreases the effective blood volume and increases the secretion of aldosterone and ADH. In addition, repeated paracentesis may produce a sodium loss syndrome with shock or renal failure. (Excessive diuretic therapy can also cause a similar syndrome.)

Patients with a *nephrotic syndrome* may or may not respond to corticosteroids. Approximately three-fourths of children will respond; approximately three-fourths of adults will not. Regardless of the response to corticosteroids, the patient should be given a high protein diet, from 2 to 3 g of protein per kg weight daily. Meat, eggs and milk are particularly valuable.

Rigid salt restriction and diuretics may be dangerous because they may cause a decrease in the circulating blood volume and a decrease in glomerular filtration rate. As a result, hypotension or shock or hyperkalemia may result. If a diuretic is needed, a loop diuretic such as furosemide, or a thiazide can be used. Spironolactone or triamterene should not be used because either one raises the serum potassium concentration.

Treatment of *idiopathic cyclic edema* is difficult. Spironolactone may be effective, although the increased aldosterone secretion that may be present is probably secondary to the decreased circulatory blood volume that results from the transudation of fluid out of the capillary walls, and from the decreased circulating blood volume that may result from excessive diuretic use. Small doses of a thiazide can also be used with or without spironolactone.

Supportive stockings or panty hose may be helpful in preventing some of the postural changes. A sympathomimetic drug such as dextroamphetamine may also lower serum aldosterone levels and decrease the tendency to fluid retention. The usual dose is 10 to 20 mg a day, in time-release capsules.

REFERENCES

Annotation: Drug therapy. Dietary sodium. Drug Therapy, August 1977, page 121.

Ascione, F.J.: Lithium with diuretics. Drug Therapy, Sept 1977, page 125.

Baggenstoss, A.H., and Wollaeger, E.E.: Portal hypertension due to chronic occlusion of the extrahepatic portion of the portal vein: Its relation to ascites. Am J Med, *21*:16, 1956.

Beyer, K.H., Jr.: The pharmacological basis for modern diuretic therapy. Rational Drug Ther, *12*:no. 2, February 1978.

Coleman, M., Horwith, M., and Brown, J.L.: Idiopathic edema. Studies demonstrating protein-leaking angiopathy. Am J Med, *49*:106, 1970.

Davis, J.O.: Mechanisms of salt and water retention in congestive heart failure. The importance of aldosterone. Am J Med, *29*:486, 1960.

Edwards, O.M., and Bayliss, R.I.S.: Idiopathic edema of women. Quart J Med, *45*:125, 1976.

Espiner, E.A., Jagger, P.I., et al.: Effect of acute diuresis on aldosterone secretion in edematous patients. N Engl J Med, *280*:1141, 1969.

Feldman, H.A., Jayakumar, S., and Puschett, J.B.: Idiopathic edema. A review of etiologic concepts and management. Cardiovasc Med, *3*:475, 1978.

Gill, J.R., Jr., et al.: Idiopathic edema resulting from occult cardiomyopathy. Am J Med, *134*:253, 1965.

Gill, J.R., Jr., Waldman, T.A., and Bartter, F.C.: Idiopathic edema. I. The occurrence of hypoalbuminemia and abnormal metabolism in women with unexplained edema. Am J Med, *52*:444 and 452, 1972.

Ginsberg, A.L.: Cirrhotic diuresis. Questions and Answers. JAMA, *247*:2152, 1982.

Gregory, P.B.: The treatment of ascites. Rational Drug Ther, *12*:no. 7, July 1978.

Liebowitz, H.R.: Pathogenesis of ascites in cirrhosis of liver. New York State J Med, *69*:1895, 1969.

Lipman, A.G.: Sodium content of commonly used parenteral antibiotics. Modern Med, May 30, 1977, page 83.

Lipman, A.G.: Sodium content of frequently used analgesics and gastrointestinal drugs. Modern Medicine, June 15, 1977, page 59.

Maffly, R.H.: How to avoid complications of potent diuretics. JAMA, *235*:2526, 1976.

Mailloux, L.V., et al.: Peritoneal dialysis for refractory congestive heart failure. JAMA, *199*:123, 1967.

Martinez-Maldonado, M., and Garcia, A.: A practical approach to the nephrotic syndrome. Drug Therapy, p. 79, March 1981.

Porter, G.A.: The role of diuretics in the treatment of heart failure. JAMA, *244*:1614, 1980.

Reineck, H.J., and Stein, J.H.: Mechanisms of action and clinical use of diuretic drugs, in Brenner, B.M. and Rector, F.C., Jr. editors. *The Kidney,* 2nd ed., Philadelphia, W.B. Saunders Co., vol 1, 1981.

Riemer, A.D.: Application of the newer corticosteroids to augment diuresis in congestive heart failure. Am J Cardiol, *1*:488, 1958.

Rubin, A.L., et al.: The use of 1-lysine monohydrochloride in combination with mercurial diuretics in the treatment of refractory fluid retention. Circulation, *21*:332, 1960.

Sanders, L.L., and Melby, J.C.: Aldosterone and the edema of congestive heart failure. Arch Intern Med, *113*:331, 1964.

Shashall, P.D.: Gross oedema in the nephrotic syndrome treated with frusemide in high dosage. Br Med J, *1*:319, 1971.

Shear, L., Ching, S., and Gabuzda, G.J.: Compartmentalization of ascites and edema in patients with hepatic cirrhosis. N Engl J Med, *282*:1391, 1970.

Sherlock, S., et al.: The complications of diuretic therapy in patients with cirrhosis. Ann New York Acad Sci, *139*:497, 1966.

Smith, F.G., et al.: The nephrotic syndrome. Current concepts. Ann Intern Med, *76*:463, 1972.

Steigmann, F., Dubin, A., and Sisson, A.: "Intractable" ascites in cirrhosis. Its management by a multiple diuretic approach. Ann J Med Sci, *245*:521, 1963.

Streeten, D.H.P.: The role of posture in idiopathic edema. S Afr Med J, *49*:462, 1975.

CHAPTER 11

SYNDROMES ASSOCIATED WITH DISTURBED OSMOLALITY

OSMOMETRY

Osmotic pressure was described in a general way in Chapter 2. In this chapter, the clinical uses of osmometry will be described., Measurement of the osmolality of the plasma (or serum) and the extracellular water is important because osmolality is related to the concentration of free particles, molecules, or ions in a solution. For example, when sodium or chloride ions, which are the chief ions in the extracellular water, are lost, the osmolality of the plasma and the extracellular water will decrease greatly. Similarly, when the concentration of glucose or blood urea nitrogen rises, this will tend to be associated with an increased osmolality of the extracellular water.

The terms "osmolarity" and "osmolality" are almost but not quite synonymous. For example, a *molar* solution contains a gram molecular weight of a substance dissolved in a solvent to make 1 liter. A *molal* solution, however, contains a gram molecular weight of a substance dissolved in 1000 g of a solvent. *Osmolality* is therefore more exact. It is determined by measuring the depression of the freezing point of a solution, compared to water, using an osmometer, and expressing the value in °C below 0°. The value can also be expressed in milliosmoles, using the factor 1000 mOsm = 186° C or 1° C = 538 mOsm. Osmolality may be quickly and easily determined on serum or plasma, urine, saliva, cerebrospinal fluid, sweat, or gastric or other juices.

The normal range of serum osmolality, as measured, is 275 to 290 mOsm/kg of water. Females show values 5 to 10 mOsm/kg less than males.

THE FREEZING POINT OSMOMETER

When a substance is dissolved in a solution, it can change many of the physical characteristics of the solution, for example, the specific gravity, refractive index, conductivity, viscosity, turbidity, and freezing point, depending on the number of particles in solution, the size of the particles, their electrical charge, the number, size and shape of undissolved particles, and the opacity of the solution.

Variations in the freezing point of the solution are dependent only on the number of the dissolved particles (that is, their osmotic concentration or osmolality) and not on their size or shape. This is why measurement of the depression of the freezing point is used to determine the osmolality of a solution.

An osmometer consists essentially of (1) a refrigerated bath to hold, cool, stir, and freeze body or other fluids, (2) an electric thermistor or probe to measure temperature, and (3) a Wheatstone bridge and galvanometer to convert variations in temperature into calibrated units of osmolality.

The sample is supercooled to several degrees below its freezing point and then is vibrated intensely for a moment. This causes many ice crystals to form, which releases their heat of fusion. The heat cannot be transferred to the surrounding ethylene glycol bath all at once and the trapped heat melts some of the new ice. The sample stays at equilibrium temperature for a few minutes while the ice is freezing and thawing. During this time the temperature measurement is made.

The electrical resistance of the thermistor probe varies directly with the temperature of the sample. This resistance is balanced with a Wheatstone bridge. The electrical resistance of the thermistor is also directly proportional to the osmolality of the sample. Therefore the variable resistance dial of the Wheatstone bridge can be calibrated directly into mOsm/kg of the sample. The greater the concentration of solute in the solution, the lower the temperature, the greater the electrical resistance, and the higher the osmolality reading.

THE RELATIONS BETWEEN SERUM OSMOLALITY AND SERUM SODIUM CONCENTRATION

Two formulas have been used to interpret serum osmolality values:
1. *Calculated Serum Osmolality.* Serum osmolality can be calculated from the serum concentrations of sodium, BUN (blood urea nitrogen), and glucose, viz:

$$\text{Calculated mOsm/kg} = 1.86\ \text{Na} + \frac{\text{Glucose}}{18} + \frac{\text{BUN}}{2.8}$$

The constant 1.86 is obtained by assuming that both sodium and chloride ions have an osmotic coefficient of 0.93. The term *osmotic coefficient* describes the % deviation from an ideal behavior of a substance. For example, ideal behavior would include complete dissociation in the solution, no water binding, and so forth. If sodium chloride completely dissociated in plasma, each molecule of the salt would yield 2 ions. However, if the osmotic coefficient of sodium chloride is 0.93, the effective osmolality of a solution of sodium chloride is 2 × 0.93 = 1.86.

Glucose is the plasma glucose concentration in mg/dl. The constant 18 is derived from the molecular weight of glucose, which is 180. (Therefore, each 180 mg% glucose in the blood will raise the serum osmolality by 10 mOsm/L.)

BUN is the plasma concentration of blood urea nitrogen in mg per dl. The constant $\frac{1}{2.8}$ is derived from the mean nitrogen content of BUN, or urea. Urea contains two nitrogen molecules and thus has a molecular weight of 14 × 2 = 28. (Therefore each 28 mg % BUN concentration in the blood will raise the serum osmolality by 10 mOsm/kg.)

Normally, the *calculated* serum osmolality is 5 to 8 mOsm/kg less than the osmolality measured by the freezing point depression method.

The above formula for the *calculated* serum osmolality can be simplified by multiplying the serum sodium concentration by 2, rather than by 1.86. The formula therefore becomes:

$$\text{Calculated serum osmolality, mOsm/kg} = 2\,\text{Na} + \frac{\text{Glucose}}{18} + \frac{\text{BUN}}{2.8}$$

Relations Between Measured and Calculated Osmolality

Normally, as was pointed out above, the *calculated* serum osmolality is less than 5 to 8 mOsm/kg of the *measured* osmolality. However, wide differences of more than 10 mOsm/kg can occur in two situations:

a. When the water content of the serum is decreased, due either to marked hyperlipidemia, or marked hyperproteinemia (paraproteinemia). (When such marked hyperlipidemia is present, the serum will be lipemic on observation. When such marked hyperproteinemia is present, the serum protein level will be 10 g per liter or higher.)

The *measured* serum osmolality will be normal, but the *calculated* serum osmolality will be about 10 to 15 mOsm/kg lower, due to the fact that the increased lipids or proteins are associated with a spurious lowering of the serum sodium concentration.

The reason for this is that the serum sodium concentration is measured in terms of mEq/L of serum volume. However, osmolality is measured in terms of the concentration of a substance per kilogram of serum or plasma water. In hyperlipemic or hyperproteinemic serum, the lipid or the protein occupies volume but displaces serum water, so that the serum concentration of sodium (and all the other electrolytes) in terms of mEq/L (total volume) is spuriously low. However, if the lipid is removed by ultracentrifugation, or if the excess protein is removed, the concentration of sodium and other electrolytes in the subnatant fluid will be normal. Albrink describes a 16-year-old boy with mild diabetes and xanthoma diabeticorum. His serum sodium concentration was 102.5 mEq/L, and his serum chloride concentration was 74.5 mEq/L. The serum was markedly lactescent. When the insoluble lipids were removed by ultracentrifugation, the electrolyte concentrations of the clear subnatant fluid were essentially normal: sodium 135 mEq/L, and chloride 102.5 mEq/L. (This is one of the reasons that serum sodium concentrations in mEq/L of serum *water* correlate better with serum osmolality than serum sodium concentration as usually measured per liter of serum volume.)

b. When non-measured low-molecular weight substances (molecular weight less than 150), such as ethanol, methanol, ethylene glycol, paraldehyde, acetone, trichlorethylene, and so on, are present in the plasma. In such cases, the *measured* serum osmolality is almost always more than 300 mOsm/kg. When such low-molecular weight substances accumulate, they greatly increase the osmolality of the plasma because osmolality depends on the number of particles in solution, rather than on their size.

2. *Effective Serum Osmolality*

Evaluation of the serum osmolality can also be done by calculating the *effective* osmolality (Gennari), using the following formula:

$$2Na + \frac{Glucose}{18}. \text{ Normally the value is 185 mOsm/kg.}$$

This is based on the fact that the sodium ions and glucose are the major solutes in the blood and extracellular water that do not permeate cells freely.

When the *effective* osmolality is increased, this generally indicates a relative water loss.

When the *effective* osmolality is decreased, this generally indicates a relative water excess.

Example: patient with renal insufficiency
Na 125 mEq/L
Glucose 90 mg per dl
Measured serum osmolality 290 mOsm/kg water

Effective serum osmolality 255 mOsm/kg water

In this case, the *measured* serum osmolality is essentially normal, 290 mOsm/kg water, (due to the high BUN of 90 mg per dl,) but the *effective* serum osmolality is low, 255 mOsm/kg water. The cause of the low effective serum osmolality was the renal insufficiency. As a result, the patient was imbibing more water than he could excrete through his kidneys. This produced a water excess.

Example: patient with diabetic acidosis.
Na 134 mEq/L
Glucose 700 mg per dl
Measured serum osmolality 312 mOsm/kg water
Effective serum osmolality 306.9 mOsm/kg water

The *measured* serum osmolality is high, 312 mOsm/kg water. However, the *effective* serum osmolality is also high, 306.9 mOsm/ kg water. This is related to the water loss due to the osmotic diuresis caused by the glucose filtering through the kidneys, lack of adequate water intake, loss of fluids by vomiting, and so on. As a result, a water loss developed.

THE CLINICAL SIGNIFICANCE OF SERUM OSMOLALITY VALUES

A high *measured* serum osmolality indicates a high osmolality of the extracellular water. Values as high as 400 mOsm/kg have been reported in adults, with higher values in children. Values above 350 mOsm/kg indicate a grave prognosis. A high serum osmolality can occur in water loss, rarely with sodium excess, or with hypernatremia produced by drugs or diseases in diabetes, azotemia, lactic acidosis, liver failure, sepsis, after intoxication with salicylates, barbiturates, alcohol and other substances, with high-protein nasogastric feedings or total parenteral nutrition, or a combination of the above conditions. Treatment should be directed to lower the high serum osmolality by the removal of the abnormal substances, if possible, and by increasing the oral or parenteral water intake.

A high *measured* serum osmolality can be associated with a normal, low, or high serum sodium concentration. These uncorrected serum sodium concentrations do not indicate whether sodium loss or sodium excess is present and these uncorrected values cannot be used as a basis for treatment. It is therefore necessary to calculate the *effective* serum osmolality (see above).

A low *measured* serum osmolality indicates a low osmolality of the extracellular water. Values as low as 230 mOsm/kg have been reported. In these patients, the serum sodium concentration is also low. A low *measured* serum osmolality can occur in water excess or sodium loss, or a combination of both conditions. Treatment consists of water restriction, increased salt in the diet, or the intravenous use of hypertonic sodium chloride solution when indications are present.

OTHER CAUSES OF A HIGH SERUM OSMOLALITY

When the pylorus does not function normally to restrain the rapid passage of partially digested food into the duodenum and jejunum, concentrated food substances may enter the circulation from the duodenum or jejunum, and may cause a sudden rise in plasma osmolality. This is associated with symptoms of sweating, flushing, warmth, tachycardia and increased pulse pressure, associated with peripheral vasodilatation (*the dumping syndrome*).

A marked rise in serum osmolality occurs with intoxication due to ethanol, methanol, trichlorethylene, ethylene glycol and other low molecular weight substances.

Methanol and ethylene glycol cause a metabolic acidosis with an elevated anion gap. Therefore, if there is a wide gap between the calculated and measured osmolalities, and if the anion gap is elevated and if alcoholic acidosis or diabetic coma are excluded, this indicates methanol or ethylene glycol poisoning.

URINE OSMOLALITY

The osmolality of the urine is a more accurate measurement of kidney function than specific gravity of the urine, because the kidneys respond to changes in the osmolality of the body fluids and not to changes in specific gravity. In addition, the specific gravity of urine depends on the weight of the substances dissolved in it, not on the concentration of these substances. Therefore, heavy molecules such as glucose or albumin will cause a rise in specific gravity out of proportion to their concentration in the urine. This can cause marked differences between urine specific gravity and urine osmolality. For example, at a specific gravity of 1.023, the urine osmolality can vary from 722 to 1166 mOsm/kg urine.

If an adult is on a medium protein diet with an average salt intake, about 1200 mOsm of solute are excreted a day. Urea comprises about 500 mOsm of this. The remainder is due mostly to sodium, potassium, and ammonium salts. If a patient receives only glucose, the urinary osmolality may fall to 200 mOsm a day. If he or she is on a high-protein diet with water restriction, the daily urine osmolality may even reach 1700 mOsm.

Normally, after a 14-hour fast, a person will show a concentrated urine with an osmolality of 850 mOsm/kg urine, or higher.

When moderate renal insufficiency is present, the urine osmolality may vary from 400 to 600 mOsm a day. When severe renal insufficiency is present, the daily urinary osmolality may be less than 400 mOsm.

THE URINE-SERUM OSMOLALITY RATIO

Normally, this ratio is greater than 1 and is usually 3 or higher. In chronic renal disease it falls to 1. In diabetes insipidus it is less than 1 because of the excretion of a large volume of water. In compulsive water drinking, the urine-serum ratio is also less than 1. However, when a patient with diabetes insipidus is deprived of water, the urine-serum ratio will continue to remain below 1 although the urine osmolality rises slightly. In compulsive water drinking, the urine-serum ratio will rise to 1 or higher after water deprivation.

In inappropriate ADH secretion syndromes, the urine osmolality is characteristically higher than the serum osmolality in spite of the presence of hyponatremia.

REFERENCES

Abele, J.E.: The physical background of freezing point osmometry and its medical-biological applications. Am J Med Electronics, *2*:32, 1963.

Albrink, M.J., Hald, P.M., Man, E.B., and Peters, J.P.: The displacement of serum water by the lipids of hyperlipemic serum. A new method for the rapid determination of serum water. J Clin Invest, *34*:1483, 1955.

Boyd, D.R., et al.: Utilization of osmometry in critically ill surgical patients. Arch Surg, *102*:363, 1971.

Champion, H.R., et al.: Alcohol intoxication and serum osmolality. Lancet, *1*:1402, 1975.

Dashe, A.M., et al.: A water deprivation test for the differential diagnosis of polyuria. JAMA, *185*:699, 1963.

Edelman, I.S., Leibman, J., O'Meara, M.P., and Birkenfeld, L.W.: Interrelations between serum sodium concentration, serum osmolarity and total exchangeable sodium, total exchangeable potassium and total body water. J Clin Invest, *37*:1236, 1958.

Galambos, J.T., Herndon, E.G., and Reynolds, G.H.: Specific gravity determination. Fact or fancy? N Engl J Med, *270*:506, 1964.

Gennari, F.J.: Serum osmolality. Uses and limitations. N Engl J Med, *310*:102, 1984.

Glasser, L., et al.: Serum osmolality and its applicability to drug overdose. Am J Clin Path, *60*:695, 1973.

Holmes, J.H.: Measurement of osmolality in serum, urine and other biologic fluids by the freezing point determination. Pre-workshop manual of the workshop on urinalysis and renal function studies. Am Soc Clin Path, 1962.

Jacobsen, D., et al.: Anion and osmolal gaps in the diagnosis of methanol and ethylene glycol poisoning. Acta Med Scandinav, *212*:17, 1982.

Jacobson, M.H., et al.: Urine osmolality. A definitive test of renal function. Arch Intern Med, *110*:121, 1962.

Ladenson, J.H., Apple, F.S., and Koch, D.D.: Misleading hyponatremia due to hyperlipemia. A method-dependent error. Ann Intern Med, *95*:707, 1981.

Olmstead, E.G., and Roth, D.A.: The relationship of serum sodium to total serum osmolarity. A method of distinguishing hyponatremic states. Am J Med Sci, *233*:392, 1957. Also Surg Gynecol Obstet, *106*:41, 1958.

Robinson, A.G., and Loeb, J.L.: Ethanol ingestion—commonest cause of elevated plasma osmolality. N Engl J Med, *284*:1253, 1971.

Rodrigo, F., et al.: Osmolality changes during hemodialysis. Ann Intern Med, *86*:554, 1977.

Sklar, A.H., and Linas, S.L.: The osmolal gap in renal failure. Ann Intern Med, 98:481, 1983.

Warhol, R.M., Eichenholz, A., and Mulhausen, R.O.: Osmolality. Arch Intern Med, 116:743, 1965.

PART 4

SYNDROMES DUE TO DISTURBANCES IN ACID-BASE BALANCE

CHAPTER 12

THE PRINCIPLES OF ACID-BASE CHEMISTRY AND PHYSIOLOGY

The subject of acid-base balance is confusing because of a confusion in terminology. For example, a cation such as sodium and an anion such as bicarbonate have been called "bases," but the chloride anion has been called an "acid" by some investigators. Others have loosely called cations "bases," and anions "acids." Much of the confusion can be eliminated if we accept the following chemical definitions of an acid and of a base:

An acid is a hydrogen ion (proton) donor.

A base is a hydrogen ion (proton) acceptor (Brønsted). For example:

Acid (hydrogen ion donor)	H$^+$ (hydrogen ion)	+	Base (hydrogen ion acceptor)
H_2CO_3	H$^+$	+	HCO_3^-
H_3PO_4	H$^+$	+	$H_2PO_4^-$

An alkali can produce hydroxyl (OH) ions (base) in aqueous solution, for example, $NaOH$, NH_4OH.

THE MEANING OF pH

Any acid, such as HCl, in a water solution dissociates wholly or partly into its component ions: $HCl \rightleftharpoons H^+ + Cl^-$. The strength of the acid depends on the degree to which it becomes dissociated in the solution and on the concentration of the hydrogen ions which it contains.

In 1909, S.P.L. Sorensen, a Danish biochemist, noted that enzyme activity was related to minute changes in the hydrogen ion concentration of a solution, for example, 0.01 to 0.0000001 mole per liter. Mathematically, these numbers can be rewritten as 10^{-2} to 10^{-7}. He called the -2 and the -7 the hydrogen ion exponent or power, or *puissance Hydrogen* (the paper was written in French), then eliminated the negative signs and further shortened the term to pH.

pH therefore represents the negative logarithm of the hydrogen ion concentration in moles (gram molecules) per liter of solution.

For example, in a 0.01 molar solution of HCl (which is almost completely dissociated), the hydrogen ion concentration is approximately 0.01 molar, or $[H^+] = 0.01 = 1 \times 10^{-2}$. The logarithm of the hydrogen ion concentration is therefore -2; and the negative logarithm, or pH, is 2.

(A molar solution contains 1 gram-molecular weight of the solute in a liter of solution. A 0.01 molar solution of HCl therefore contains 0.01 of 36.5 g [the molecular weight of HCl] in a liter of water.)

Water dissociates into H and OH ions, as follows: $H_2O \rightleftharpoons H^+ + OH$. The equilibrium of this reaction at room temperature has been found to be $[H^+] \times [OH^+] = 10^{-14}$. Since pure water yields equivalent amounts of H and OH ions, it follows that the hydrogen ion concentration of pure water is 10^{-7}, and the pH of water is 7.

Since acids have a greater hydrogen ion concentration than water, the pH of an acid will be lower than 7. Since bases have a lower concentration of hydrogen ions than water, the pH of a base will be greater than 7. Since the normal pH of the blood is 7.4, this means that the blood normally has a faintly basic or alkaline reaction.

Hydrogen ion concentration can also be described in terms of its actual concentration, rather than in terms of pH. Since the hydrogen ion concentration in plasma or other body fluids is very low, measurements are made in terms of *nanoequivalents* (or nanomoles) per liter. One nanoequivalent equals 10^{-9} equivalent per liter. The relationship between nanoequivalents per liter (nEq/L) (or nanomoles per liter, nM/L) and pH is shown in Figure 12–1.

Kassirer and Bleich have described the following simple rule to correlate pH and H^+ (hydrogen ion) concentrations: A pH of 7.40 is equivalent to a H^+ concentration of 40 nEq/L. Each increase (or decrease) in pH of 0.01 unit from 7.40 corresponds to a decrease (or increase) of H^+ concentration of 1 nEq/L.

For example, a pH of 7.37 is 0.03 unit more acid than 7.40. Therefore, the equivalent H^+ concentration is 43 nEq/L (3 more than 40). A pH of 7.44 is 0.04 more alkaline than 7.40. Therefore, the equivalent H^+ concentration is 36 nEq/L (4 less than 40).

This rule is approximately accurate between pH values of 7.28 and 7.45. However, when the pH falls below 7.28 or rises above 7.45, the estimated H^+ concentration is always lower than its actual value (see Fig. 12–1).

Theoretically, it is preferable to use nEq/L rather than pH to describe changes in acidity or alkalinity. One reason is that a decrease of 1 unit pH below 7.4 indicates a much larger change in hydrogen ion concentration (expressed in nEq/L) than an equal rise of pH above 7.4. For example, a decrease of pH from 7.2 to 7.1 represents a large increase in hydrogen ion concentration of 17 nEq/L, but a rise in pH from 7.5 to 7.6 represents only a small decrease in hydrogen ion concentration

Fig. 12–1.   Relationship between hydrogen ion activity (nEq/L) and pH.

of 7 nEq/L (Fig. 12–1). However, the term pH is so well known that I shall continue to use it.

THE CHEMICAL AND PHYSIOLOGICAL REGULATION OF THE pH OF THE BODY

In the past century, physiologists have learned that the reaction of the extracellular water must be maintained slightly to the base side of the neutral point, in order for an organism to live. In other words, the pH of the extracellular water must be slightly above 7.

Three factors help maintain this pH:

1. Chemical buffers of the body fluids and cells can neutralize strong acids and bases that are produced within the body, or which enter the body. Extracellular chemical buffering occurs instantaneously. Cellular buf-

fering (which consists of the diffusion of hydrogen ions into the cells and their neutralization) occurs in a period of several hours.

2. Respiratory regulatory mechanisms help eliminate and regulate the concentration of carbonic acid, which is the major acid end-product of metabolism.

   Respiratory buffering occurs in a period of minutes.

3. The kidneys also help eliminate excess acids and bases. The kidneys are the most important of these three mechanisms, because they compensate for any defects in the action of the buffer salts, or of respiratory action. The sulfuric and phosphoric acids produced by the catabolism of proteins and phospholipids, as well as any acid that cannot be metabolized to carbonic acid, can be eliminated from the body only by the kidneys.

   Renal buffering occurs in a period of hours to days.

The Chemical Buffers of the Body

The term *buffer* describes a chemical substance which, by its presence in a solution, decreases the pH change caused by the addition of an acid or a base. A buffer is a mixture either of a weak acid and its alkali salt or of a weak base and its acid salt. In the body, the buffers of physiological importance are mixtures of weak acids and their alkali salts—carbonic acid and sodium (or potassium) bicarbonate, monohydrogen and dihydrogen phosphate salts, and the proteins with their alkali salts, H protein and B protein. The B represents a cation such as sodium or potassium.

The importance of buffers can be appreciated when one realizes that all of the base which is available for the immediate neutralization of acid of the body is in the form of buffer salts. Salts of strong acids, such as sodium chloride, have no neutralizing power, and a strong alkali, such as sodium hydroxide, cannot exist in the living body.

There are four main buffer systems in the body, which help maintain the constancy of the pH:

1. The bicarbonate-carbonic acid buffer system. This is quantitatively the largest in the body. It operates in the extracellular water.
2. The phosphate buffer system. This is important in the red blood cells and in other cells, especially in the cells of the kidney tubules, where it enables the kidneys to excrete hydrogen ions.
3. The protein buffer system. This is predominant in the tissue cells. It also operates in the plasma.
4. The hemoglobin buffer system of the red blood cells.

The Bicarbonate-Carbonic Acid Buffer System. During the course of the normal metabolic activities of the body, most of the organic and inorganic acids which are formed are stronger than carbonic acid. This causes the following type of reaction:

$HCl + NaHCO_3 \rightarrow H_2CO_3 + NaCl \cdot H_2CO_3 \rightarrow H_2O + CO_2 \uparrow$.

The bicarbonate ion is not the only one that is able to neutralize acids, as I have already pointed out. However, bicarbonate is unique because its acid is volatile. Therefore, when the bicarbonate salt reacts with an acid, the carbon dioxide set free from the reaction can be removed from the body at once by the lungs. A foreign acid can therefore be completely neutralized by bicarbonate. The foreign acid is converted into a neutral salt, and into carbon dixoide, which is expelled in the expired air.

On the other hand, when a base such as sodium hydroxide enters the body, or is formed in the body, it combines with carbon dioxide to form bicarbonate in the following way:

$NaOH + H_2CO_3 \rightarrow NaHCO_3 + H_2O$

Carbon dixoide is continually produced in the body by the processes of metabolism and is always available. Therefore, any base which enters the body can be immediately and automatically converted into bicarbonate.

Because of the importance of bicarbonate ions and carbon dioxide in the regulation of acid or base excesses or deficits, the pH of the blood is dependent on the bicarbonate/carbonic acid ratio in the plasma and extracellular water. Under normal conditions, the bicarbonate/carbonic acid ratio is 20/1 and the pH is 7.4. This value is derived as follows.

Henderson, Hasselbalch, and others have shown that the pH of the body fluids can be expressed by the following equation:

$$pH = 6.1 + \log \frac{HCO_3^-}{H_2CO_3} + CO_2$$

where HCO_3^- represents bicarbonate. The CO_2 and H_2CO_3 represent the concentrations of dissolved carbon dixoide plus carbonic acid. For example, at a pH of 6.1, the concentrations of bicarbonate and carbonic acid in the body are equal (and the logarithm of $\frac{1}{1} = 0$).

Normally, the concentration of bicarbonate in the plasma and extracellular water is 27 mEq/L, and the concentration of carbonic acid is 1.35 mEq/L.

The pH can now be calculated as follows:

$$pH = 6.1 + \log \frac{27}{1.35}$$

Since $27/1.35 = 20$, the equation becomes $pH = 6.1 + \log 20$.

Using a table of logarithms, one finds that the logarithm of 20 is 1.3. Therefore, the pH is $6.1 + 1.3 = 7.4$.

When the bicarbonate concentration of the blood rises, or the carbonic acid concentration falls, the bicarbonate-carbonic acid ratio increases, and the pH becomes greater than the normal value of 7.35 to 7.45. This is described as alkalosis.

When the bicarbonate concentration of the blood falls, or the carbonic acid concentration rises, the bicarbonate-carbonic acid ratio decreases, and the pH becomes less than the normal value of 7.35 to 7.45. This is described as acidosis, even though the pH is still slightly on the alkaline side of neutrality.

The Phosphate Buffer System. This is important in red blood cells and in other cells, especially in the cells of the kidney tubules, where it enables the kidneys to excrete hydrogen ions.

Phosphate ions exist in the body in two forms, monohydrogen phosphate ions, HPO_4, and dihydrogen phosphate ions, H_2PO_4. At the normal pH of 7.4, there is about 5 times as much monohydrogen phosphate as dihydrogen phosphate in the body. Therefore, if a strong acid such as hydrochloric acid is introduced into the body, the following reaction would occur: $HCl + Na_2HPO_4 \rightarrow NaCl + NaH_2PO_4$. In other words, a strong acid is converted to a neutral salt, sodium chloride, by a phosphate buffer salt, which undergoes a change from a mildly basic form to a mildly acid form.

Similarly, if a strong base such as sodium hydroxide is introduced into the body, the following reaction would occur: $NaOH + NaH_2PO_4 \rightarrow Na_2HPO_4 + H_2O$. In other words, a strong base is converted into water by a phosphate buffer salt, which undergoes a change from a mildly acid form to a mildly basic form.

The Protein Buffer System. This is predominant in the tissue calls. It also operates in the plasma. The proteins of the body act as anions in the alkaline pH of the body. They may exist in the form of acids (H protein), or as alkaline salts (B protein). In this way they are able to bind or release excess hydrogen ions as needed.

The Hemoglobin Buffer System. Only about 5% of the carbon dioxide is carried in the plasma in simple solution. Another 20% is transported in the red blood cells as a carbamino compound with hemoglobin. The remaining 75% of the carbon dioxide is carried by the blood as bicarbonate. The process by which this occurs can be briefly described as follows.

Carbon dioxide is formed during the processes of cellular metabolism. It then diffuses into the tissue spaces and into the plasma. As its concentration in the plasma increases, it diffuses into the red blood cells. Here the enzyme carbonic anhydrase (ca) converts the carbon dioxide to carbonic acid: $CO_2 + H_2O \rightarrow H_2CO_3$. This immediately dissociates into H^+ and HCO_3^- ions. The H^+ ion reacts with reduced hemoglobin, *viz:* $H^+ + Hb^- \rightarrow HHb$. The bicarbonate ion reacts with potassium ions in the red blood cells to form $KHCO_3$.

The bicarbonate ion accumulates within the red blood cells. When its concentration increases above that in the plasma, it diffuses into the plasma and is replaced by a chloride ion, to form potassium chloride to maintain electroneutrality.

red blood cell:$KHCO_3 \rightarrow K^+ + (HCO_3^-)$ to plasma.
    plasma:$Cl^- \rightarrow$ to red blood cell $\rightarrow KCl$.

In the alveolar capillaries of the lungs, the reduced hemoglobin, HHb, is oxygenated and becomes $HHbO_2$. It reacts with bicarbonate salts to form carbonic acid ($HHbO_2 + KHCO_3 \rightarrow H_2CO_3 + KHbO_2$). As the carbonic acid is formed, the chloride which had previously entered the cells passes back into the plasma again, and the potassium ion reacts with bicarbonate to form potassium bicarbonate again. The carbonic acid which has been formed is converted into carbon dioxide and water by means of carbonic anhydrase. The carbon dioxide then passes from the red blood cells to the plasma and into the alveolar capillaries where it is eliminated.

Respiratory Regulation of pH

The chemical and physiological actions of a gas depend on the pressure it exerts. This pressure which a gas exerts is called the *partial pressure* of the gas. It is usually represented by the symbol P. Thus, P_{CO_2} represents the partial pressure of carbon dioxide. The partial pressure of a gas depends only on the number of moles of the gas in a given volume, and on the termperature. It is completely independent of the presence or absence of other gases in the same volume.

The partial pressure of a gas may be determined by chemical or physical means. When physical means are used, the result is given as millimeters of mercury (mm Hg) pressure. When chemical means are used, the result is given as volumes % (vol. %). At normal (760 mm Hg) barometric pressure, the following formula can be used to convert vol. % CO_2 to mm Hg CO_2:

1 vol. % CO_2 = 7 (approx.) mm Hg pressure.

The term *torr* is a unit of pressure, named in honor of Torricelli, the inventor of the barometer. It can be used to describe P_{CO_2}, P_{O_2}, blood pressure, or other pressure measurements. A torr is the unit of pressure equal to 1/760 of normal atmospheric pressure or the pressure necessary to support a column of mercury 1 mm high at 0°C and standard gravity. Therefore, pressure values can be described as either mm Hg or torr.

Respiration is regulated by sensors located in the central nervous system and in the systemic circulatory system. The CNS receptors located in the medulla, which are in contact with the CSF (cerebrospinal fluid) are sensitive to small changes in pH and P_{CO_2}. Small increments in P_{CO_2} or decrements in pH result in dramatic increases in ventilation triggered by these CNS receptors. Since the CSF is far more permeable to CO_2 than to HCO_3, acute changes in P_{CO_2} are sensed within minutes, whereas changes in HCO_3 concentration may not be sensed for hours.

The peripheral chemoreceptors located in the aortic arch and carotid sinus are also stimulated by an increase in P_{CO_2} or decrease in pH. In addition, hypoxemia stimulates the carotid sinus. Stimulation of these chemoreceptors results in increased ventilation, so that an acid load, a rise in P_{CO_2} or hypoxemia will be counteracted by a rapid ventilatory response.

Conversely, an alkaline load or a decline in P_{CO_2} will result in reduced ventilation mediated by the central and peripheral chemoreceptors.

It should be stressed that these respiratory compensations are capable of returning the pH of the blood toward normal, but do not result in complete restoration of normal pH.

Carbon dioxide excess or lack is the most important stimulant of the respiratory center. However, if the P_{CO_2} of the alveolar air rises above 9 vol. % (approximately 65 mm Hg), this acts as a depressant to the central nervous system and can result in *carbon dioxide narcosis.* This occurs in patients with severe respiratory acidosis.

Oxygen does not normally act as a stimulus for the respiratory center so long as normal oxygenation occurs in the alveoli. However, if anoxemia is present and the amount of available oxygen is reduced, the decreased oxygen concentration of the blood acts as a respiratory stimulant, and hyperventilation results. If a patient with cor pulmonale, who may show such a condition, is given excessive concentrations of oxygen to inhale (more than 50%), the inhaled oxygen can cause the respiratory center to stop functioning. As a result, excessive carbon dioxide accumulates in the body and the patient may become comatose and die (see carbon dioxide narcosis, Chap 16).

Changes in pH also affect respiration. For example, marked hyperventilation occurs when the pH falls to 7.2. This becomes maximal when a pH of about 7 is reached. However, when the pH falls below 7, the hyperventilation disappears. This is one reason that so-called *air hunger* (the Kussmaul type of hyperventilation with exaggerated respiratory action, particularly an exaggerated depth of respiration) is not always present in patients with acidosis.

The partial pressure of carbon dioxide in the alveolar air is in equilibrium with the partial pressure of the carbon dioxide of the arterial blood, and this is in equilibrium with the carbonic acid content of the blood. Therefore, a change in the P_{CO_2} of the alveolar air will cause a corresponding change in the P_{CO_2} and in the H_2CO_3 content of the blood.

Normally, the P_{CO_2} of the alveolar air is about 40 mm Hg (5.5 vol. %). If the concentration of carbonic acid in the blood increases, this will cause an increase in the P_{CO_2} of the alveolar air, and will stimulate the respiratory center. Hyperventilation will occur and will lower the P_{CO_2} of the alveolar air, by causing carbon dioxide to be exhaled faster than it is produced. The most extreme voluntary hyperventilation can lower the P_{CO_2} to about 15 mm Hg.

Hyperventilation can also affect the P_{CO_2} of the alveolar air in the following way. The partial pressure of a gas is proportional to the volume in which it is enclosed. The lung volume can increase by means of deep respiration. As a result, the P_{CO_2} of the alveolar air and the CO_2 content of the arterial blood will decrease, even though the rate of respiration remains unchanged. Conversely, a decreased depth of respiration causes a decreased lung volume, an increased P_{CO_2} of alveolar air, and an increased CO_2 content of arterial blood.

Primary changes in the bicarbonate concentration of the blood can also be regulated by the respiratory mechanisms. For example, a patient is given a massive dose of sodium bicarbonate, and the bicarbonate concentration rises from 27 mEq/L to twice its concentration, 54 mEq/L. The respiratory center responds by decreasing the respiratory rate and depth. In this way, the lung volume is decreased and the P_{CO_2} of the alveolar air increases from the normal value of 40 to 80 mm Hg. The carbonic acid content of the blood, which is normally 1.35 mEq/L will also rise to twice its value, 2.70 mEq/L. In this way, the bicarbonate-carbonic acid ratio and the pH remain unchanged. (The bicarbonate-carbonic acid ratio of 54/2.70 is the same as 27/1.35 or 20/1.)

Conversely, if the bicarbonate concentration of the blood decreases, the respiratory rate and depth will increase. This causes the lung volume to increase and the P_{CO_2} of the alveolar air and the carbonic acid content of the blood to decrease. As a result, the pH remains at its former level.

Since the partial pressure of carbon dioxide in the plasma (P_{CO_2}) is proportional to the concentration of carbonic acid and dissolved carbon dioxide in the plasma, the Henderson-Hasselbalch equation (page 123) can be rewritten:

$$pH = 6.1 + \log \frac{HCO_3^-}{P_{CO_2} \times 0.03}$$

where 0.03 represents a constant. (This is the basis for the Astrup method of describing acid-base disturbances—see Chap 15.)

At this point it should be stressed again that both the buffer and respiratory compensations are essentially temporary mechanisms. They are often not completely successful in restoring or maintaining the pH of the blood and extracellular water. The kidneys, however, are able to make permanent adjustments.

Regulation of pH by the Kidneys

During the course of normal metabolism, the kidneys contribute to acid base homeostasis in two ways. The bicarbonate ions that are filtered by the glomeruli must be reabsorbed by mechanisms described below. Over 24 hours, in a person with a normal GFR (glomerular filtration rate) of 120 ml/min, and a normal serum HCO_3 concentration of 24 mEq/L, over 4,000 mEq of HCO_3 must be reabsorbed. Secondly, during normal metabolism, the body produces approximately 1 mEq/kg body weight per day of nonvolatile acids (such as phosphoric, sulfuric, etc.). This excess acid is excreted by the kidneys by acidification of buffer salts and by the excretion of NH_4^+. These two processes, which are also described below, account for the acid pH of the urine. The capacity of these processes can be dramatically increased during abnormal states of excess metabolic acid production (e.g. diabetic ketoacidosis or lactic acidosis).

The Reabsorption of Bicarbonate Ions. Normally, all the bicarbonate ions which pass the glomeruli and enter the tubular urine (glomerular filtrate) are reabsorbed. This occurs by means of an exchange of hydrogen ions (which the renal tubular cells secrete) for sodium ions in the tubular urine.

Hydrogen ions are available in the tubular cells because the enzyme carbonic anhydrase (ca) is able to convert carbon dioxide (which is present in all cells) and water into carbonic acid. This ionizes into H^+ and HCO_3^+ ions, *viz:*

$$CO_2 + H_2O \xrightarrow{\text{ca}} H_2CO_3 \rightarrow H^+ + HCO_3^-.$$

In the tubular urine, the hydrogen ions combine with the bicarbonate ions of the tubular urine to form carbonic acid. This then forms water and carbon dioxide. The water is excreted and the carbon dioxide is reabsorbed by the tubular cells. At the same time, sodium ions pass from the tubular urine into the tubular cells where they unite with the bicarbonate ions there, to form sodium bicarbonate. The bicarbonate then passes into the plasma and extracellular water where its concentration is maintained (Fig. 12–2).

Acidification of Buffer Salts. A similar exchange mechanism occurs between hydrogen ions of the renal tubular cells and the (sodium) salts of various buffer anions, which appear in the urine. Quantitatively, monohydrogen phosphate, Na_2HPO_4 is overwhelmingly the major buffer. This salt dissociates into Na and $NaHPO_4$ ions. As a sodium ion is reabsorbed, a hydrogen ions moves into the tubular urine to unite with the $NaHPO_4$ ion to form a dihydrogen phosphate salt, NaH_2PO_4, which is excreted. In this way, a hydrogen ion is removed from the body.

The Secretion of Ammonia. Ammonia, NH_3, is formed in the renal

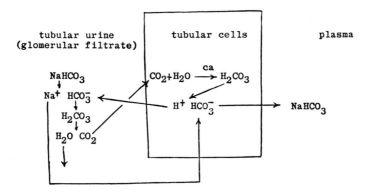

Fig. 12–2. Diagram showing the mechanism by which bicarbonate ions are conserved by the kidneys. See text.

tubular cells from the oxidation of the amino acid, glutamine, by the enzyme, glutaminase, and by oxidation of other amino acids. The free ammonia is converted into an ammonium ion, NH_4^+, by uniting with a hydrogen ion and is excreted as ammonium chloride, NH_4Cl. In this way, another hydrogen ion is removed from the body. (The ammonia can also be converted to urea by the liver and then excreted by the kidneys.)

In acidosis, all these renal regulatory mechanisms are exaggerated. For example, the urine shows a pH which may be as low as 4.5. Bicarbonate excretion may diminish or disappear. Titratable acid and ammonium excretion increase dramatically.

On the other hand, in alkalosis, these regulatory mechanisms either decrease or stop. The urine shows a pH which may rise as high as 7.8. (In alkalosis due to potassium deficiency, the urinary pH may remain low [see Chap 27].) Bicarbonate ion secretion increases. Ammonium salt excretion decreases, and the excretion of cations such as sodium and potassium increases. Titratable acid and chloride ion excretion also decrease and chloride ions may disappear from the urine.

(The term *titratable acid* is used to describe the amount of hydrogen ions in the urine which are bound to phosphate and organic buffers. Its value is measured by determining the milliequivalents of sodium hydroxide that have to be added to urine to raise the pH to 7.4, which is the pH of the plasma from which the glomerular filtrate originated.)

REFERENCES

Barker, E.S., and Elkinton, J.R.: Hydrogen ions and buffer base. Am J Med, 25:1, 1958.
Bates, R.G.: *Determination of pH. Theory and Practice.* New York, John Wiley & Sons, 1964.
Bear, R.A., and Gribik, M.: Assessing acid-base imbalances through laboratory parameters. Hosp Pract, 9:157, 1974.
Brønsted, J.N.: Acid and base catalysis. Chem Rev, 5:231, 1928.

Brown, E.B., Jr.: Blood and tissue buffers. Arch Intern Med, *116*:665, 1965.

Campbell, E.J.M.: R I pH. Lancet, *1*:681, 1962.

Christensen, H.N.: Anions versus cations? Am J Med, *23*:163, 1957.

Christensen, H.N.: *Body Fluids and the Acid-Base Balance.* Philadelphia, W.B. Saunders Co., 1964.

Cohen, J.J., and Kassirer, J.P.: Acid-base metabolism. In *Clinical Disorders of Fluid and Electrolyte Metabolism.* 3rd ed. (Maxwell, M.H., and Kleeman, C.R., editors). New York, McGraw-Hill Book Co., 1980.

Creese, R., Neil, M.W., Ledingham, J.M., and Vere, D.W.: The terminology of acid-base regulation. Lancet, *1*:419, 1962.

Davenport, H.W.: *The ABC of Acid-Base Chemistry,* 6th ed. Chicago, The University of Chicago Press, 1974.

Finston, H.L., and Rychtman, A.C.: *A New View of Current Acid-Base Theories.* New York, Wiley-Interscience, 1982.

Gamble, J.L., Jr.: *Acid-Base Physiology. A Direct Approach.* Baltimore, Johns Hopkins University, 1982.

Gamble, J.L., Jr.: Sodium and chloride and acid-base physiology. Bull Hopkins Hosp, *105*:247, 1960.

Garfinkel, H.B., and Gelfman, N.A.: Bicarbonate, not CO_2. Editorial. Arch Intern Med, *143*:2063, 1983.

Gilbert, D.L.: Buffering of blood plasma. Yale J Biol Med, *32*:378, 1960.

Hood, I., and Campbell, E.J.M.: Is pK OK? Editorial. N Engl J Med, *306*:864, 1982.

Kassirer, J.P., and Bleich, H.L.: Rapid estimation of plasma carbon dioxide tension from pH and total carbon dioxide content. N Engl J Med, *272*:1067, 1965.

Kaufman, H.E.: and Rosen, S.W.: Clinical acid base regulation—the Brønsted schema. Surg Gynecol Obstet, *103*:101, 1956.

Nuttall, F.Q.: Serum electrolytes and their relation to acid-base balance. Arch Intern Med, *116*:670, 1965.

Peters, J.P., and Van Slyke, D.D.: *Quantitative Clinical Chemistry.* Vol. I: Interpretations. Baltimore, Williams & Wilkins, 1932.

Pitts, R.F.: Mechanisms for stabilizing the alkaline reserves of the body. Harvey Lect, *48*:72, 1952–1953.

Seal, U.S.: The chemistry of buffers. Arch Intern Med, *116*:658, 1965.

Smith, T.C. (Editorial): Toward better management. J Anesthesiol, *30*:125, 1969.

Weisberg, H.F.: *Water, Electrolyte and Acid-Base Balance.* Baltimore, Williams & Wilkins, 1953.

Weisberg, H.F.: Respiratory factors in disturbance of acid-base balance. Am J Clin Path, *23*:1082, 1953.

CHAPTER 13

ACIDOSIS AND ALKALOSIS

The terms *acidosis* and *alkalosis* are used to describe changes in acid-base balance of the body fluids. The normal range of the plasma (or serum) pH is 7.36 to 7.44. The extreme range of pH compatible with life is 6.7 to 7.9.

ACIDOSIS

Acidosis is a term used to describe patients with an increased hydrogen ion concentration in the blood—in other words, with a pH below 7.36.

The increased hydrogen ion concentration may occur as a result of a primary respiratory disturbance (*primary respiratory acidosis, carbonic acid excess*), or as a result of primary metabolic disturbance (*primary metabolic acidosis, primary nonrespiratory acidosis*). Here it may be due to an excess of inorganic or organic acids, or to a decreased amount of base in the body.

ALKALOSIS

Alkalosis is a term used to describe patients with a hydrogen ion concentration in the blood below normal—in other words, with a pH above 7.44.

The decreased hydrogen ion concentration may occur as a result of a primary respiratory disturbance (*primary respiratory alkalosis, carbonic acid loss*), or as a result of a primary metabolic disturbance (*primary metabolic alkalosis, primary nonrespiratory alkalosis*). Here it may be due to an increased amount of base, or a loss of acid from the body.

UNCOMPENSATED AND COMPENSATED ACIDOSIS AND ALKALOSIS

In the previous chapter, the chemical and physiological mechanisms by which the pH of the body is maintained at a more or less constant level are described. When an acidosis or an alkalosis develops, these

131

Table 13–1.   Uncompensated and Compensated Respiratory Acidosis

	Normal	Uncompensated respiratory acidosis	Partially compensated respiratory acidosis
Bicarbonate	24 mEq/L	24 mEq/L	38 mEq/L
Carbonic acid	1.2 mEq/L	2.7 mEq/L	2.7 mEq/L
Bicarbonate-carbonic acid ratio	20:1	8.8:1	14:1
P_{CO_2}	40 mm Hg	90 mm Hg	90 mm Hg
pH	7.4	7.04	7.32

compensatory mechanisms help restore the pH toward its previous normal level. However, in the process, marked changes in the concentrations of carbonic acid, partial pressure of carbon dioxide (P_{CO_2}) and bicarbonate may occur, even though the pH is restored to normal.

These changes can be demonstrated in four main types of acid-base disturbances.

Respiratory Acidosis

In a patient with respiratory acidosis, an accumulation of carbonic acid occurs due to hypoventilation. This causes the P_{CO_2} of the plasma to rise, and the bicarbonate-carbonic acid ratio and the pH to fall. This can be called an *uncompensated* respiratory acidosis (Table 13–1).

However, as a result of the compensatory mechanisms described in Chapter 12, bicarbonate is retained in the body, and the bicarbonate-carbonic acid ratio and the pH rise and may return to normal, even though the concentration of both carbonic acid and bicarbonate are now greater than normal. The P_{CO_2} remains high and unchanged. This can be called a *compensated* respiratory acidosis (Table 13–1).

Respiratory Alkalosis

In a patient with respiratory alkalosis, there is a loss of carbonic acid due to hyperventilation. As a result, the P_{CO_2} falls, and the bicarbonate-carbonic acid ratio and the pH rise. This can be called an *uncompensated* respiratory alkalosis (Table 13–2).

However, as a result of compensatory mechanisms described in Chapter 12, bicarbonate is excreted by the kidneys, and the bicarbonate-carbonic acid ratio and the pH fall toward normal, even though the concentrations of bicarbonate and carbonic acid are now less than normal. The P_{CO_2} remains low and unchanged. This can be called a *compensated* respiratory alkalosis (Table 13–2).

Table 13–2. *Uncompensated and Compensated Respiratory Alkalosis*

	Normal	Uncompensated respiratory alkalosis	Partially compensated respiratory alkalosis
Bicarbonate	24 mEq/L	24 mEq/L	20 mEq/L
Carbonic acid	1.2 mEq/L	0.6 mEq/L	0.6 mEq/L
Bicarbonate-carbonic acid ratio	20:1	40:1	33.3:1
P_{CO_2}	40 mm Hg	20 mm Hg	20 mm Hg
pH	7.4	7.55	7.50

Metabolic Acidosis

In a patient with metabolic acidosis, an excess of acid or a loss of base is present. This causes the bicarbonate-carbonic acid ratio and the pH to fall. No change occurs in the P_{CO_2} (*uncompensated* metabolic acidosis, Table 13–3).

However, compensatory mechanisms described in Chapter 12 may occur. As a result, carbonic acid is excreted by the lungs in the form of carbon dioxide, and bicarbonate is retained by the kidneys. Therefore, the P_{CO_2} falls, and the bicarbonate-carbonic acid ratio and the pH rise toward normal, even though the concentrations of bicarbonate and carbonic acid are now less than normal (*compensated* metabolic acidosis, Table 13–3).

Metabolic Alkalosis

In a patient with metabolic alkalosis, there is an excess of base or a loss of acid. This causes the bicarbonate-carbonic acid ratio and the pH to rise. No change occurs in the P_{CO_2} (*uncompensated* metabolic alkalosis, Table 13–4).

However, compensatory mechanisms described in Chapter 12 may develop. The compensatory respiratory acidosis may be so marked that the P_{CO_2} may rise higher than 55 mm Hg (see Chap 26). In addition, bicarbonate ions are excreted by the kidneys. This is associated with a decrease in the bicarbonate-carbonic acid ratio and the pH, even

Table 13–3. *Uncompensated and Compensated Metabolic Acidosis*

	Normal	Uncompensated metabolic acidosis	Partially compensated metabolic acidosis
Bicarbonate	24 mEq/L	15 mEq/L	15 mEq/L
Carbonic acid	1.2 mEq/L	1.2 mEq/L	0.75 mEq/L
Bicarbonate-carbonic acid ratio	20:1	12.5:1	20:1
P_{CO_2}	40 mm Hg	40 mm Hg	25 mm Hg
pH	7.4	7.2	7.3

Table 13–4. Uncompensated and Compensated Metabolic Alkalosis

	Normal	Uncompensated metabolic acidosis	Partially compensated metabolic acidosis
Bicarbonate	24 mEq/L	28 mEq/L	34.5 mEq/L
Carbonic acid	1.2 mEq/L	1.2 mEq/L	1.35 mEq/L
Bicarbonate-carbonic acid ratio	20:1	31.6:1	25.6:1
P_{CO_2}	40 mm Hg	40 mm Hg	45 mm Hg
pH	7.4	7.6	7.55

though the serum concentrations of bicarbonate and carbonic acid are still greater than normal (*compensated* metabolic alkalosis, Table 13–4).

IMPORTANCE OF COMPENSATION

These observations are important for several reasons. Notice that in a severe respiratory acidosis, a normal bicarbonate concentration may be present. In addition, the bicarbonate rises to an abnormal value when compensation occurs and the pH returns toward normal (Table 13–1). Conversely, in a severe metabolic acidosis, the bicarbonate concentration is low and it remains very low even when compensation occurs and the pH rises toward normal (Table 13–3). Similar observations can be made for respiratory and metabolic alkalosis.

Overcompensation may also develop. For example, the respiratory compensation which occurs in a diabetic acidosis may continue after the metabolic acidosis has been corrected, so that a respiratory alkalosis, with a high pH and a low P_{CO_2}, may develop. Similarly, the metabolic compensation that occurs in a chronic respiratory acidosis may be so marked that a metabolic alkalosis with a high pH occurs.

In other words, an acid-base disturbance must be described in terms of both the primary or compensatory *respiratory* changes and the primary or compensatory *metabolic* changes which may occur, in addition to changes in pH. Clinically, the *respiratory* changes are indicated by the P_{CO_2} and other measurements. The *metabolic* changes are indicated by the serum bicarbonate concentration and other measurements (see Chaps 14 and 15).

Some physicians have used the terms *acidemia* or *alkalemia* to describe an abnormally low or high pH, *hypocapnia* or *hypercapnia* to describe an abnormally low or high P_{CO_2}, and *hypobasemia* or *hyperbasemia* to describe an abnormally low or high serum bicarbonate concentration.

Ordinarily, a hospital laboratory technician will determine the serum bicarbonate concentration indirectly by means of the CO_2 content test.

Fig. 13–1. 95% confidence bands of acidosis and alkalosis patients. (Adapted from Goldberg and associates.)

However, this test merely indicates the metabolic component of an acid-base disturbance (see Chap 14).

Simple methods of obtaining the Pco_2, serum bicarbonate concentration, and pH are described in Chapters 14 and 15.

THE USE OF 95% CONFIDENCE BANDS

Investigators have found that when they have studied large groups of patients with acidosis and alkalosis, the pH-Pco_2 changes of 95% of these patients are located within certain limits (95% confidence bands) (Fig. 13–1). These confidence bands have been used as guides, particularly in the computer diagnosis of acid-base disturbances. They are generally helpful, but the fact that the pH-Pco_2 values of a patient are located within a confidence band does not necessarily indicate that the patient has only a simple, uncomplicated acid-base disturbance. One must consider pH-Pco_2 values in terms of a patient's history, clinical course, medication or other therapy that has been used, and other previous and present laboratory data.

REFERENCES

Camien, M.N., Simmons, D.H., and Gonick, H.C.: A critical reappraisal of "acid-base" balance. J Clin Nutr, 22:786, 1969.

Campbell, E.J.M.: R I pH. Lancet, 1:681, 1962.

Creese, R., Neil, M.W., Ledingham, J.M., and Vere, D.W.: The terminology of acid-base regulation. Lancet, 1:419, 1962.

Davenport, H.W.: The ABC of Acid-Base Chemistry. 6th ed. Chicago, The University of Chicago Press, 1974.

Goldberg, M., et al.: Computer-based instruction and diagnosis of acid-base disorders. A systemic approach. JAMA, 223:269, 1973.

Huckabee, W.E.: Henderson vs. Hasselbalch. Clin Res, 9:117, 1961.

MacConnachie, H.F.: An old-fashioned approach to acid-base balance. Am J Med, 49:504, 1970.

Masoro, E.J., and Siegel, P.D.: Acid-Base Regulation. Philadelphia, W.B. Saunders Co., 1971.

Nahas, G.G., et al.: Current concepts of acid-base measurement. Ann New York Acad Sci, 133:1, 1966.

Weisberg, H.F.: Water and electrolyte balance. Bull Mt Sinai Hosp, 2:65, 85, 112, 154, 1950.

CHAPTER 14

CLINICAL MEASUREMENT OF ACID-BASE BALANCE

In Chapter 12, it is pointed out that

$$pH = 6.1 + \log \frac{\text{bicarbonate}}{\text{carbonic acid} + \text{carbon dioxide}}$$

This can be rewritten by stating that the pH is equivalent to the bicarbonate-carbonic acid ratio. To express this schematically,

$$pH \equiv \frac{\text{bicarbonate}}{\text{carbonic acid}}$$

Similarly, $pH \equiv \dfrac{\text{bicarbonate}}{P_{CO_2}}$ (page 127).

Therefore, in order to describe an acid-base disturbance accurately and completely, it is necessary to know the pH, the serum bicarbonate concentration, and the serum carbonic acid concentration, or P_{CO_2}. When any two of these values are known, the third can be determined from an appropriate nomogram. When the physician measures only one value, such as the serum bicarbonate concentration (which is indicated indirectly in the CO_2 content), he or she may make serious errors in diagnosis. For example, Tables 13–2 and 13–3 show that a low bicarbonate concentration may occur in a patient with respiratory alkalosis with a high pH, or in a patient with metabolic acidosis with a low pH.

In the past, measurements of pH and P_{CO_2} were not done routinely because of technical difficulties. However, accurate pH and P_{CO_2} meters are not available.

MEASUREMENT OF THE pH

The pH can be measured directly, using a pH meter equipped with a glass electrode. Theoretically, the pH should be determined on heparinized arterial blood, or arterialized blood, such as from a warmed ear lobe or fingertip. Venous blood, drawn without stasis, can also be used. The determination should be done as quickly as possible to prevent changes in pH due to loss of carbon dioxide and to the formation of lactic acid from the breakdown of glucose. The latter can be prevented by adding sodium fluoride to the blood.

Normally, the pH varies from 7.36 to 7.44. The ideal pH is 7.40.

pH determinations should also be done at body temperature 37° or 38° C to obtain accurate results, because the pH becomes more basic when blood is drawn at one temperature and the pH is measured at a lower temperature, such as room temperature and vice versa. Rosenthal has described the following formula to indicate this difference: $pH (38°) = pH_t - 0.0147 (38° - t)$, or $pH (37°) = pH_t - 0.0147 (37° - t)$, where t is the temperature at which the pH is measured. However, other investigators have noted variations from this formula.

The reverse situation occurs in patients who are undergoing surgical operations under hypothermia. Here, the true pH of the patient will be different from the measured pH. The relations between the true and measured pHs are: $True\ pH = pH (37°) + (37° - t) \times 0.0147$, where t is the patient's temperature.

Edmark has pointed out that when cardiac and other surgical procedures are done under hypothermia, a pH of 7.4 is not optimal. He has therefore suggested that the patient's pH should be reduced 0.0147 of a pH unit for each °C below 37°. Carson has varied the percentage of carbon dioxide in the pump-oxygenator gas mixture to obtain and maintain a desired pH. Frequent pH measurement should be done during the operation, and the necessary correction factors used, because, as was pointed out above, the measured pH is not identical with the true pH of the patient. The following ilustrates this:

Example:

Patient's body temperature 25° C. Measured pH (at 37° C) 7.0. The true pH of the patient is therefore:

$$True\ pH = pH (37°) + (37 - t) \times 0.0147$$
$$= 7.00 + (37 - 25) \times 0.0147$$
$$= 7.176$$

Since the patient's temperature has been lowered 12° (37° − 25°), the pH should be decreased to $7.40 - 12 (0.0147) = 7.22$. However, the patient's true pH is now 7.176. Therefore, it should be raised slightly.

MEASUREMENT OF THE PLASMA CARBONIC ACID CONCENTRATION AND THE P_{CO_2}

The carbonic acid concentrations cannot be measured directly in a hospital laboratory. However, the concentration of carbonic acid in the blood is proportional to the partial pressure of the carbon dioxide (P_{CO_2}) in the blood and in alveolar air. This can be measured with suitable P_{CO_2} meters.

In addition, when the pH and plasma bicarbonate (or the total carbon

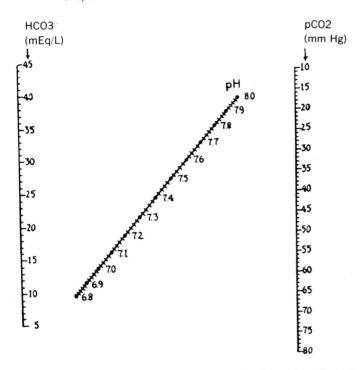

Fig. 14–1. Nomogram by which the P_{CO_2} can be determined from the pH and the serum bicarbonate concentration. (After McLean.)

dioxide content) are known, the P_{CO_2} can be determined from appropriate nomograms (Figs. 14–1 and 15–3, page 148).

MEASUREMENT OF THE PLASMA BICARBONATE ION CONCENTRATION

This is not measured directly. However, it can be calculated either from the nomogram in Figure 14–1 or the nomogram in Figure 15–3 (page 148).

The approximate bicarbonate ion concentration can also be determined by subtracting 1 mEq/L from the CO_2 content value (see below). The bicarbonate ion concentration can also be obtained from the following formula: Bicarbonate = CO_2 content − $(0.03 \times P_{CO_2})$. Similarly, the CO_2 content = bicarbonate + $(0.03 \times P_{CO_2})$ (see page 145).

MEASUREMENT OF THE CO₂ CONTENT

This measures the total carbon dioxide which is liberated by acidification of the plasma or serum. It therefore represents the sum of all forms of carbon dioxide in the blood, namely, the carbon dioxide dissolved in the plasma, the carbon dioxide derived from bicarbonate, and the carbon dioxide derived from plasma carbonic acid. It is measured on true plasma, that is, plasma obtained from blood which is collected anaerobically. Venous blood should be collected without stasis, allowed to clot, and centrifuged without exposure to air.

In the past, it was suggested that the blood be collected under mineral oil and that the tube be stoppered before centrifugation to avoid loss of carbon dioxide. However, Paulsen has shown that collecting the blood under mineral oil is not satisfactory, because the oil can absorb a large amount of carbon dioxide. He points out that a satisfactory method is to collect the blood in an ordinary way, fill a small test tube, and stopper the tube. The tube can then be refrigerated for several hours. When the tube is refrigerated for 5 hours at 4° C, it loses only 0.3 to 0.5 mEq/L carbon dioxide. When refrigeration for 5 hours is done at 23° C, 1 mEq/L carbon dioxide is lost. Paulsen further points out that centrifugation at 2000 r.p.m. for 5 minutes at room temperature causes a loss of 0.3 mEq/L carbon dioxide.

Originally, the CO_2 content was measured using a Van Slyke blood gas apparatus. It can now be measured automatically by introducing a precise volume of plasma into a reaction cup containing an electrode that responds to the rate of pH change as the CO_2 passes through a silicone rubber membrane covering the pH electrode. The diffusing CO_2 lowers the pH of a bicarbonate solution between the membrane and the pH electrode. The rate of the pH changes is directly proportional to the CO_2 concentration of the sample.

If the CO_2 content is measured on whole blood, higher values will be obtained because the whole blood has a greater buffering capacity than either plasma or serum.

Measurement of the CO_2 content is valuable, for example, when one is trying to determine whether a diuretic is producing a metabolic alkalosis as a side effect. This will be noted by a rise in CO_2 content (and a fall in serum potassium and chloride concentrations). However, one must be constantly aware that the CO_2 content merely measures the sum of the bicarbonate (HCO_3^-) ions and the carbonic acid (H_2CO_3) concentration in the blood and extracellular water, and that a value for the CO_2 content may indicate a high bicarbonate ion concentration with a low or normal carbonic acid concentration, a normal bicarbonate ion and normal carbonic acid concentration, or a low bicarbonate ion concentration with a normal or high carbonic acid concentration. Therefore, determining the value of the CO_2 content without measuring the value of the pH is like trying to interpret the meaning of a white blood cell count without determining the differential cell count (Gambino).

THE CO_2 CAPACITY AND THE CO_2 COMBINING POWER

Each of these tests measures the carbon dioxide concentration of plasma or serum which has been equilibrated with 5.5% carbon dioxide, which has a partial pressure of 40 mm Hg. However, there are important differences between these two tests.

The CO_2 Capacity Test

Whole blood is equilibrated at 38° C (body temperature) with a 5.5% carbon dioxide gas mixture. (This has a partial pressure [Pco_2] of 40 mm Hg, which is identical with the Pco_2 of alveolar air.) Then the plasma (true plasma) is separated from the red blood cells anaerobically, so that no carbon dioxide is lost in the process. The carbon dioxide concentration is then determined. This method is not used now. The CO_2 content test is used instead.

The CO_2 Combining Power Test

Plasma or serum is separated from the red blood cells (separated plasma), and then is equilibrated at room temperature with the technician's alveolar air, which presumably has a Pco_2 of 40 mm Hg. The carbon dioxide concentration is then determined. This is the method which had been used in hospital laboratories, and what is meant when the term "carbon dioxide combining power," or "alkali reserve" is mentioned in the literature.

The CO_2 combining power is less accurate than the CO_2 capacity because the test is done on separated plasma rather than on the true plasma, and at room temperature rather than at body temperature, and with the technician's air, which may not represent true alveolar air, rather than with a 5.5% carbon dixoide gas mixture.

For these reasons, the carbon dioxide combining power test is not used and the CO_2 content test is used instead.

In most patients, the history and clinical course are usually sufficient to determine whether the respiratory or metabolic disturbance is primary. However, if a complex problem is present, the pH must be measured.

MEASUREMENT OF Pco_2

The Pco_2 of arterial or arterialized blood (or alveolar air) can now be easily and quickly determined with special Pco_2 meters. In addition, the Pco_2 can be determined from the pH and CO_2 content (or the bicarbonate concentration), using the nomogram in Figure 14–1, or from the Siggaard-Andersen nomogram (Fig. 15–3), page 148.

The normal Pco_2 varies from 35 to 48 mm Hg. The ideal Pco_2 is 40 mm Hg.

DESCRIPTION OF AN ACID-BASE DISTURBANCE IN TERMS OF THE RELATIONS AMONG Pco_2, pH, AND CO_2 CONTENT

A high Pco_2 indicates underventilation and a respiratory acidosis. A low Pco_2 indicates overventilation and a respiratory alkalosis. A normal Pco_2 represents *respiratory balance.* It may be present normally, or with a metabolic acidosis or alkalosis, or may occur as the result of respiratory acidosis which has been superimposed on a respiratory alkalosis, or *vice versa.*

An uncompensated respiratory acidosis is characterized by a low pH, a high CO_2 content, and a high P_{CO_2}.

An uncompensated respiratory alkalosis is characterized by a high pH, a low CO_2 content, and a low P_{CO_2}.

An uncompensated metabolic acidosis is characterized by a low pH, a low CO_2 content, and a normal P_{CO_2}.

An uncompensated metabolic alkalosis is characterized by a high pH, a high CO_2 content, and a normal P_{CO_2}.

When a respiratory acidosis is compensated by a metabolic alkalosis, the pH tends to return to normal, but the CO_2 content becomes higher. The P_{CO_2} remains unchanged.

When a respiratory alkalosis is compensated by a metabolic acidosis, the pH tends to become normal, but the CO_2 content becomes lower. The P_{CO_2} remains unchanged.

When a metabolic acidosis is compensated by a respiratory alkalosis, the pH tends to return to normal, but the CO_2 content becomes lower, and the P_{CO_2} becomes low.

When a metabolic alkalosis is compensated by a respiratory acidosis, the pH tends to return to normal, but the CO_2 content becomes higher, and the P_{CO_2} becomes high. However, this does not ordinarily occur (Chap 26).

Another method of describing the respiratory component of an acid-base disturbance in terms of P_{CO_2} and pH is described in Chapter 15.

THE USE OF VENOUS BLOOD TO MEASURE pH, P_{CO_2}, AND CO_2 CONTENT

Theoretically, arterial or capillary blood should be used. However, venous blood drawn without stasis can also be used. The difference between the pH of arterial and venous blood ranges from 0.01 to 0.03 unit.

A tourniquet should be placed lightly around the extremity to avoid compressing the artery. If the arm or hand is cold, warm towels will improve the reliability of the blood sample. The tourniquet should be kept in place while the blood is drawn, and the first tube of blood should be used for measuring the pH. If the tourniquet is removed, one should wait 2 minutes before drawing the blood. The blood is drawn preferably into heparinized vacuum tubes.

Capillary blood from a warmed surface can also be used. If an ear or finger is heated with 40° to 45° C water or a lamp for 3 to 5 minutes, the capillary blood will become arterialized. The skin can be punctured with a #11 blade. Drops of blood can then be collected into a large heparinized capillary blood collecting tube, or into a heparinized Astrup capillary tube.

If the blood is kept at a room temperature below 27° C, the pH will change less than 0.015 pH unit in one-half hour. However, if the blood has to stand more than one-half hour, it should be placed in ice water, where it can be kept as long as 4 hours. If blood is placed in ice water, it should not be centrifuged when it is ice cold, if the pH is to be measured, because a pH reading too alkaline will be obtained. The error may be greater than 0.1 pH unit.

Studies by Phillip and Peretz indicate that measurements from central venous blood give reliable values for metabolic disturbances, but are not as reliable in determining respiratory disturbances.

REFERENCES

American Society of Clinical Pathologists: Workshop Manual on Blood pH, pCO_2 Oxygen Saturation and pO_2, 1963.

Austin, W.H.: Acid-base balance. Am Heart J, *69*:691, 1965.

Bedford, R.H., and Woolman, H.: Questions and Answers. Arterial puncture for blood gas studies. Sites, complications, personnel. JAMA, *228*:763, 1974.

Campbell, E.J.M., and Howell, J.B.L.: The determination of mixed venous and arterial CO_2 tension by rebreathing techniques. In Woolmer, R.F. (see below).

Chung, T.O.: Central venous versus arterial blood gas values. Ann Intern Med, *71*:870, 1969.

Cohen, J.J.: A new acid-base nomogram featuring hydrogen ion concentration. Ann Intern Med, *66*:159, 1967.

Davenport, H.W.: *The ABC of Acid-Base Chemistry*, 3rd ed. Chicago, University of Chicago Press, 1950.

Edmark, W.: Continuous blood pH mesurement with extracorporeal cooling. Surg Gynecol Obstet, *109*:743, 1959.

Fagan, T.J.: Estimation of hydrogen ion concentration. N Engl J Med, *288*:915, 1973.

Faulkner, W.R.: Evaluation of error in measurement of pH in blood at room temperature. Cleveland Clin Quart, *28*:116, 1961.

Fuh, Y-J: Acid-base disorders. JAMA, *223*:330, 1973.

Gambino, S.R.: The clinical value of routine determinations of venous plasma pH in acid base problems. Am J Clin Path, *32*:301, 1959.

Gambino, S.R.: Workshop Manual on Blood pH, pCO_2, Oxygen Saturation and pO_2. Am Soc Clin Path, 1963.

Gambino, S.R.: Comparison of pH in human arterial, venous, and capillary blood. Am J Clin Path, *32*:298, 1959. Also Ann New York Acad Sci, *133*:235, 1966.

Gleason, D.F.: pH measurements. Arch Intern Med, *116*:649, 1965.

Hills, A.G., and Reid, E.L.: More on pH. Ann Intern Med, *66*:238, 1967.

Hofford, J.M., Dowling, A.S., and Pell, S.: More about arterialized capillary blood measurements. JAMA, *224*:1297, 1973.

Huckabee, W.E.: Henderson vs. Hasselbalch, Clin Res, *9*:116, 1961.

Henderson, L.J.: *Blood.* New Haven, Yale University Press, 1929.

Kaufman, H.E., and Rosen, S.W.: Clinical acid-base regulation—the Bronsted schema. Surg Gynecol Obstet, *103*:101, 1956.

Long, A.P.: Venous or arterial blood gas measurements. JAMA, *217*:1706, 1971.

McLean, F.C.: Application of law of chemical equilibrium (law of mass action) to biological problems. Physiol Rev, *18*:495, 1938.

Olivia, J.V., et al.: Earlobe capillary blood for estimating arterial oxygen tension. JAMA, *223*:1388, 1973.

Paine, E.G., Boutwell, J.H., and Stoloff, L.A.: The reliability of "arterialized" venous blood for measuring arterial pH and pCO_2. Am J Med Sci, *242*:431, 1961.

Paulsen, L.: Comparison between total carbon dioxide content in plasma or serum from blood collected with or without paraffine oil. Scand J Clin Lab Invest, 9:402, 1957.

Peters, J.P., and Van Slyke, D.D.: *Quantitative Clinical Chemistry,* Vol. 1, and Vol. 2. Baltimore, Williams & Wilkins, 1932.

Petty, T.L., Cheng, T.O., Sharp, J.T., Peretz, D.I., and Grossfeld, J.I.: Questions and Answers. Source of blood samples for blood gas studies in critically ill patients. JAMA, 216:1042, 1971.

Phillips, B., and Peretz, D.I.: A comparison of central venous and arterial blood gas values in the critically ill. Ann Intern Med, 70:745, 1969.

Rosenthal, T.B.: The effect of temperature on the pH of blood and plasma in vitro. J Biol Chem, 173:25, 1948.

Severinghaus, J.W.: Recent developments in blood O_2 and CO_2 electrodes. In Woolmer, R.F. (see below).

Singer, R.B., and Hastings, A.B.: Improved clinical method for estimation of disturbances of acid-base balance of human blood. Medicine, 27:223, 1948.

Stadie, W.C., and Van Slyke, D.D.: Studies on acidosis. XV. Content and capacity in arterial and venous blood plasma. J Biol Chem, 41:191, 1920.

Ullian, R.B., Kogos, I.G., Golub, M., and Stein, M.: Calculation of pH with the use of venous blood. N Engl J Med, 265:235, 1961.

Van Slyke, D.D., and Cullen, G.E.: Studies on acidosis. I. J Biol Chem, 30:289, 1917.

Weisberg, H.F.: pH of venous blood. Queries and minor notes. JAMA, 194:688, 1968.

Wilson, R.F., and Walt, A.J.: Differences in acid base levels and oxygen saturation between central venous and arterial blood. Lancet, 2:748, 1967.

Woolmer, R.F., Editor: *A Symposium on pH and Blood Gas Measurement: Methods and Interpretation.* Boston, Little, Brown and Co., 1959.

CHAPTER 15

CLINICAL MEASUREMENT OF ACID-BASE BALANCE (Continued)

THE ASTRUP METHOD OF DETERMINING ACID-BASE DISTURBANCES

Astrup and his colleagues invented an apparatus (manufactured by the Radiometer Co., Copenhagen), with which one can determine the pH and P_{CO_2} of blood quickly and simply. They also developed several new ways of describing acid-base disturbances and introduced the terms *standard bicarbonate concentration* and *base excess concentration*. Some physicians have objected to the use of base excess values, for example, as a means of treating patients. However, even if these objections are valid, this does not invalidate the use of the Astrup apparatus. Furthermore, I have shown below how these objections can be overcome.

PRINCIPLES OF THE ASTRUP METHOD

In Chapter 12 it was pointed out that

$$pH = 6.10 + \log \frac{HCO_3^-}{H_2CO_3 + CO_3}$$

However, when a gas such as carbon dioxide dissolves in a liquid, the concentration of the gas in the liquid is directly proportional to the partial pressure of the gas P_{CO_2}. In addition, the concentration of carbonic acid (H_2CO_3) is proportional to the concentration of the dissolved carbon dioxide. Therefore, the term P_{CO_2} can be substituted for the denominator of the above equation, which becomes:

$$pH = 6.10 + \log \frac{HCO_3^-}{P_{CO_2} \times 0.03}$$

where 0.03 represents a proportionality constant between dissolved CO_2 and P_{CO_2}. The pH, therefore, varies with the P_{CO_2}.

145

pCO₂ mm Hg

Fig. 15–1. The pH-log Pco₂ line for a blood sample. (After Astrup.) Point A indicates the measured pH value of 7.12 after equilibration of the blood at a Pco₂ tension of 60 mm Hg. Similarly, point B indicates a pH of 7.30 at a Pco₂ tension of 30 mm Hg. The line between points A and B is the pH-log Pco₂ line. Since the actual pH of the anaerobically drawn blood is 7.24 (point C), the actual Pco₂ of this blood sample is 38 mm Hg (see text for details).

If pH values are plotted against Pco_2 values on fully oxygenated blood with a normal hemoglobin concentration, their relations will be denoted by a curved line. However, when pH values are plotted aginst the logarithms of Pco_2 values, a straight (diagonal) line results. (The actual slope of this line will vary with the hemoglobin concentration of the blood sample.)

Therefore, if a sample of blood is equilibrated with two known CO_2 tensions, and the pH for each of these tensions is measured, if these values are plotted on a graph, as in Figure 15–1, the line joining these two pH values describes the relations between all pH and Pco_2 values of this particular blood sample. This can be called the pH-log Pco_2 line.

If the actual pH of the blood sample is then determined, the Pco_2 of this sample can be read directly from the graph (Fig. 15–1). In addition, the pH-log Pco_2 line itself intersects several scales which give values for buffer base concentration, actual bicarbonate concentration, standard bicarbonate concentration, and base excess concentration (Fig. 15–3). The total CO_2 concentration can also be obtained by adding

Fig. 15–2.   The Siggaard-Andersen nomogram. See text for details.

actual bicarbonate concentration to ($PCO_2 \times 0.03$). (The meaning of these terms is described on page 150.)

The values obtained can be checked with actual measurement of the hemoglobin, because *the slope of the pH-log PCO_2 line is a function of the hemoglobin concentration.* (When the hemoglobin value remains constant, varying pH and PCO_2 values will shift the *location* of the line, but its slope will remain unchanged.) The theoretical hemoglobin concentration in g per dl can be determined from a scale on the nomogram in Figure 15–2, where the pH-log PCO_2 line meets the buffer base curve. This can then be checked with the actual measured value of the hemoglobin.

For example, in Figure 15–3

Buffer base − base excess = normal buffer base
  41.4   −   (−6.1)   =   47.5

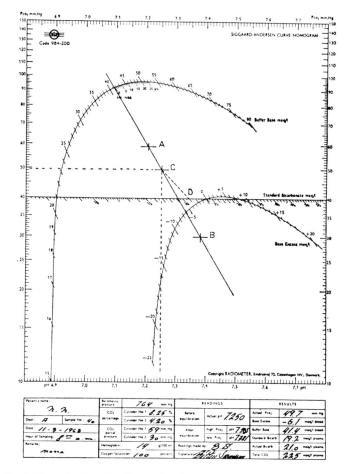

Fig. 15–3. Method of using the Siggaard-Andersen nomogram. See text for detials. The data indicate that the patient is suffering from a simultaneous respiratory acidosis and metabolic acidosis (see Chap 29).

Opposite 47.5 on the buffer base curve is the value 14.5 g/dl hemoglobin. This should compare with the actual hemoglobin value by ± 3 g/dl.

The term *normal buffer base* describes the buffer base of blood with a pH of 7.40 at a P_{CO_2} of 40 mm Hg. It varies with the hemoglobin concentration as follows: Normal buffer base = 41.6 + 0.42 × hemoglobin concentration (g/dl).

METHOD OF USING THE ASTRUP APPARATUS

Three ml of arterial blood or 100 μl arterialized capillary blood can be used. Arterialized capillary blood from an ear lobe puncture is satisfactory. This gives acid-base values which are identical to those obtained from arterial blood. The ear lobe is first warmed to increase the circulation and to arterialize the capillary bed. An incision, large enough to form large drops of blood, is made in the lower tip of the lobe. A preheparinized collecting tube is inserted into the center of the droplet, to fill the tube rapidly. A small piece of iron wire is inserted into the tube; the ends are then sealed with plasticine, for anaerobic storage of the blood sample. The blood and heparin are mixed by the small iron wire insert, from the external movement of a small magnet. Samples can be drawn at the bedside and measured within 15 minutes if stored at room temperature, or within 3 hours if stored in ice water.

For measurement, the end of the tube is cut off and the blood is placed directly into a micro blood pH meter, which is maintained at a constant temperature of 38° C.

The blood sample is then equilibrated to two artificial levels of P_{CO_2}, by equilibrating it for 3 minutes with a CO_2–O_2 mixture from calibrated gas tanks. The corresponding levels of pH are then measured.

These latter two pH values are marked on the nomogram devised by Siggaard-Andersen and Engel, and a straight line is drawn between them (Figs. 15–2 and 15–3).

The actual P_{CO_2} of the blood sample is then determined from the nomogram in the following way:

In Figure 15–3, the actual pH of a blood sample is 7.250. After equilibrating the sample with a high P_{CO_2} mixture (59 mm Hg) obtained from a tank, the pH measures 7.205. After equilibrating another portion of the sample with a low P_{CO_2} mixture (30 mm Hg), obtained from another tank, the pH measures 7.381. These values are marked on the nomogram (points A and B). A straight line is then drawn between these two points.

The actual pH of 7.250 is noted on the abscissa of the nomogram. A perpendicular is drawn upward from this point until it meets the diagonal line joining A and B, at point C. A horizontal line drawn from point C meets the P_{CO_2} ordinate at 49.7 mm Hg.

The values of buffer base, standard bicarbonate, and base excess are obtained from the nomogram, at the intersections of the line AB with the respective buffer base, standard bicarbonate, and base excess curves. These values are as follows:

Buffer base, 41.4 mEq/L blood.
Standard bicarbonate, 19.2 mEq/L plasma.
Base excess, −6.1 mEq/L blood.

Actual bicarbonate concentration is obtained by drawing a line at an angle of −45° from point C until it meets the standard bicarbonate line, at point D. Its value is 21 mEq/L plasma.

Total CO_2 (CO_2 content) is obtained by adding (P_{CO_2} × 0.03) to the actual bicarbonate concentration. Its value is:

$(P_{CO_2} \times 0.03)$ + Actual bicarbonate
(49.7×0.03) +   21   = 22.5 mEq/L plasma.

The use of the nomogram assumes that the oxygen saturation of the patient is 90% or higher. The nomogram is also accurate for most clinical purposes even when the oxygen saturation is lower than 90%, even though the pH and the P_{CO_2} rise as the oxygen saturation falls.

INTERPRETATION OF THE DATA OBTAINED WITH THE ASTRUP METHOD AND THE SIGGAARD-ANDERSEN NOMOGRAM

The values of P_{CO_2}, buffer base concentration, actual bicarbonate concentration and total CO_2 concentration can be interpreted in the usual way, regardless of whether these values are obtained directly or indirectly, with any macro- or micromethods. However, Astrup has described two new measurements, which are obtained from the Siggaard-Andersen nomogram, namely, standard bicarbonate concentration and base excess. These are related to the term buffer base in the following way.

The term *whole blood buffer base* was first used in 1948 by Singer and Hastings. They defined it as the sum of the concentrations of the buffer anions (in mEq/L) which were contained in whole blood. These buffer anions include the bicarbonate in plasma and in red blood cells, hemoglobin, plasma proteins, and the phosphates in plasma and red blood cells. Nearly all this buffering action is due to the hemoglobin and the bicarbonate. The total quantity of these buffer anions in normal blood (determined by the titration of whole blood with strong acid) is about 45 to 50 mEq/L.

If respiration is impaired and CO_2 accumulates, it dissolves in the blood and forms carbonic acid (H_2CO_3). However, this excess acid can be buffered by hemoglobin, for example, to form acid hemoglobin and bicarbonate:

$$H_2CO_3 + Hb \rightarrow HHb + HCO_3^-$$

The decreased amount of hemoglobin buffer which results from this reaction is equal to the increased amount of bicarbonate ions which are released by the reaction. Therefore, the total buffer anion content of the whole blood will not be altered by changes in CO_2 content or P_{CO_2}. *Buffer base changes, therefore, represent the effect of metabolic (nonrespiratory) disturbances in the body.* Buffer base can be determined using Singer and Hasting's original nomogram, or the Siggaard-Andersen nomogram (Figs. 15–2 and 15–3).

Astrup's terms *standard bicarbonate* and *base excess* represent these metabolic changes in a slightly different way:

Standard bicarbonate represents the bicarbonate concentration in the plasma of blood which has been equilibrated at a P_{CO_2} of 40 mm Hg, and with oxygen, in order to fully saturate the hemoglobin. Since most of the buffering of blood is carried out by the hemoglobin, unsaturated blood will show a deficient buffering activity. The normal value of standard bicarbonate is 24 (22 to 26) mEq/L. *Base excess* describes the presence in the blood of an excess of base (or deficit of fixed acid), or a deficit of base (or an excess of fixed acid). (Fixed acid does not include carbonic acid.) It is defined as zero for blood with a pH of 7.4 at a P_{CO_2} of 40 mm Hg. *Positive* values indicate an excess of base (or deficit of fixed acid). *Negative* values indicate a deficit of base (or an excess of fixed acid).

Base excess represents the amount of strong base or acid per liter of blood, which has been added as a result of metabolic disturbances (which may be primary or compensatory). Its value is determined from the Siggaard-Andersen nomogram. It is derived by multiplying the deviation in standard bicarbonate from normal by an empirical factor of 1.2. This factor represents the greater buffer action of red blood cells, compared to plasma. The exact correction actually depends on the hemoglobin concentration of the blood sample, but relatively large changes in hemoglobin cause small changes in this value.

The normal value of base excess is 0 (+ 2.5 to −2.5) mEq/L.

There are two advantages of using standard bicarbonate and base excess rather than buffer base values: these values can be rapidly and accurately determined with the Astrup method, and they are not influenced by the oxygen saturation of the original blood sample, unlike buffer base.

Astrup has suggested that the values of base excess can be used not only for diagnosis but also for the treatment of metabolic acidosis or alkalosis patients using the following formula:

mEq base required to correct a metabolic acidosis = body weight (kg) × 0.3 × −base excess, where 0.3 represents a factor which Astrup and his associates determined experimentally.

Similarly: mEq acid required to correct a metabolic alkalosis = body weight (kg) × 0.3 × +base excess.

Clinically, this formula has been found useful in treating metabolic acidosis or alkalosis. However, these values can be misleading when used to treat respiratory acidosis or respiratory alkalosis.

I have already pointed out (Chap 13) that a patient with uncompensated respiratory acidosis or respiratory alkalosis may show a normal actual bicarbonate concentration. Similarly, such a patient will show a normal standard bicarbonate concentration, and a normal base excess value. In addition, a patient who shows a primary respiratory *acidosis* complicated by a primary (independent) metabolic *acidosis,* or a patient with primary respiratory *alkalosis* who develops a primary (independent) metabolic *alkalosis,* may also show normal actual bicarbonate,

Table 15–1.   Complicated Acid-Base Changes which May Theoretically Occur.
(After Schwartz and Relman.)

	pH	P$_{CO_2}$	Actual bicarbonate[1]	Standard bicarbonate[2]	Base excess[3]
1	7.18	80	29	24	0
2	7.58	20	18	24	0

1. Chronic primary respiratory acidosis (emphysema) with a complicating primary (independent) (diabetic) metabolic acidosis.
2. Primary respiratory alkalosis induced by a mechanical respirator, with a complicating primary (independent) metabolic alkalosis, induced by severe vomiting.

[1]Defined on pages 149 and 150.
[2]Defined on pages 150 and 151.
[3]Defined on page 151.

standard bicarbonate, and base excess concentrations (Table 15–1), despite the serious acidosis or alkalosis which is present. In such patients, the normal base excess concentration cannot be used as a guide to treatment.

This difficulty of understanding the significance of base excess values can be resolved if one remembers the following:

In Chapter 12, it was pointed out that a disturbance in pH can be associated with compensatory changes which occur in three different regulatory systems, namely, buffer compensation, respiratory compensation, and renal compensation. As a result of the interaction of these three systems, a pH abnormality seldom indicates a simple disturbance, but, instead, represents the interaction of primary or compensatory metabolic disturbances, associated with primary or compensatory respiratory disturbances.

Similarly, a P$_{CO_2}$ value which is obtained represents a *balance* between respiratory acidosis and alkalosis processes which may be present simultaneously in a patient. For example, a patient with respiratory acidosis will usually develop a compensatory metabolic alkalosis. However, if for any reason a metabolic acidosis develops independently, there will be a tendency for a compensatory respiratory alkalosis to develop. Also, a patient with chronic respiratory acidosis may be placed in a respirator. A "normal" P$_{CO_2}$ in such a patient, therefore, merely indicates that *respiratory balance* is present, and does not necessarily indicate that no respiratory disturbance is present.

Similarly, the standard bicarbonate and base excess values represent a *balance* between metabolic acidosis and metabolic alkalosis processes which may be present simultaneously in a patient. For example, a patient with metabolic acidosis will usually develop a compensatory respiratory alkalosis. However, if for any reason a respiratory acidosis develops independently, there will be a tendency for a compensatory metabolic alkalosis to develop. "Normal" standard bicarbonate and base excess values in such a patient, therefore, merely indicate that *metabolic balance* is present, and do not necessarily indicate that no metabolic disturbance is present (see Table 15–1).

The importance of this is that a physician must always use the base excess value in association with a description of the *patient,* the P_{CO_2} and pH, to obtain a full description of the total acid-base balance (in the extracellular water).

This information can also be obtained by inspection, by merely plotting the points of intersection of the pH abscissa and the log P_{CO_2} ordinate on the Siggaard-Andersen nomogram (Fig. 15–4).

Figure 15–5 is a more detailed analysis of Figure 15–4.

DESCRIPTION OF AN ACID-BASE DISTURBANCE IN TERMS OF THE RELATIONS BETWEEN THE ACTUAL BICARBONATE AND THE STANDARD BICARBONATE CONCENTRATIONS

In previous editions of the book, I described how the relationships between the values of the CO_2 content and the CO_2 capacity could be used to describe various acid-base disturbances. Since the CO_2 capacity is infrequently calculated now, I have deleted discussion of the CO_2 capacity from this edition. However, similar information can be obtained by using the values of the standard bicarbonate and actual bicarbonate, popularized by Astrup, because the CO_2 capacity is similar to that of the standard bicarbonate, and the CO_2 content is similar to that of the actual bicarbonate. This is described in the next chapter. I should like to stress that the nomogram of Siggaard-Andersen which is used to calculate the actual and standard bicarbonate values can be used when the pH and pCO_2 are determined with any method.

Under ideal conditions, the standard bicarbonate and the actual bicarbonate should show equal values. The reason for this is that normally the pCO_2 of the blood is 40 mm Hg, and the standard bicarbonate represents the bicarbonate value when the blood plasma has been equilibrated at a pCO_2 of 40 mm Hg.

If a respiratory acidosis is present, the actual bicarbonate will be higher than the standard bicarbonate value for the following reason: standard bicarbonate is determined from a pCO_2 of 40 mm Hg. When a respiratory acidosis is present, the pCO_2 is higher than 40 mm Hg. Therefore, when the blood is equilibrated with a gas mixture of 40 mm Hg, some of the carbon dioxide will leave the blood as equilibration occurs. As a result, the actual bicarbonate value will be higher than the standard bicarbonate.

If a respiratory alkalosis is present, the actual bicarbonate will be lower than the standard bicarbonate for the following reason: Standard bicarbonate is determined from a pCO_2 of 40 mm Hg. When a respiratory alkalosis is present, the pCO_2 is lower than 40 mm Hg. Therefore, when the blood is equilibrated with a gas mixture of 40 mm Hg, the blood

Fig. 15–4.   Chart (devised by the author) showing how the respiratory and metabolic components of an acid-base disturbance can be described by inspection, by finding the point of intersection of the pH abscissa and the log P_{CO_2} ordinate on the Siggaard-Andersen nomogram.

The *zone of respiratory balance* is drawn to indicate the normal range of P_{CO_2} from 34 to 46 mm Hg. The *zone of metabolic balance* is drawn to indicate the normal range of standard bicarbonate concentration from 22 to 26 mEq/l. The slope of the metabolic balance zone is drawn to indicate hemoglobin contents of 15 g and 10 g per dl blood. The *pH zone* is drawn to indicate a normal pH range from 7.36 to 7.44. The polygon formed by the intersection of these three zones indicates the normal zone of both respiratory and metabolic balance.

Point A represents an example of a metabolic acidosis patient with a partially compensatory respiratory alkalosis. The pH is 7.29 and the P_{CO_2} is 20.54 mm Hg. The location of point A in Figure 15–4 visually indicates that a metabolic acidosis and a respiratory alkalosis are present.

Point B represents an unusual example of a respiratory acidosis patient with an independent metabolic acidosis (example 1 in Table 15–1). The pH is 7.18 and the P_{CO_2} is 80 mm Hg. The location of point B in Figure 15–4 visually indicates that a respiratory acidosis and a metabolic balance are present. This can occur in two types of patients: (1) when an acute respiratory acidosis is present without any compensatory metabolic alkalosis, or (2) when a respiratory acidosis is complicated by an independent metabolic acidosis.

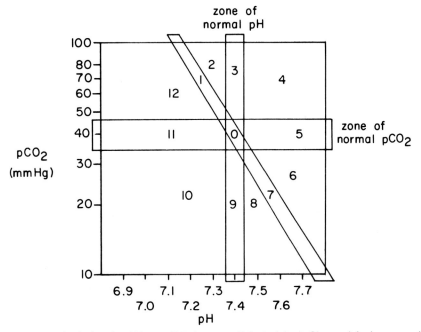

Fig. 15–5. Analysis of acid-base disturbances. (Adapted from Siggaard-Andersen and Engle, 1960). Each area in the diagram represents a specific acid-base disturbance.
0 Normal region; *1* Uncompensated respiratory acidosis; *2* Partly compensated respiratory acidosis; *3* Fully compensated respiratory acidosis; *4* Partly compensated metabolic alkalosis; *5* Uncompensated metabolic alkalosis; *6* Combined metabolic and respiratory alkalosis; *7* Uncompensated respiratory alkalosis; *8* Partly compensated respiratory alkalosis; *9* Fully compensated respiratory alkalosis; *10* Partly compensated metabolic acidosis; *11* Uncompensated metabolic acidosis; *12* Combined metabolic and respiratory acidosis.

will absorb some of the carbon dioxide as equilibration occurs. As a result, the actual bicarbonate will be lower than the standard bicarbonate.

When these relationships are used, one should remember that normally the standard and actual bicarbonate values may vary as much as ±2 mEq/L.

1. The standard bicarbonate indicates a metabolic acidosis or alkalosis.
   a. When the standard bicarbonate is low, this is a sign of a metabolic acidosis.
   b. When the standard bicarbonate is high, this is a sign of a metabolic alkalosis.
2. The difference between the actual bicarbonate and the standard bicarbonate concentrations indicates a respiratory acidosis or alkalosis.
   a. When the actual bicarbonate is higher than the standard bicarbonate, this is a sign of a respiratory acidosis.
   b. When the actual bicarbonate is lower than the standard bicarbonate, this is a sign of respiratory alkalosis.
3. When the actual bicarbonate and standard bicarbonate are equal, this indicates respiratory balance.

    a. When the actual bicarbonate and standard bicarbonate are low and equal, this indicates an uncompensated metabolic acidosis.

    b. When they are high and equal, this indicates an uncompensated metabolic alkalosis.

4. When the standard bicarbonate is high or low, the actual bicarbonate must also be high or low. However, a low, normal, or high actual bicarbonate may occur with a normal standard bicarbonate concentration.

REFERENCES

Astrup, P.: Acid-base disorders. Correspondence. N Engl J Med, *268*:817, 1963.

Astrup, P.A.: A new approach to acid-base metabolism. Clin Chem, *7*:1, 1961.

Astrup, P., Jørgensen, K., Siggaard-Andersen, O., and Engle, K.: Acid-base metabolism. New approach. Lancet, *1*:1035, 1960.

Maas, A.H.J., and van Heijst, A.N.P.: A comparison of the pH of arterial blood with arterialized blood from the ear lobe with Astrup's microglasselectrode. Clin Chim Acta, *6*:31, 34, 1961.

McDonald, J.S., Laughlin, D.E., and Bedell, G.N.: Direct approach to evaluation of patients with acid-base imbalance. JAMA, *188*:9, 1964.

Mellengaard, K., and Astrup, P.: Quantitative determination of surplus amounts of acid or base in the human body. Scand J Clin Lab Invest, *12*:172, 1960.

Nahas, G.G., Consulting Editor: Current concepts of acid-base measurement. Ann New York Acad Sci, *133*:1, 1966.

Relman, A.R., and Schwartz, W.B.: Primum pH. N Engl J Med, *272*:541, 1965.

Schwartz, W.B., and Relman, A.S.: A critique of the parameters used in the evaluation of acid-base disorders. N Engl J Med, *268*:1382, 1963.

Schwartz, W.B.: Archives of acid-base balance. N Engl J Med, *272*:318, 1965.

Siggaard-Andersen, O.: A graphic representation of changes of the acid-base status. Scand J Clin Lab Invest, *12*:311, 1960.

Siggaard-Andersen, O.: Sampling and storing of blood for determination of acid-base status. Scand J Clin Lab Invest, *13*:196, 1961.

Siggaard-Andersen, O.: The pH-log pCO_2 blood acid-base nomogram revised. Scand J Clin Lab Invest, *14*:598, 1962.

Siggaard-Andersen, O.: *The Acid-Base Status of the Blood,* 2nd ed. Baltimore, Williams & Wilkins, 1964.

Siggaard-Andersen, O., and Engle, K.: A new acid-base nomogram. Scand J Clin Lab Invest, *12*:186, 1960.

Singer, R.B., and Hastings, A.B.: Improved clinical method for estimation of disturbances of acid-base balance of human blood. Medicine, *27*:223, 1948.

CHAPTER 16

PRIMARY RESPIRATORY ACIDOSIS

Primary respiratory acidosis is due to the accumulation of carbon dioxide and carbonic acid in the body. This may occur in one of two ways: (1) when the patient breathes air with a carbon dioxide content above normal, or (2) most commonly, when a pulmonary or neuro-muscular lesion is present which interferes with respiration and with the elimination of carbon dioxide by the lungs.

Synonym: Carbonic acid excess, hypercapnia.

PATHOPHYSIOLOGY

The primary characteristic of respiratory acidosis is an increase (above 46 mm Hg) in the partial pressure of CO_2 in arterial blood. As a result of this, the normal bicarbonate-carbonic acid ratio of 27:1.35 (20:1) decreases, because the carbonic acid concentration may rise to 2.70 or higher. The pH of the blood may therefore fall to 7.0 or lower, as the P_{CO_2} rises (see Chap 13).

When this happens the following compensatory mechanisms develop:

1. The blood buffers react with the carbonic acid and form more basic salts (Chap 12).
2. The following compensatory mechanisms develop in the kidneys (Chap 12).
   a. An increased secretion and excretion of hydrogen ions occur.
   b. Ammonium formation is stimulated, and ammonium ions are excreted.
   c. Bicarbonate is retained, and chloride ions are excreted instead. This causes an increased serum bicarbonate concentration and a decreased serum chloride concentration. The increase in serum bicarbonate concentration is approximately the same as the decrease in serum chloride concentration. Therefore, respiratory acidosis does not affect the anion gap (see Chap 1).
   d. There is also a slight decrease in sodium excretion because of the conservation and retention of bicarbonate. As a result, the serum sodium concentration may rise slightly.
   e. Monohydrogen phosphate is converted into dihydrogen phosphate and is excreted.
3. The acidosis also causes a shift of electrolytes. Hydrogen and sodium

157

ions move into the cells, and potassium ions move from the cells into the extracellular water and blood, causing the serum potassium concentration to rise. This also helps elevate the pH. However, the serum potassium concentration may rise rapidly to a toxic level and may cause ventricular fibrillation and death.

As a result of all these compensatory changes, the bicarbonate concentration and the pH rise toward normal, to produce a partially compensated respiratory acidosis (see Chap 13). However, compensation is apparently always incomplete in patients with severe respiratory acidosis (when the Pco_2 is 80 mm Hg or higher).

If acute respiratory acidosis is produced experimentally in dogs or in human volunteers by having them inhale carbon dioxide gas and the actual *in vitro* compensation is compared to the compensation as determined from blood samples, the two sets of values will not agree, particularly when the Pco_2 is 70 mm Hg or higher. The reason for this is that, during the experimental production of the respiratory acidosis, there is a migration of bicarbonate ions out of the blood into the extravascular extracellular water. As a result, calculations using the blood of these subjects may show a low bicarbonate concentration and a "base deficit," which erroneously suggests that a metabolic acidosis is regularly associated with a respiratory acidosis.

Methods for describing respiratory acidosis in terms of whole body compensation, rather than in terms of blood values, have been described by Brackett, Schwartz, Armstrong, and others.

Many patients may actually overcompensate so that the pH rises above normal. Such patients therefore show a respiratory acidosis (with a high Pco_2) and an overcompensatory metabolic alkalosis, associated with a decreased serum potassium concentration, and the other characteristics of a metabolic alkalosis, namely, high standard bicarbonate concentration, a positive base excess, and a pH above 7.46.

An overcompensatory metabolic alkalosis with an elevated pH can occur in patients with chronic respiratory acidosis in several ways:

1. It has already been pointed out that the respiratory acidosis causes a decreased serum chloride concentration because the kidneys excrete chloride ions at the same time as bicarbonate ions are retained. When the Pco_2 falls to normal, the lost chloride ions must be replaced before the serum bicarbonate concentration can also fall to normal. If this does not occur, a metabolic alkalosis will develop. This is the rationale for the use of potassium chloride as part of the treatment of respiratory acidosis.
2. A metabolic alkalosis may also develop because of the loss of potassium ions after the Pco_2 has been lowered, especially in patients who have received corticosteroids, or the thiazide, or other diuretics.
3. Normally the Pco_2 rises during sleep and falls when one wakens in the morning. When the Pco_2 falls, it decreases the renal tubular reabsorption of bicarbonate ions, which are excreted in the urine. However, this mechanism may be absent in patients with chronic respiratory acidosis.

ETIOLOGY

Acute respiratory acidosis can be caused by acute pulmonary lesions such as acute pulmonary edema, severe pulmonary infections, bronchial obstruction, foreign bodies, mechanical respirators, atelectasis, pneumothorax, hemothorax or open chest wounds, severe abdominal distension, positions on an operating room table which interfere with respiration, central nervous system lesions involving the respiratory center in the medulla, poliomyelitis, rarely extreme loss of potassium ions which interferes with the function of the respiratory muscles, an overdosage of opiates, anesthetics, alcohol, or sedatives which depress respiration.

Acute respiratory acidosis can also result if air with a high carbon dioxide content is inhaled for any length of time. This can occur during surgical anesthesia.

Chronic respiratory acidosis can be caused by chronic pulmonary lesions, such as pulmonary fibrosis, emphysema, bronchiectasis, multiple pulmonary embolizations, bronchial asthma, kyphoscoliosis and chronic cor pulmonale from any cause. Hypoventilation also occurs in some obese patients as part of the Pickwickian syndrome, which is characterized by hypercapnia, cyanosis, somnolence, polycythemia and cor pulmonale. Chronic respiratory acidosis can also occur in brain tumors and when the respiratory nerves are damaged, as in poliomyelitis.

SYMPTOMS AND SIGNS

Acute Respiratory Acidosis

There may not be any evident signs of an acute respiratory acidosis. For example, during an operation, a patient who has a normal color and apparently good oxygenation may develop acute respiratory acidosis if respiratory movements are not sufficient to cause the elimination of carbon dioxide from the lungs. The first sign of respiratory acidosis may therefore be the development of ventricular fibrillation. Ventricular fibrillation may also occur if an acute respiratory acidosis is suddenly corrected.

Carbon dioxide narcosis may occur as a sign of acute respiratory acidosis when a patient with chronic pulmonary disease is given an excessive amount of oxygen.

Carbon Dioxide Narcosis. This syndrome is due to the development of acute respiratory acidosis in a patient with chronic pulmonary disease. It is serious and may be fatal. It is produced in the following way.

The respiratory center is normally sensitive to changes in arterial carbon dioxide content. However, when the partial arterial carbon dioxide pressure (P_{CO_2}) rises above approximately 65 mm Hg, the respiratory center becomes insensitive to carbon dioxide. As a result, hypoxia (anoxia) becomes the main stimulus to respiration, by way of aortic and carotid chemoreceptors, which respond to the lowered arterial *oxygen* saturation. When oxygen is given in a sufficient concentration to raise the arterial oxygen saturation (Pa_{O_2}), this stimulus is removed. Ventilation decreases, and the rate of carbon dioxide elimination is decreased. As a result, increased amounts of carbon dioxide are retained in the blood. This causes the carbon dioxide concentration and carbonic acid concentration of the blood to rise, and the pH to fall. Therefore, the respiratory acidosis deepens, and coma and death may occur.

(The mechanism for carbon dioxide narcosis is probably more complex than this, because it has been shown that patients with emphysema with a normal P_{CO_2} may show a decreased respiratory response when they inhale carbon dioxide.)

The clinical signs of carbon dioxide narcosis are varied. Psychological disturbances are common. There is impairment of consciousness, ranging from drowsiness to deep coma. The patient may be irritable, depressed, euphoric, manic, show paranoid tendencies, or have hallucinations.

Common neurological findings include muscle twitching and tremors of the face or limbs. Flaccid or spastic paralysis of the extremities may occur, as may myoclonus or generalized convulsions. The deep tendon reflexes may be unequal, diminished, or absent. *Asterixis* (an abnormal involuntary jerking movement of the hands which occurs when the patient is asked to put the wrist in dorsiflexion and then extend and spread the fingers) is common. The electroencephalogram may show increased or decreased voltage with prominent theta waves or abnormal alpha waves.

The corneal reflexes may disappear during deep coma. The pupils may be small or dilated, unequal, or sluggish in reaction. Blurring of vision may occur, in association with increased cerebrospinal pressure (pseudotumor cerebri).

Slight respiratory depression, or even apnea, may be present. Cardiovascular signs such as tachycardia and a warm flushed skin with excessive perspiration (due to acidosis) may be present. The blood pressure varies. It may be elevated, or hypotension or signs of shock may appear.

When carbon dioxide narcosis develops slowly, coma does not usually appear until the P_{CO_2} is 80 mm Hg or higher. However, if it develops rapidly, coma may develop when the P_{CO_2} is only 60 mm Hg.

Chronic Respiratory Acidosis

A patient with chronic respiratory acidosis usually has severe chronic pulmonary disease, especially bronchiectasis, chronic bronchitis, or pulmonary fibrosis. He or she may show hyperpnea, a chronic productive cough, cyanosis, polycythemia, and a typical emphysematous barrel chest. However, the decreased oxygenation of the blood (low PaO_2) which is present, or even cyanosis which may be present, does not itself indicate that respiratory acidosis (high PCO_2) is also present in these patients.

General symptoms, such as weakness and a dull headache, may also be present. When the respiratory acidosis becomes acute, stupor or coma may develop (see Carbon Dioxide Narcosis, above).

The depression of the central nervous system that occurs in acidosis is due more to a decreased pH of the spinal fluid than to a decreased pH of the blood. Therefore, symptoms are more common and more profound in respiratory acidosis than in metabolic acidosis, because respiratory acidosis is associated with a retention of carbon dioxide which quickly and easily diffuses across the blood-brain barrier. (A metabolic acidosis is not primarily associated with a retention of carbon dioxide, but with the retention of hydrogen ions from metabolic disturbances. In these patients, the increased hydrogen ions do not easily move across the blood-brain barrier.)

Cardiac arrhythmias, such as shifting pacemaker, atrial tachycardia, atrial or ventricular premature beats, may occur.

LABORATORY FINDINGS

These depend on whether the respiratory acidosis is acute or chronic.

Acute Respiratory Acidosis

The typical compensatory changes are not yet apparent. Therefore, the characteristic findings are:

pH.—This falls to the lower level of normal. However, it may reach 7 or lower, in a few minutes.

PCO_2.—This is above the upper level of normal (about 46 mm Hg) and may rise to 120 mm Hg or higher.

CO_2 content.—This rises to the upper normal level of 28 mEq/L and may exceed this.

Standard bicarbonate and base excess.—These remain normal.

Actual bicarbonate.—This rises to the upper limit of normal (26 mEq/L) and may reach 29 mEq/L, but it does not exceed this.

Notice that the actual bicarbonate is higher than the standard bicarbonate. This is a characteristic finding in respiratory acidosis. The normal base excess indicates that metabolic balance is present.

95% Confidence Bands. Figure 13–1, page 135, shows the pH and PCO_2 ranges in both acute and chronic respiratory acidosis. Notice that the high PCO_2 values of acute respiratory acidosis are associated with lower pH values than occur in chronic respiratory acidosis.

These confidence bands can be used for diagnosis. For example, if a patient with respiratory acidosis shows a pH of 7.2 and a PCO_2 of 70 mm Hg, and if these values are plotted on Figure 13–1, they meet within the confidence band of acute respiratory acidosis. This highly suggests that the patient has an acute respiratory acidosis.

Serum Electrolytes. The cation-anion balance is normal. The serum sodium concentration may rise slightly as a result of the respiratory acidosis. The serum potassium concentration may become high. If the PCO_2 is lowered by treatment, the serum potassium concentration may fall even below normal, and signs of hypokalemia may develop.

Example: Acute respiratory acidosis in a patient during surgical anesthesia.
pH, 7.22
PCO_2, 80 mm Hg
CO_2 content, 33.9 mEq/L
Standard bicarbonate, 26 mEq/L
Actual bicarbonate, 31.5 mEq/L
Base excess, +2.5 mEq/L
Serum potassium concentration, 6 mEq/L

The pH is low, indicating an acidosis. The PCO_2 is high, indicating that a respiratory acidosis is present. Similarly, the actual bicarbonate is higher than the standard bicarbonate, because of the respiratory acidosis. The base excess is normal, indicating that metabolic balance is present.

When the pH and PCO_2 values are plotted on the diagram of Figure 15–4, page 154, this also indicates that a respiratory acidosis with metabolic balance is present.

Chronic Respiratory Acidosis

The changes in pH, PCO_2 and CO_2 content, described for acute respiratory acidosis patients, are present. However, the kidneys have been able to retain bicarbonate, so that the CO_2 capacity and the pH rise. This is associated with a reciprocal fall in serum chloride concentration. The serum sodium concentration may be slightly elevated, and the serum potassium concentration is also elevated.

The 95% confidence band of chronic respiratory acidosis patients is discussed in Chapter 13.

Example: Patient with chronic respiratory acidosis.
pH, 7.4
PCO_2, 66 mm Hg
CO_2 content, 33.9 mEq/L
Standard bicarbonate, 31 mEq/L
Actual bicarbonate, 39.5 mEq/L
Base excess, +8 mEq/L

The pH is normal. This indicates that if any acid-base disturbance is present, it is compensated. The P_{CO_2} is high. This indicates a respiratory acidosis. Similarly, the actual bicarbonate is higher than the standard bicarbonate. The base excess is high. This indicates that a metabolic alkalosis is present.

When the pH and P_{CO_2} values are plotted on the diagram of Figure 15–4, this also indicates that a respiratory acidosis and a metabolic alkalosis are present.

However, these values do not indicate whether the respiratory acidosis or the metabolic alkalosis is primary. One indirect clue is the P_{CO_2} of 66 mm Hg because it is rare for the P_{CO_2} to rise higher than 55 or 60 mm Hg when a compensatory respiratory acidosis develops in a patient with a primary metabolic alkalosis (see Chap 26). In most patients, a knowledge of the history and clinical course is necessary to determine whether the respiratory or the metabolic disturbance is primary (or whether two independent acid-base disturbances are present; see Chap 29).

Example: Same patient.
Cation-anion balance
Na 143;   K 5.5; HCO_3 39.5   Cl 85 mEq/L

   Anion gap = (Na + K) − (HCO_3 + Cl)
         = (143 + 5.5) − (39.5 + 85)
         = 148.5 − 124.5
         = 24 mEq/L. This is a slight elevation of the anion gap (normal 16 mEq/L or less). It is due to the chronic hypoxemia which is present. This causes an accumulation of lactic and other acid metabolites.

DIAGNOSIS

Respiratory acidosis (P_{CO_2} above 50 mm Hg) is almost always associated with hypoxemia (Pa_{O_2} below 60 mm Hg) unless a patient with normal ventilation has been inhaling carbon dioxide. However, hypoxemia can exist with or without respiratory acidosis, for example:

Hypoxemia *with* respiratory acidosis (*ventilatory failure*) occurs in patients with chronic obstructive pulmonary disease (COPD), neuromuscular diseases affecting the respiratory muscles, as a result of the depressant effect of drugs on breathing, and so on.

Hypoxemia *without* respiratory acidosis (*gas exchange failure*) occurs in patients with acute pulmonary edema, shock, massive pulmonary embolism, interstitial fibrosis and other causes of alveolar-capillary block, and so on. (Discussion of hypoxemia without respiratory acidosis is outside the scope of this book.)

(Normally, the arterial oxygen content is more than 80 mm Hg [corresponding to a hemoglobin oxygen saturation of approximately 95%]. [Normal elderly persons have slightly lower values.] Hypoxemia is minimal until the Pa_{O_2} falls to approximately 55 mm Hg, but becomes serious when the PaO_2 falls below 45 mm Hg, and dangerous to life when it falls to approximately 30 mm Hg.

Acute respiratory acidosis should be suspected or anticipated when inadequate respiratory ventilation or signs of shock occur in any acutely ill or injured patient, or during an operation. The patient may show good color, and is usually not cyanosed. One of the earliest signs of acute respiratory acidosis may be the development of electrocardiographic signs of hyperkalemia.

Characteristic laboratory findings of a respiratory acidosis are a low pH and a high Pco_2. However, metabolic compensation often occurs in a chronic respiratory acidosis. The pH may not only return to normal but may even become high due to the metabolic alkalosis which has developed. However, this does not occur in patients with severe respiratory acidosis, who show a Pco_2 greater than 80 mm Hg (also see page 134).

COURSE AND PROGNOSIS

If pulmonary obstruction is suddenly released by tracheotomy, for example, in an acute respiratory acidosis, the patient may begin to hyperventilate and may eliminate a large amount of carbon dioxide. However, bicarbonate concentration may remain temporarily high. As a result, an acute respiratory alkalosis and tetany may develop. Death in acute respiratory acidosis is often due to ventricular fibrillation. This is probably caused by the sudden development of hyperkalemia.

In patients with chronic respiratory acidosis, most of the pulmonary changes are chronic and irreversible. Therefore, the prognosis for such a patient is poor.

TREATMENT

Acute Respiratory Acidosis

If acute respiratory acidosis is suspected in a surgical patient, assisted respiration or intubation should be used. Moore has pointed out that there is no time to wait for chemical confirmation, because pH can be lowered to 7.2 within 8 minutes of rebreathing, or breathing a carbon dioxide enriched mixture, even in a normal subject.

If hyperkalemia and ventricular fibrillation occur in a patient with acute respiratory acidosis, the intravenous use of the sodium bicarbonate may be lifesaving. One to two or more ampuls of the concentrated 7.5% solution (Chap 35) can be given undiluted intravenously, in association with cardiopulmonary resuscitation.

ACUTE RESPIRATORY ACIDOSIS COMPLICATING CHRONIC OBSTRUCTIVE PULMONARY DISEASE (COPD)

This can be treated in the following way:

1. Treat hypoxemia, if necessary. If the PaO_2 is 50 mm Hg or higher, oxygen therapy is generally not needed (Keighley and Mithoefer). If the PaO_2 is less than 50 mm Hg oxygen should be given with a Venturi type of mask, rather than with nasal cannulas, to ensure sustained adequate oxygenation. A flow rate of 28% (rarely 35%) is adequate. The PaO_2 should be raised only to 60 mm Hg, to prevent carbon dioxide narcosis.

   Oxygen can also be given at a concentration not exceeding 40%, using nasal catheters or cannulas, at a flow rate of 1 to 2 liters per minute, or less. However, this requires a special flowmeter.

   The PCO_2 should be checked periodically. If it rises when oxygen is given, this may be a sign of impending carbon dioxide narcosis. Stop the oxygen.

2. Eliminate thick secretions. An increased fluid intake (oral or parenteral) helps decrease the viscosity of bronchial secretions. In addition, the inspired air should be humidified to 100% saturation with water. A solution of acetylcysteine can also be given, either with a nebulizer or with intermittent positive pressure breathing apparatus, to help liquefy the thick mucus. (Acetylcysteine must be used cautiously in patients with bronchial asthma because it can induce bronchospasm.)

   If the patient's cough reflex is adequate, deep breathing exercises and postural drainage may also be helpful. If the cough reflex is ineffective, nasotracheal suctioning or bronchoscopy may be indicated.

3. Treat bronchospasm. A bronchodilator such as racemic epinephrine (Vaponefrin) (2.25% solution) can be given by nebulizer. Aminophylline can be given intravenously. Oral bronchodilators such as theophylline or other xanthines or terbutaline a beta-2 agonist, albuterol, isoetharine, metaproterenol, or isoproterenol, are also of value. Corticosteroids can be used if life-threatening bronchospasm persists. Some patients may require long-term therapy with oral corticosteroids.

4. Treat respiratory infection, if present, with an appropriate antibiotic.

5. Maintain an adequate airway. Endotracheal intubation or tracheostomy may be needed if the PaO_2 does not rise with medical treatment. Mechanical ventilation should be used only if the patient is apneic, or has not responded to treatment.

6. Alkalinizing drugs. Sodium bicarbonate should be used to raise the pH only when it is not possible to lower the PCO_2 promptly, and when the pH is less than 7.20. If an excessive amount of sodium bicarbonate is given concomitantly with treatment which decreases the PCO_2, the patient may develop an acute metabolic alkalosis, even with tetany. (If sodium bicarbonate is given to a patient with respiratory acidosis, the pH must be carefully monitored and the amount of sodium bicarbonate given should be calculated to raise the pH only to 7.30 [see page 180 for method of calculating sodium bicarbonate dosage].)

Chronic Respiratory Acidosis

The treatment of chronic respiratory acidosis depends on many factors—the degree of hypoxemia, presence of infection, bronchospasm, and so on.

Oxygen therapy is not needed in every patient with chronic respiratory acidosis. For example, a patient with chronic obstructive pulmonary disease can continue to be ambulatory even when the PaO_2 is persistently 40 mm Hg and the PCO_2 50 mm Hg or higher. However, when oxygen is indicated, it should be used as described above.

General therapy is as follows. The patient must stop smoking. Antihistamines should be avoided because they cause thickening of the bronchial mucus. Sedatives should also be avoided because they may depress respiration. Bronchial or pulmonary infections should be treated promptly with appropriate antibiotics. Bronchospasm can be treated with theophylline or other preparations described above. Corticosteroids should be avoided unless other medication is not effective; then they should be given in minimally effective doses. When given on a long-term basis, the patient may also need isoniazid to prevent reactivation of a quiescent tuberculosis infection. IPPB has been used in patients with chronic obstructive pulmonary disease, but its value has been questioned. Cough and thick bronchial secretions can be treated by adequate hydration and by the use of water vapor inhalation, postural drainage, and physical therapy with chest percussion. Potassium iodide drops have also been used to loosen thick bronchial secretions.

One should remember that chronic respiratory acidosis, itself, does not require treatment. However, severe hypoxemia must always be treated.

Vigorous treatment of chronic respiratory acidosis patients with mechanical ventilation may be associated with the development of generalized convulsions and other signs of central nervous system excitation, and coma, along with the development of a respiratory alkalosis. Because of this, the elevated PCO_2 should be decreased slowly.

A carbonic anhydrase inhibitor such as Diamox may be helpful, with small doses of digitalis, if the patient has chronic cor pulmonale and congestive heart failure. The mechanism by which a carbonic anhydrase inhibitor is able to lower the arterial carbon dioxide tension and improve the mental state of patients with chronic respiratory acidosis is not known. A metabolic acidosis may develop from the use of the drug and this may cause a compensatory hyperventilation.

If a metabolic alkalosis, with a high pH, is present in chronic respiratory acidosis, the patient should be given potassium chloride to correct the alkalosis, in addition to the other treatment for the respiratory acidosis.

REFERENCES

Aberman, A., and Fulop, M.: The metabolic and respiratory acidosis of acute pulmonary edema. Ann Intern Med, *76*:173, 1972.

Addis, G.J.: Bicarbonate buffering in acute exacerbation of chronic respiratory failure. Thorax, *20*:337, 1965.

Armstrong, B.W., Mohler, J.G., et al.: The in-vivo carbon dioxide titration curve. Lancet, *1*:759, 1966.

Bader, M.E., and Bader, R.A.: Respiratory stimulants in obstructive lung disease. Am J Med, *38*:165, 1965.

Beale, H.D., Schiller, I.W., Halperin, M.H., Franklin, W., and Lowell, F.C.: Delirium and coma precipitated by oxygen in bronchial asthma complicated by respiratory acidosis. N Engl J Med, *244*:710, 1951.

Bedon, G.A., Block, A.J., and Ball, W.C., Jr.: The "28%" Venturi mask in obstructive airway disease. Arch Intern Med, *125*:106, 1970.

Berliner, R.W., and Orloff, J.: Carbonic anhydrase inhibitors. Pharmacol Rev, *8*:137, 1956.

Brackett, N.C., Jr., Cohen, J.J., and Schwartz, W.B.: Carbon dioxide titration curve of normal man: Effect of increasing degrees of acute hypercapnia on acid-base equilibrium. N Engl J Med, *272*:6, 1965. Also ibid. *280*:124, 1969.

Campbell, E.J.M.: Respiratory failure. Br Med J, *1*:1451, 1965.

Carter, N.W., Seldin, D.W., and Teng, H.C.: Tissue and renal response to chronic respiratory acidosis. J Clin Invest, *38*:949, 1959.

Cochran, R.T., Jr.: Pulmonary insufficiency and hypercapnia complicated by potassium-responsive alkalosis. N Engl J Med, *268*:521, 1963.

Comroe, J.H., Jr., Bahnson, E.R., and Coates, E.O., Jr.: Mental changes occurring in chronically ill anoxemia patients during oxygen therapy. JAMA, *143*:1044, 1950.

Editorial: Convulsions after therapy for alveolar hypoventilation, JAMA, *189*:993, 1964.

Editorial: Carbon dioxide in body fluids. N Engl J Med, *280*:162, 1969.

Eichenholz, A., Blumentals, A.S., and Walker, F.E.: The pattern of compensatory response to chronic hypercapnia in patients with chronic obstructive pulmonary disease. J Lab Clin Med, *68*:265, 1966.

Foulds, H.P.S., Mendel, D., and deMowbray, R.R.: Changes in serum potassium level and in pH of arterial blood in respiratory acidosis. Lancet, *1*:405, 1958.

Gaensler, E.A.: Respiratory acidosis as seen following surgery. Am J Surg, *103*:289, 1962.

Giebisch, G., Berger, L., and Pitts, R.F.: The extrarenal response to acute acid-base disturbances of respiratory origin. J Clin Invest, *27*:231, 1955.

Haynie, G.D., et al.: Recovery from chronic hypercapnia. The critical role of chloride in restoration of normal acid-base equilibrium. J Clin Invest, *40*:1047, 1961.

Hunter, C.C.: Errors in management of patients dying of chronic obstructive lung disease. JAMA, *199*:488, 1967.

Keighley, J.V.H., and Mithoefer, J.C.: The management of arterial hypoxia in chronic obstructive pulmonary disease. Chest, *62*:45S, 1972.

Kettel, L.J.: Acute respiratory acidosis. Hospital Med, *12*:31, 1976.

Kettel, L.J., et al.: Treatment of acute respiratory acidosis in chronic obstructive lung disease. JAMA, *217*:1503, 1971.

Levitin, H., Branscome, W., and Epstein, E.H.: The pathogenesis of hypochloremia in respiratory acidosis. J Clin Invest, *37*:166, 1958.

MacDonald, F.M.: Respiratory acidosis. Arch Intern Med, *116*:681, 1965.

Maier, H.C., Rich, G.S., and Eichen, S.: Clinical significance of respiratory acidosis during operations. Ann Surg, *134*:653, 1951.

Makoff, D.L., and Rosenbaum, B.J.: Potassium depletion and hypercapnia. N Engl J Med, *280*:669, 1969.

Makoff, D.: Compensatory patterns in acid-base disorders. Geriatrics, *26*:107, 1971.

McCurdy, D.K.: Mixed metabolic and respiratory acid-base disturbances. Diagnosis and treatment. Chest, *62*:35S, 1972.

Miller, A., Bader, R., and Bader, M.E.: The neurologic syndrome due to marked hypercapnia with papilledema. Am J Med, *33*:309, 1962.

Moore, F.D.: Common patterns of water and electrolyte change in injury, surgery and disease. N Engl J Med, *258*:277, 325, 377, 427, 1958.

Nordqvist, P., et al.: Two hospital cases with CO_2 retention from insufficient ventilation requiring tracheostomy. Acta Med Scand, *166*:189, 1960.

O'Reilley, R.J.: The clinical recognition of carbon dioxide intoxication. Dis Chest, *37*:185, 1960.

O'Donohue, W.J., Jr., and Baker, J.P.: Controlled low-flow oxygen in the management of acute respiratory failure. Chest, *63*:818, 1973.

Pitt, B., et al.: Respiratory failure with focal neurological signs. Arch Intern Med, *115*:714, 1965.

Rastegar, A., and Thier, S.O.: Physiological consequences and bodily adaptations to hyper- and hypocapnia. Chest, *62*:28S, 1972.

Robin, E.D.: Abnormalities of acid-base regulation in chronic pulmonary disease, with special reference to hypercapnia and extracellular alkalosis. N Engl J Med, *268*:917, 1963.

Rodman, T., and Close, H.P.: Primary hypoventilation syndrome. Am J Med, *26*:808, 1959.

Schwartz, W.B.: Defense of extracellular pH during acute and chronic hypercapnia. Ann New York Acad Sci, *133*:125, 131, 1966. Also N Engl J Med, *272*:319, 1965.

Sealy, W.C., Young, W.G., Jr., and Harris, J.S.: Studies on cardiac arrest: The relationship of hypercapnia to ventricular fibrillation. J Thorac Surg, *28*:477, 1954.

Vandenlberg, R., et al.: Oxygen therapy in acute respiratory failure. Med J Aust, *2*:874, 1970.

Weiss, E.B., and Dulfano, M.J.: Quantitative acid-base dynamics in chronic pulmonary disease. Defense of pH during acute respiratory acidosis superimposed upon chronic hypercapnia. Ann Intern Med, *69*:263, 1968.

CHAPTER 17

METABOLIC ACIDOSIS SYNDROMES

The term *metabolic acidosis* describes acidosis resulting from a relative excess of inorganic or organic acids which are not freely excreted by the kidneys, or from a loss of base from the body.

Synonyms: Base deficit, bicarbonate deficit.

PATHOPHYSIOLOGY

We know that a metabolic acidosis develops because of an increased amount of acid or a decreased amount of base in the body. As a result of this, the normal bicarbonate-carbonic acid ratio of 27/1.35 (20/1) decreases, and the pH falls below 7.36 and may fall to 7.0 or lower (see Chap 22).

The decreased pH stimulates the respiratory center, and increased depth and rate of respiration occur in an attempt to lower the carbonic acid concentration and restore the pH to its normal value. (Pulmonary compensation is usually not complete.) In addition, the renal compensatory mechanisms described in Chapter 16 for respiratory acidosis may develop, and bicarbonate ions may be retained.

As a result of these compensatory changes, namely, the pulmonary elimination of carbon dioxide and the renal retention of bicarbonate, the bicarbonate-carbonic acid ratio and the pH rise toward normal.

When renal insufficiency is the cause of the acidosis, the renal compensatory mechanisms will be inadequate. In addition, pulmonary compensation may be markedly inadequate if the patient has chronic pulmonary disease and a respiratory acidosis. Such a patient will not be able to hyperventilate sufficiently to remove the excess carbonic acid.

The compensatory hyperventilation which occurs as a result of the metabolic acidosis may persist even after the patient is no longer acidotic. The reason for this is not known. However, this observation is important because the patient who is recovering from metabolic acidosis can develop a serious respiratory alkalosis due to the hyperventilation which continues.

This can lead to great confusion particularly if an alkaline salt such as sodium bicarbonate or sodium lactate has been given to correct the metabolic acidosis. The reason for this is as follows: The original metabolic acidosis causes a low actual bicarbonate and standard bicarbonate. The sodium bicarbonate or lactate causes the pH and the bicarbonate values to rise. However, the compensatory respiratory alkalosis, due to hyperventilation, persists even when the metabolic acidosis is corrected. This causes the pH to rise and the actual bicarbonate to fall. The standard bicarbonate also tends to remain low to compensate for the respiratory alkalosis which has developed. Therefore, if the patient's progress is being checked only by determination of the CO_2 content, it will be noted that, as the alkalinizing salt is given, the rise in CO_2 values will be deceptively low in relation to the rise in pH, and will be deceptively high in relation to the rise in P_{CO_2}.

The following example illustrates this. Bock, Field, and Adair described a 14-year-old boy (case 4) who was admitted to the hospital with typical signs of diabetic acidosis and stupor. Immediate treatment consisted of small doses of insulin, subcutaneous saline, and orange juice by mouth. After 6 hours, his condition was only slightly improved. Therefore, he was given 4 g of sodium bicarbonate in a rectal enema of 6 ounces of 5% dextrose every 3 hours, a total of 32 g a day. This was continued for 3 days. The following are some of the electrolyte concentrations:

Date	CO_2 Content	P_{CO_2}	pH
Jan. 29	4.37 mm Eq/L	9.7 mm Hg	7.03
Jan. 31	16.0	21.4	7.46

Notice that the CO_2 content had risen more than 3 times, but that the P_{CO_2} had risen less than 3 times its previous value. The rise in the CO_2 content indicates that the patient's metabolic acidosis was being corrected. Theoretically, when this happened, the compensatory hyperventilation and the respiratory alkalosis should have stopped and the P_{CO_2} should have risen almost to normal. This did not occur. The hyperventilation and the respiratory alkalosis continued, even though the original stimulus, namely, the low pH of 7.03, was no longer present, and even though an alkalosis with a pH of 7.46 had developed.

ETIOLOGY

Patients with metabolic acidosis can be classified in several ways. For example, they can be divided into two groups: those with a normal anion gap (Na + K) − (HCO$_3$ + Cl) of approximately 16 mEq/L or less (Chap 1), and those with an abnormally large anion gap (22 mEq/L or more), due to the accumulation of abnormal acid anions.

The serum bicarbonate concentration is reduced in both groups of patients. However, when the anion gap is normal, the serum chloride concentration becomes reciprocally elevated to fill the gap produced by the decreased serum bicarbonate concentration (hyperchloremic metabolic acidosis). When the anion gap is increased, unmeasured anions fill this gap.

Metabolic Acidosis Associated with a Normal Anion Gap

These patients show an increased serum chloride concentration (*hyperchloremic metabolic acidosis*).

1. Administration of ammonium chloride or other chloride salts (see below).
2. Carbonic anhydrase inhibitor administration (see below).
3. Other drugs, such as sulfamylon, cholestyramine.
4. "Dilution" acidosis (see below).
5. Diarrheas or draining gastrointestinal (particularly pancreatic) fistulas (see below).
6. Proximal or distal renal tubular acidosis (Chap 18).
7. Intravenous hyperalimentation.
8. Post-hypocapnia.

Metabolic Acidosis Associated with an Abnormal (Large) Anion Gap

These patients show a normal serum chloride concentration, but an accumulation of unmeasured acid anions.

1. Diabetic ketoacidosis (Chap 22).
2. Azotemia (Chap 20).
3. Lactic acidosis (Chap 19).
4. Salicylate (salicylic acid) intoxication (Chap 23).
5. Ethyl alcohol nondiabetic ketoacidosis (Chap 22).
6. Intoxication due to the accumulation of other acids, for example methanol (methyl alcohol), formic acid, paraldehyde, various organic acids, boric acid, ethylene glycol, oxalic acid and other acids.

Further, patients with metabolic acidosis can be described based on the presence of an acid excess or a base (bicarbonate ion) deficit.

Metabolic Acidosis Due to Acid Excess (Acid Gain Acidosis)

This occurs from an increase in the absolute amount of acids in the blood. Normally, the catabolism of proteins and nucleic acids produces amino acids, phosphoric, sulfuric and uric acids. Similarly, lactic, pyruvic, and succinic acids are produced in the course of carbohydrate catabolism, and ketone and fatty acids are produced from the hydrolysis and oxidation of fats. However, these acids may accumulate in the body in the following way:

1. Diabetic acidosis (Chap 22).
2. Starvation. When there is a deficient intake of carbohydrate, an increased

catabolism of body protein and fat occurs. This causes an increase in ketone acids.
3. Surgical anesthesia.
4. High fever, infectious diseases, and anorexia. The increased metabolic needs of the body in association with decreased food intake, as well as anoxia, causes an increased production of metabolic acids.
5. Thyrotoxicosis. The increased metabolic demands on the body may deplete the carbohydrate stores. As a result, energy is supplied from the catabolism of protein and fat. This causes an excessive amount of ketone acids.
6. Violent exercise, and convulsions.
7. Shock.
8. Lactic acidosis (Chap 19).

Metabolic Acidosis Due to Dietary or Parenteral Intake of Excessive Acids

This can occur in the following ways:

Chloride Acidosis. This is the result of the oral or parenteral administration of acids, such as hydrochloric acid, or salts containing chloride ions, such as sodium chloride (when given in excessive amounts parenterally), calcium chloride, ammonium chloride, cation exchange resins, arginine HCl, or carbonic anhydrase inhibitors.

Ammonium Chloride. Ammonium chloride acidosis usually occurs in patients with severe congestive heart failure who have been receiving large amounts of ammonium chloride as a diuretic. The ammonium ion NH_4 reaches the liver and is converted to ammonia, NH_3, releasing a hydrogen ion and producing an acidosis. The ammonia is later converted to urea and excreted. Part of the chloride is also excreted by the kidneys with sodium and water. (It acts as a diuretic in this way.)

When the ammonium chloride is given for only 3 or 4 days at a time, it merely produces a mild asymptomatic acidosis. However, if it is given continuously for weeks at a time, particularly to patients who already are acidotic due to renal disease, or if an excessive amount of ammonium chloride is given intravenously, it can cause a severe metabolic acidosis with symptoms and signs of ammonia toxicity, such as pallor, sweating, retching, Kussmaul type of hyperventilation or irregular breathing, bradycardia, cardiac arrhythmias, local and general muscle twitching, tonic convulsions, and coma. (Electrolyte determinations show a high chloride and low bicarbonate (page 178).)

A high BUN concentration may develop with ammonium chloride acidosis. The cause of this is obscure. It disappears when the metabolic acidosis is corrected.

Carbonic Anhydrase Inhibitors. On page 128 it was pointed out that all the bicarbonate ions which pass the glomeruli and enter the tubular urine (glomerular filtrate) are reabsorbed. This occurs because the hydrogen and bicarbonate ions are produced in the tubule cells by means of carbonic anhydrase. The hydrogen ions pass into the urine and react with sodium bicarbonate to form carbonic acid, which is excreted. The sodium ions pass back into the tubular cells, react with the bicarbonate, and then pass back into the plasma as sodium bicarbonate.

When a carbonic anhydrase inhibitor such as Diamox is given, carbonic acid is not formed in the kidney tubule cells, and a large amount of sodium bicarbonate and water is excreted in the urine. This causes a diuresis and also an acidosis, due to the loss of bicarbonate. In addition, a large amount of potassium ions is also excreted in the urine. (There is an exchange mechanism for potassium and hydrogen ions in the kidney tubule cells. This causes hydrogen and potassium ions to be excreted in inverse proportional concentrations in the urine.)

Sodium Chloride. Large doses of sodium chloride parenterally (especially in the form of hypertonic saline) can cause a metabolic acidosis in the following way: Normally, the extracellular water contains more sodium ions than chloride ions, Na 142 mEq/L to Cl, 100 Eq/L. Isotonic saline solution contains approximately 150 mEq of sodium and chloride per liter. Therefore, when a large amount of sodium chloride is administered and kidney function is not normal, an excess of chloride ions is added to the body. The sodium ions are excreted as sodium bicarbonate and the chloride ions are retained with hydrogen ions. This can produce a metabolic acidosis.

An increased volume of extracellular water can itself produce a metabolic acidosis in the following way: If one adds some neutral fluid, such as isotonic saline solution, to a buffer solution which contains sodium bicarbonate and carbonic acid in a normal bicarbonate-carbonic acid ratio of 20:1 (see Chap 12), the buffering capacity of the solution, per unit volume, will decrease, but the pH will not change, because the bicarbonate-carbonic acid ratio does not change. However, if a large volume of isotonic saline solution is infused into a patient and the extracellular water volume is increased in this way, the pH will fall, because carbon dioxide and carbonic acid are constantly being produced in the body and the bicarbonate-carbonic acid ratio becomes smaller. The metabolic acidosis produced in this way has been called a *dilution (or expansion) acidosis.*

Calcium Chloride. When calcium chloride is given orally, the calcium is not able to penetrate the intestinal mucosa, but the chloride ions are absorbed as hydrochloric acid.

Cation Exchange Resins. These resins exchange cations, such as hydrogen, ammonium, and potassium, for sodium, in the intestinal tract, the sodium being excreted in the stool. However, excessive use of the resins may remove large amounts of sodium, and also potassium, calcium and magnesium, replacing these ions with hydrogen ions. As a result, a severe metabolic acidosis may develop.

Boric Acid Poisoning. This may cause metabolic acidosis.

Salicylic Acid Poisoning (Chap 23).

Methanol Poisoning. Acidosis occurs as a result of the formation of formic and other organic acids.

Ethylene Glycol Poisoning. Ethylene glycol is the active ingredient in permanent antifreeze solutions. If it is imbibed, a metabolic acidosis, acute renal failure and death may develop. The metabolic acidosis is due to the breakdown of the ethylene glycol to oxalic acid which crystallizes in the kidneys. In addition, other metabolic acids are formed.

Metabolic Acidosis Due to Retention of Acids Normally Produced

This occurs in renal disease where sulfuric and phosphoric acids particularly, as well as other metabolic acids, are retained in the body (see Chap 20).

Metabolic Acidosis Due to Loss of Base (Bicarbonate Ions)

This can occur with loss of intestinal secretions, due to severe diarrheas, small bowel fistulas, or severe biliary fistulas. (This type of acidosis can also occur in patients with renal tubular acidosis [Chap 18].)

The mechanism by which a metabolic acidosis occurs with a loss of intestinal secretions is as follows: In the stomach, the parietal cells form carbonic acid from carbon dioxide and water by means of the enzyme carbonic anhydrase. The carbonic acid dissociates into hydrogen and bicarbonate ions. The hydrogen ions enter the stomach lumen along with chloride to form hydrochloric acid and the bicarbonate enters the bloodstream. (This produces the transient "alkaline tide" noted after meals.)

In the alkaline medium of the intestines, the intestinal epithelial cells also form carbonic acid from carbon dioxide and water, by means of carbonic anhydrase. However, here, the hydrogen ions pass back into the bloodstream and the bicarbonate ions pass into the lumen of the gut. This restores the neutrality of the blood.

When a diarrhea occurs, large amounts of bicarbonate are secreted into the gut and excreted. In addition, more hydrogen ions enter the blood than are needed to neutralize the bicarbonate which entered the blood from the stomach when hydrochloric acid was formed. The hydrogen ions react with sodium bicarbonate in the blood, forming carbonic acid. This dissociates into water and carbon dioxide, which is eliminated by the lungs. As a result, the bicarbonate concentration and the bicarbonate-carbonic acid ratio fall, causing a decreased pH and an acidosis. Sodium ions are also excreted into the gut along with bicarbonate as sodium bicarbonate. Therefore, the serum sodium concentration may be lowered.

SYMPTOMS AND SIGNS

A mild metabolic acidosis may be asymptomatic. Symptoms usually appear when the CO_2 content falls to 18.2 mEq/L (40 vol %), or lower. The patient may complain of weakness or general malaise, or dull headache. In addition, nausea, vomiting, and abdominal pain may be present. Characteristic *deep* respirations (Kussmaul breathing, air hunger) are often present. This is more common in acute metabolic acidosis than in chronic metabolic acidosis. The respiratory rate is also usually increased, but may be slow. The increased depth of respiration is more characteristic of acidosis than the increased respiratory rate.

These signs are usually present when the CO_2 content falls below 9.1 mEq/L and the pH is 7.2 or lower. When the pH falls to 7.0, respiratory depression may occur.

Peripheral vasodilatation may be present. This produces a warm and flushed skin, a wide pulse pressure with a bounding pulse and active apical impulse.

Osteomalacia may develop as a complication of chronic metabolic acidosis, because calcium salts may be withdrawn from bone for use as buffers to neutralize the excessive hydrogen ions.

The clinical picture also depends on the cause of the acidosis. Diabetic acidosis patients may have a fruity, acetone odor to the breath, and may show signs of severe water loss, such as thirst and dry mucous membranes, or signs of severe sodium loss, such as loss of skin turgor and shock. In addition, hyperglycemia, ketonemia, ketonuria and glycosuria are present.

Uremic patients also have a fruity odor to the breath and may show signs of water or sodium loss. Muscle twitching may occur because of a decreased concentration of ionized serum calcium. Convulsions may occur, usually due to hypertensive encephalopathy and not to uremia or acidosis.

When the pH falls below 7.0, the cardiac output decreases and bradycardia may develop; the circulatory system becomes unresponsive to catecholamines. This is particularly important when a patient develops metabolic acidosis associated with cardiogenic shock, or particularly cardiac arrest. In such a patient, it is imperative to raise the pH to 7.30 if possible, in association with other treatment.

When the pH in a diabetic acidosis patient decreases to 7.0 or less, the acidosis interferes with carbohydrate metabolism and with the effectiveness of insulin. The pH in such a patient should also be raised with intravenous sodium bicarbonate.

Electrocardiogram

Hyperkalemia is often associated with acidosis, for reasons already discussed. However, the electrocardiogram may or may not show signs

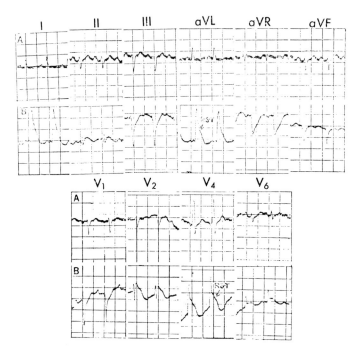

Fig. 17–1. Electrocardiogram in acidosis. A metabolic acidosis was produced in this patient by 700 ml of 5% NaCl, which was given because of a severe sodium loss syndrome and shock, which had been treated with an excessive amount of norepinephrine in dextrose in water. *A:* Minimal changes in lead aVL. The patient has been digitalized. *B:* Twelve hours later, marked ST elevations, characteristic of myocardial injury, in leads I, II aVL, $V_{2,4,5}$. At autopsy, no signs of myocardial or pericardial injury were present.

of hyperkalemia (Chap 24). Patients with diabetic acidosis may show signs of hypokalemia (Chap 27), and these signs may become more marked with treatment (if the serum potassium concentration becomes lowered). When azotemic acidosis is present, the electrocardiogram may show signs of hypocalcemia as well as hyperkalemia (prolongation of the Q-T interval and peaked T waves).

Severe acidosis can cause ST deviations of the type usually found in myocardial injury (Fig. 17–1).

LABORATORY FINDINGS

The laboratory findings are somewhat different in uncompensated and compensated metabolic acidosis.

Uncompensated Metabolic Acidosis

In a patient with uncompensated metabolic acidosis, renal and pulmonary compensatory mechanisms have not yet developed. Therefore, the pH is low and the P_{CO_2} is normal. The standard bicarbonate is low and equal to the actual bicarbonate, and the base excess shows a negative value (Chap 15).

Serum electrolytes will show a low bicarbonate and a reciprocal elevation of chloride. Serum sodium concentration may be normal, high, or low, depending on the cause of the acidosis.

A large abnormal anion gap may or may not be present, depending on the cause of the acidosis (see above).

Compensated Metabolic Acidosis

When compensation occurs, the pH rises slightly but may remain lower than normal. The P_{CO_2} falls as a result of the hyperventilation. This produces a compensatory respiratory alkalosis. The bicarbonate concentration (the standard bicarbonate) may also rise toward normal, if the kidneys are able to conserve bicarbonate ions. The actual bicarbonate also rises but also remains below normal.

Because of the respiratory alkalosis the actual bicarbonate is lower than the standard bicarbonate.

Serum electrolytes show a low bicarbonate and a normal, low, or high chloride concentration. Serum sodium may be normal or low. It will be low when sodium loss is associated with the development of the acidosis, as in diarrheas, diabetic acidosis, or renal disease. Serum potassium concentration is elevated because of the acidosis (Chap 24). However, if a severe potassium depletion is present, the serum potassium concentration may be normal.

(A normal or low potassium concentration in the presence of acidosis is a sign of potassium depletion.)

A large abnormal anion gap may or may not be present, depending on the cause of the acidosis (see above).

White Blood Count

A leukocytosis may be present.

Urine

The urine has a high ammonia content and is acid (pH 4.6 to 6.2). However, in acidosis due to chronic kidney disease, the renal compensatory mechanisms for combatting acidosis are not effective. In such patients, the urinary pH may be normal, in spite of the acidosis.

Example: Partially compensated metabolic acidosis in chronic nephritis.
pH 7.28
P_{CO_2} 26.4 mm Hg
CO_2 content 12.8 mEq/L
Standard bicarbonate 15 mEq/L
Actual bicarbonate 12 mEq/L
Base excess -13 mEq/L

The pH is low. This indicates an acidosis. The negative base excess and the low standard bicarbonate indicate that a metabolic acidosis is present. The low P_{CO_2} and the fact that the actual bicarbonate is lower than the standard bicarbonate indicate that a respiratory alkalosis is present. Therefore, a primary metabolic acidosis is present with a partially compensatory respiratory alkalosis (see Chap 15).

This information can also be determined from the pH and P_{CO_2} by inspection of Figure 15–4, page 154.

Cation-anion balance:
Na 132   K 6   Cl 87 HCO_3 12 mEq/L
Anion Gap = (Na + K) − (HCO_2 + Cl)
          = (132 + 6) − (12 + 87)
          = 138 − 99
          = 39 mEq/L. This is abnormal and is due to the retention of sulfuric, phosphoric, and other metabolic acids.

Example: Partially compensated metabolic acidosis due to ammonium chloride poisoning.
pH 7.3
P_{CO_2} 30 mm Hg
CO_2 content 14.9 mEq/L
Standard bicarbonate 16.5 mEq/L
Actual bicarbonate 14 mEq/L
Base excess -10.5 mEq/L

The pH is low, indicating an acidosis. The negative base excess and the low standard bicarbonate indicate that a metabolic acidosis is present. The low P_{CO_2} and the fact that the actual bicarbonate is lower than the standard bicarbonate indicate that a respiratory alkalosis is present. Therefore, a primary metabolic acidosis is present with a partially compensatory alkalosis (Chap 15).

This information can also be determined from the pH and P_{CO_2} by inspection of Figure 15–4, page 154.

Cation-anion balance:
Na 131   K 4.5 HCO_3 14   Cl 113 mEq/L
Anion Gap = (Na + K) − (HCO_3 + Cl)
          = (131 + 4.5) − (14 + 113)
          = 135.5 − 117
          = 18.5 mEq/L. This is normal.

The serum sodium concentration is low, because sodium has been excreted as a result of the diuresis produced by diuretics and the ammonium chloride.

COURSE AND PROGNOSIS

This depends on the cause of the metabolic acidosis. If it occurs in a patient with chronic renal disease, it may continue for months or years. However, if it occurs in a diabetic patient, for example, or as a result of salicylic acid poisoning, it may cause death quickly unless the patient is energetically treated.

TREATMENT

The aims of treatment are to stop the metabolic disturbance which has produced the acidosis and to restore the electrolytes which have been lost. When this is done, the acid-base balance is automatically restored.

If the acidosis is due to chloride excess, the chloride salt should be stopped immediately. In most patients the kidneys will be able to excrete the excessive amount of chloride. In patients with diabetic acidosis, insulin, sodium chloride solutions, and often potassium chloride will be needed (see Chap 22). In acute renal failure, water excess should be avoided, sodium balance should be maintained, and hyperkalemia should be treated (see Chap 21). In metabolic acidosis due to severe losses of intestinal fluids, sodium, potassium, and other electrolytes and water must be replaced.

One should always remember that as the metabolic acidosis is treated, the serum potassium concentration will usually decrease, due to the movement of potassium ions out of the extracellular water and into the cells (Chap 24). As a result, serious hypokalemia may develop in some patients, and it may be necessary to give potassium chloride, as has been mentioned above. However, this should be done only after the metabolic acidosis has started to improve, and in conjunction with serial observations of the serum potassium concentration (also see page 240).

Detailed therapy of metabolic acidosis is described in the chapters which follow.

The Use of Alkalinizing Salts

The use of an alkalinizing salt, such as sodium bicarbonate or sodium lactate, is usually not necessary, and may be dangerous because it may cause a complicating metabolic alkalosis, and it can aggravate the respiratory alkalosis which usually is present (page 239). Alkalinizing solutions should be reserved for seriously ill patients, or when the etiological agent which has caused the acidosis cannot be directly treated.

Type of Solution Needed. Alkalinizing solutions, such as sodium bicarbonate or sodium racemic lactate, are used. The lactate is rapidly oxidized to carbonic acide (by the liver), allowing the sodium to react with the carbonic acid to form sodium bicarbonate. The lactate solution also provides a small amount of calories. It cannot be used if shock, severe congestive heart failure, or respiratory alkalosis is present, or in any patient with impaired liver function. In such cases, the blood lactate concentration is high, and the liver is not able to metabolize the lactate.

Either isotonic sodium bicarbonate or lactate is usually used. However, if the water intake must be kept low, hypertonic sodium bicarbonate or lactate can be used (Chap 35).

Volume of Solution Needed. When sodium bicarbonate or lactate is given, part of the sodium will remain in the extracellular water space to correct the acidosis. An unpredictable part of the sodium will pass into the cells. For this reason, no completely satisfactory formula for determining the volume of needed sodium bicarbonate or lactate has yet been devised.

In order to prevent the development of a metabolic alkalosis from the bicarbonate or lactate. I suggest that the CO_2 content should be raised to only 18 mEq/L.

The following methods of calculating the necessary volume of sodium bicarbonate or lactate are satisfactory.

Method 1. Calculate the unit CO_2 content deficit, and multiply by the volume of extracellular water (which is 20% of the body weight). (Similar calculations can be made using the serum HCO_3^- concentration.)

> *Example:* Patient weighing 70 kg; CO_2 content 10 mEq/L
> It is desired to raise the CO_2 content to 18 mEq/L
> Extracellular water: $70 \times 0.2 = 14$ liters
> Unit CO_2 deficit: $18 - 10 = 8$ mEq/L
> Total CO_2 deficit: $8 \times 14 = 112$ milliequivalents

Therefore, treatment consists of giving 112 mEq bicarbonate ions, either as sodium bicarbonate or sodium lactate, intravenously. The following solutions can be used: (1) The volume of hypertonic (7.5%) sodium bicarbonate needed to supply 112 mEq CO_2 is $112 \times 50/45 = 124$ ml (Chap 35). (2) The volume of isotonic (1.5%) sodium bicarbonate needed to supply 112 mEq CO_2 is $112/178 \times 1000 = 630$ ml (Chap 35). (3) The volume of 1/6 molar sodium lactate needed to supply 112 mEq CO_2 is $112/167 \times 1000 = 670$ ml (see Chap 35). (4) The volume of molar (11%) sodium lactate needed to supply 112 mEq CO_2 is 112 ml (see Chap 35).

Experiments by Elkinton, Singer, Garetta, and others have indicated that when sodium bicarbonate is administered, it is distributed intracellularly as well as extracellularly in a space equivalent to 50% or more of the body weight (particularly if the metabolic acidosis is severe and the serum HCO_3^- concentration is less than 5 mEq/L). If this is correct, one would have to multiply the body weight (in kg) by the constant 0.5, and then multiply this value by the unit HCO_3^- or CO_2 content deficit instead of using the constant 0.2.

It is preferable to multiply by the lower constant of 0.2 for the following reasons. When a metabolic acidosis is present, a compensatory respiratory alkalosis develops (due to hyperventilation). Both the metabolic acidosis and the respiratory alkalosis produce a low serum HCO_3^- concentration and low CO_2 content. Therefore, the measured HCO_3^- concentration or CO_2 content represents the combined effects of an acidosis (metabolic) and an alkalosis (respiratory). If enough sodium bicarbonate (or lactate) is given to control the metabolic acidosis and to raise the HCO_3^- or CO_2 content to normal, a severe alkalosis may develop, because the compensatory respiratory alkalosis often persists for several hours or longer after the metabolic acidosis disappears. The respiratory alkalosis does not primarily affect the serum HCO_3^- concentration. However, if the HCO_3^- concentration is raised to normal, and the respiratory alkalosis persists, a severe alkalosis may develop.

Therefore, one should try to raise the serum HCO_3^- concentration or the CO_2 content to approximately 18 to 20 mEq/L, instead of to a normal value of 27 mEq/L, or the pH should be raised only to 7.30 with sodium bicarbonate or lactate.

Method 2. To raise the CO_2 content 1 mEq/L, give 1.2 ml of 1/6 molar sodium lactate per kg body weight.

Example: Patient weighing 70 kg; CO_2 content 10 mEq/L
It is desired to raise the CO_2 content 8 mEq/L to 18 mEq/L
Volume of 1/6 molar sodium lactate need is
    70 × 8 (the CO_2 deficit) × 1.2 = 672 ml

This rule is derived as follows: The extracellular water content of an adult is 20% of the body weight. Therefore, there is 0.2 kg, or 0.2 L, of extracellular water for every 1 kg body weight. If an ion such as lactate has a concentration in the extracellular water of 1 mEq/L, this represents 0.2 mEq/kg body weight.

If one uses a solution of 1/6 molar sodium lactate, which contains 167 mEq/L, 1 ml of the solution contains 0.167 mEq of the lactate ions. Therefore, 1.2 ml of the 1/6 molar solution contains 0.2 mEq.

If 1.2 ml of the 1/6 molar sodium lactate solution per kg body weight is given, this raises the lactate concentration 0.2 mEq/kg body weight, or 1 mEq/L of extracellular water. The bicarbonate concentration is raised similarly, because 1 mEq sodium lactate is converted into 1 mEq sodium bicarbonate.

Method Using pH and P$_{CO_2}$ Values. Calculate the unit HCO_3^- deficit and multiply by the volume of extracellular water (20% of the body weight).

Example: Patient weighing 60 kg, with a respiratory acidosis complicated by a metabolic acidosis.*
pH 7.02   P$_{CO_2}$ 80 mm Hg HCO_3 21 mEq/L
    It is desired to raise the pH immediately to 7.20, using intravenous sodium bicarbonate (in addition to treating the respiratory acidosis [see Chap 16]). (1) Determine the serum HCO_3 concentration that would be present when the pH is raised to 7.20 (assuming that the high P$_{CO_2}$ remains unchanged). This is done by using the nomogram (Fig. 14–1, page 139). Place a ruler edge on the pH 7.20 point and simultaneously on the P$_{CO_2}$ 80 mm Hg point. It intersects the HCO_3 point at 30 mEq/L. (2) Calculate the extracellular water volume: 60 × 0.2 = 12 liters. (3) Calculate the unit HCO_3 deficit: 30 − 21 = 9 mEq/L. Calculate the total HCO_3 deficit: 9 × 12 = 108 mEq.
    Therefore, treatment consists of giving 108 mEq bicarbonate ions (see above).

Method Using Negative Base Excess Values. Astrup's original formula is described on page 151. However, if the extracellular water is considered to be 20% of the body weight, the formula can be modified as follows:

mEq base needed = body weight (kg) × 0.2 × −base excess (mEq/L).

Route of Administration of the Solution. A mild metabolic acidosis can be treated with oral sodium bicarbonate in a dose of 5 g a day (one level teaspoonful contains 1.5 to 2 g). However, in a patient seriously ill with metabolic acidosis, sodium bicarbonate or lactate should be given intravenously. If gastric lavage is done, 200 ml of a 5% sodium bicarbonate solution can be placed in the stomach.

Rate of Administration of the Solution. Isotonic sodium bicarbonate or lactate can be given at a rate which does not exceed 1 liter per hour (see page 352). Hypertonic sodium bicarbonate or lactate should be diluted with at least an equal volume of water or glucose in water, and given at a rate which does not exceed 100 ml per hour (see page 352).

    When alkalinizing salts are given to an acidotic patient, calcium gluconate should be given in a dose of 1 to 3 g daily intravenously to prevent tetany.

REFERENCES

Albert, M.S., Dell, R.B., and Winters, R.W.: Quantitative displacement of acid-base equilibrium in metabolic acidosis. Ann Intern Med, *66*:312, 1967.
Altschule, M.D., and Sulzbach, W.M.: Tolerance of the human heart to acidosis: reversible

---

*This simultaneous respiratory and metabolic acidosis is easily recognized when the pH and P$_{CO_2}$ values are plotted on Figure 15–4, page 154.

changes in RS-T segment during severe acidosis caused by administration of carbon dioxide. Am Heart J, *33*:453, 1947.

Block, A.V., Field, H., Jr., and Adair, G.S.: The acid-base equilibrium in diabetic coma, being a study of five cases treated with insulin. J Metab Res, *4*:27, 1923.

Chazan, J.A., Stenson, R., and Kurland, G.S.: The acidosis of cardiac arrest. N Engl J Med, *278*:360, 1968.

Dow, R.P.: Metabolic acidosis, non-diabetic. Arch Intern Med, *116*:717, 1965.

Fraley, D.S., et al.: Metabolic acidosis after hyperalimentation with casein hydrolysate. Occurrence in a starved patient. Ann Intern Med, *88*:352, 1978.

Garella, S., Dana, C.L., and Chazan, J.A.: Severity of metabolic acidosis as a determinant of bicarbonate requirements. N Engl J Med, *289*:121, 1973.

Kauffman, H.E., and Rosen, S.W.: Clinical acid-base regulation—the Bronsted schema. Surg Gynecol Obstet, *103*:101, 1956.

Lennon, E.J., and Lemann, J., Jr.: Defense of hydrogen ion concentration in chronic metabolic acidosis. A new evaluation of an old approach. Ann Intern Med, *65*:265, 1966.

Miller, P.D., Heinig, R.E., and Waterhouse, C.: Treatment of alcoholic acidosis. The role of dextrose and phosphorus. Arch Intern Med, *138*:67, 1978.

Nahas, G.G., et al.: Control of acidosis and the use of titrated ACD blood in open-heart surgery. Ann Surg, *160*:1049, 1964.

Neaverson, M.A.: Metabolic acidosis in acute myocardial infarction. Br Med J, *2*:383, 1966.

Peters, J.P., and Van Slyke, D.D.: *Quantitative Clinical Chemistry,* Vol. I Interpretations. Baltimore, Williams & Wilkins, 1931.

Poppell, J.W., Vanamee, P., Roberts, K.E., and Randall, H.T.: The effect of ventilatory insufficiency on respiratory compensations in metabolic acidosis and alkalosis. J Lab Clin Med, *47*:885, 1956.

Relman, A.S., Shelburne, P.F., and Talman, A.: Profound acidosis resulting from excessive ammonium chloride in previously healthy subjects. N Engl J Med, *264*:848, 1961.

Russell, C.D.: Response to bicarbonate in severe acidosis. N Engl J Med, *289*:755, 1973.

Shires, G.T., and Holman, J.: Dilution acidosis. Ann Intern Med, *28*:557, 1948.

Shugoll, G.I.: Transient QRS changes simulating myocardial infarction associated with shock and severe metabolic stress. Am Heart J, *74*:402, 1967.

Singer, R.B., et al.: The acute effects in man of rapid intravenous infusion of hypertonic sodium bicarbonate solution. Medicine, *34*:51, 1955.

Singer, R.B., and Hastings, A.B.: An improved clinical method for the estimation of disturbances of the acid-base balance of human blood. Medicine, *27*:223, 1948.

Stewart, J.S.S., Stewart, W.K., and Gillies, H.G.: Cardiac arrest and acidosis. Lancet, *2*:964, 1962.

Trudnowski, R.T., et al.: Effect of Ringer's lactate solution and sodium bicarbonate on surgical acidosis. Surg. Gynecol Obstet, *125*:814, 1967.

Winters, R.W., Lowder, J.A., and Ordway, N.K.: Observations on carbon dioxide tension during recovery from metabolic acidosis. J Clin Invest, *37*:640, 1958.

CHAPTER 18

METABOLIC ACIDOSIS SYNDROMES (Continued)

RENAL TUBULAR ACIDOSIS

Most patients with acidosis due to renal failure have either acute renal tubular failure or chronic renal disease. In these patients, glomerular function and tubular function are both decreased. Since glomerular function is decreased more than tubular function, the patient becomes not only acidotic but azotemic. This common type of renal acidosis has been called *uremic* or *azotemic acidosis.* However, there is a less common type of renal acidosis known as *renal tubular acidosis* (RTA). Here the renal tubular function is decreased even though glomerular function is usually normal.

The renal tubules are capable of reabsorbing numerous ions and substances from the tubular urine (glomerular filtrate), including water, glucose, phosphate, bicarbonate, calcium, amino acids such as cystine. Any one or several of these functions may become disturbed. For example, a genetic defect in tubular reabsorption of water causes the *renal diabetes insipidus syndrome.* A genetic deficiency of renal tubular reabsorption of glucose causes the *renal glycosuria syndrome.* This is asymptomatic except for the glycosuria. A genetic defect of tubular reabsorption of the amino acid, cystine, causes *cystinuria* with recurrent renal calculi composed of cystine. A genetic defect in the tubular reabsorption of phosphate alone is probably the cause of vitamin D-resistant hypophosphatemic rickets. A genetic defect of tubular reabsorption of glucose, cystine and other amino acids and phosphate produces the classical *Fanconi syndrome* (page 189). A deficient renal tubular reabsorption of bicarbonate ions and/or a deficiency in tubular ability to excrete hydrogen ions causes the syndrome of *renal tubular acidosis.*

ETIOLOGY

In adults, renal tubular acidosis may occur in many ways and may be associated with either functional or pathological changes in either the distal or proximal renal tubules.

Distal renal tubular acidosis (Type I, classic) can occur in the following common conditions (adapted from Morris and associates):

1. Metabolic syndromes: hyperthyroidism with nephrocalcinosis, primary hyperparathyroidism with nephrocalcinosis.
2. Drug-induced problems: amphotericin B, vitamin D-induced nephrocalcinosis.
3. Hypergammaglobulinemic syndromes: cryoglobulinemia, Sjögren's syndrome, lupoid hepatitis, lupus erythematosus and so on.
4. Cirrhosis of the liver.
5. Pyelonephritis (rare).
6. Rejection of renal transplant.

Proximal renal tubular acidosis (Type II) can occur in the following conditions (adapted from Morris and associates):

1. Syndromes associated with disturbances of protein metabolism: nephrotic syndrome, multiple myeloma, Sjögren's syndrome, amyloidosis, and so on.
2. Drug-induced problems: from deteriorated (outdated) tetracycline, from 6-mercaptopurine, sulfonamides and so on.
3. Heavy metals: lead, cadmium.
4. Metabolic syndromes: vitamin D deficiency, secondary hyperparathyroidism.
5. Medullary cystic disease.
6. Rejection of renal transplant.
7. Genetically transmitted syndromes (adult Fanconi syndrome, hereditary or acquired, and other rare syndromes).

Type III shows signs of both distal and proximal renal tubular acidosis.

Hyperkalemic RTA—type IV (frequently with associated hyporeninemia and hypoaldosteronism) can occur in the following:

1. Chronic interstitial nephritis of any cause.
2. Obstructive uropathy.
3. Lead nephropathy.
4. Sickle hemoglobinopathies.
5. SLE (systemic lupus erythematosus).

PATHOPHYSIOLOGY

Renal tubular acidosis is characterized by a hyperchloremic metabolic acidosis, and almost invariably by hypokalemia. However, in some forms, hyperkalemia may be present. In many patients, nephrocalcinosis and hypophosphatemia with osteomalacia may also occur.

The function of the kidneys in acid-base balance is to regulate the concentration of plasma bicarbonate ions. Normally, in the proximal renal tubules, approximately 85 to 90% of the bicarbonate ions that have been filtered by the glomeruli are reabsorbed, and hydrogen ions are excreted into the tubular urine in their place. In the distal renal tubules, the residual 10 to 15% of bicarbonate are absorbed. In addition, the distal tubules are responsible for the secretion of the daily load of nonvolatile acids (phosphoric, organic, etc.). This is accomplished by the secretion of hydrogen ions and by the secretion of NH_4^+.

In the distal (classic) type of RTA, there is a defect in hydrogen ion secretion. Since the daily acid load produced by metabolism cannot be excreted, a metabolic acidosis develops. The anions of these metabolic acids (phosphates, sulfates, etc.) are excreted as sodium salts, with resultant mild volume depletion due to sodium loss. This in turn stimulates marked sodium and chloride reabsorption. The net effect is a hyperchloremic acidosis. Excessive urinary loss of potassium ions is almost invariable, and may be linked to the distal defects in hydrogen ion excretion and/or to hyperaldosteronism (which results from sodium depletion).

In the proximal type of RTA, there is reduction in the threshold of bicarbonate reabsorption, i.e. when serum bicarbonate is less than 12 to 15 mEq/L, there is complete bicarbonate reabsorption. However, as serum bicarbonate concentration rises, the tubules show their inability to reabsorb bicarbonate ions, so that large amounts of bicarbonate escape the proximal tubules, overwhelm the limited distal capacity for bicarbonate reabsorption, and appear in the urine. The result is a large loss of $NaHCO_3$, which results in a hyperchloremic metabolic acidosis. The distal tubules attempt to reclaim some of this $NaHCO_3$, which results in a large K loss. The urine of a patient with proximal RTA will be alkaline when efforts are made to maintain a normal serum bicarbonate level. However, as the serum bicarbonate falls to the threshold value, bicarbonate reabsorption becomes complete, and the urine will have an acid pH.

It should be recognized that a great percentage of patients with RTA have defects of a mixed nature, with diminished distal acidification and mild bicarbonate wasting.

In type IV RTA, a mild to moderate hyperchloremic metabolic acidosis associated with hyperkalemia occurs in patients with moderate renal insufficiency due to a variety of interstitial injuries. Defective distal tubular or collecting duct hydrogen ion and potassium excretion result from aldosterone deficiency or tubular resistance to aldosterone.

HYPOPHOSPHATEMIA

a. In proximal RTA, phosphate wasting may occur as a result of an associated defect in phosphate reabsorption.

b. In some instances, hypophosphatemia is a sign of the underlying cause of the RTA, for example, in vitamin D deficiency, hypocalcemia induces secondary hyperparathyroidism, with resultant phosphate wasting.

c. In all patients with RTA, chronic acidosis causes hypercalciuria.

This causes hypocalcemia with a resultant secondary hyperparathyroidism, which contributes to the hypophosphatemia.

NEPHROCALCINOSIS

Nephrocalcinosis or nephrolithiasis is seen primarily with distal RTA and results from several factors:

1. Hypercalciuria due to chronic acidosis.
2. Chronically alkaline urine, in which calcium salts are less soluble.
3. Hypocitraturia, which occurs in hypokalemia states. (Citrate is an inhibitor of stone formation and its absence promotes stone formation.)

SYMPTOMS AND SIGNS

These depend on the age of the patient and on the electrolytes and other substances which are lost in the urine. Weakness may be present, due to potassium loss. Disturbances in gait and bone pain are due to osteomalacia. X-ray examination will show signs of the rickets, osteomalacia or nephrocalcinosis, and pseudofractures, first described by Milkman, which are due to the osteomalacia. A Kussmaul type of hyperventilation may be present, when the acidosis is severe.

LABORATORY FINDINGS

Blood

The findings vary greatly. However, the pH is low due to the acidosis, and the serum chloride concentration is high (110 to 120 mEq/L). The serum bicarbonate concentration usually ranges from 20 to 12 mEq/L.

Hypophosphatemia is usually present. Occasionally, the serum phosphate concentration is normal. The serum calcium concentration is normal or slightly low. Hypokalemia is frequently present. Azotemia is either absent or minimal.

Urine

Patients with distal tubular acidosis characteristically show a urine with a high pH (6.0 to 7.0) regardless of the serum bicarbonate concentration. Patients with proximal renal tubular acidosis may show a urine with a normal pH (even less than 6.0) when the metabolic acidosis is severe and the serum bicarbonate concentration is low. (The reason is that reabsorption of bicarbonate ions in the proximal tubules may become complete in these patients, when the serum bicarbonate concentration is low.)

In type IV RTA, the urine pH may be inappropriately high, but it can be low, particularly in those patients with aldosterone deficiency.

The specific gravity tends to become low and fixed. Hypercalciuria is often present. Glycosuria, ketonuria, or proteinuria may also be present.

Example: Patient with renal tubular acidosis.
pH 7.19
Pco_2 33 mm Hg
CO_2 content 14 mEq/L
Standard bicarbonate 14 mEq/L
Actual bicarbonate 13 mEq/L
Base excess −14 mEq/L

The pH is low. This indicates an acidosis. The negative base excess and the low standard bicarbonate indicate that a metabolic acidosis is present. The Pco_2 is within normal. This indicates respiratory balance. However, the actual bicarbonate is lower than the standard bicarbonate. This indicates that some degree of respiratory alkalosis is present. Therefore, a primary metabolic acidosis is present with a partially compensatory respiratory alkalosis.

This information can also be determined from the pH and Pco_2 by inspection of Figure 15–4, page 154.

Cation-anion balance:
Na 140   K 2.7 HCO_3 13   Cl 120
Anion Gap = (Na + K) − (HCO_3 + Cl)
$\quad\quad\quad\quad$ = (140 + 2.7) − (13 + 120)
$\quad\quad\quad\quad$ = 142.7 − 133
$\quad\quad\quad\quad$ = 9.7 mEq/L. This is normal.

DIAGNOSIS

Renal tubular acidosis can be suspected if a patient shows a hyperchloremic metabolic acidosis (serum chloride concentration 110 to 120 mEq/L, in association with nephrocalcinosis or severe hypokalemia or osteomalacia or pseudofractures.

Several methods have been described to differentiate distal from proximal renal tubular acidosis. The following tests are simple to perform:

1. In the patient with significant spontaneous acidotic (serum bicarbonate <18), the urine pH can be checked with a pH meter. In distal renal tubular acidosis, the urine pH will be consistently high (6.5 to 7.0), as has been pointed out above. A urine pH less than 6.0 excludes distal renal tubular acidosis is present. (This rule does not apply if a urinary tract infection, due to urease-producing bacteria, is present, because this will cause the urine pH to be higher than 7.0.)
2. In the patient who is not spontaneously acidotic, ammonium chloride is given orally by the method of Wrong and Davies (0.1 g per kg body weight,

given over a period of 1 hour, and using either ammonium chloride solution or ammonium chloride in capsules). A fall of urine pH to less than 5.5 (in a period of 5 hours) indicates proximal tubular acidosis. (If the ammonium chloride loading test falls to produce a fall to less than 5.5, this suggests but does not necessarily indicate distal renal tubular acidosis.)

Recently, measurement of urinary pH during Na_2SO_4 loading, and measurement of urine-blood Pco_2 during $NaHCO_3$ loading have been used as sophisticated tools for assessing the precise nature of certain distal acidification defects.

The combination of nephrocalcinosis and osteomalacia, with pseudofractures, is nearly specific for distal renal tubular acidosis, when hypervitaminosis D is excluded by the patient's history (Courney and Pfister).

If ketonuria and glucosuria are present, this can simulate diabetes mellitus. However, in renal tubular acidosis, the blood sugar concentration is normal.

Renal tubular acidosis can be differentiated from renal rickets, because in renal rickets there is azotemia and an elevated serum phosphate concentration.

A metabolic acidosis similar to that found in renal tubular acidosis often occurs in the Fanconi syndrome. This usually is due to a genetic disturbance of renal tubular function for glucose, cystine and other amino acids, and phosphate. It is seen mostly in infants and children. The clinical picture is similar to that of renal tubular acidosis. However, the patient characteristically shows renal glycosuria, urinary excretion of cystine and other amino acids, and an increased urinary phosphate excretion. The blood shows normal serum glucose and amino acid concentrations, hypophosphatemia, normal serum calcium concentration, low serum bicarbonate and high chloride concentrations if acidosis is present, and a normal or slightly elevated blood urea nitrogen concentration. Nephrocalcinosis does not occur. In the later stages, glomerular function becomes decreased. This may cause retention of phosphate ions in the blood.

COURSE AND PROGNOSIS

Death may occur in children and young adults from progressive renal insufficiency. However, adults may show some of the electrolyte changes but no signs of renal insufficiency. Control of the metabolic abnormalities may help to avoid progressive renal insufficiency.

TREATMENT

The aim of treatment is to replace the bicarbonate ions which have been lost, and to stop the progress of the osteomalacia or rickets.

Patients with distal renal tubular acidosis can be treated with sodium bicarbonate orally in a dose of 4 to 6 g (48 to 72 mEq bicarbonate ions). However, if the serum bicarbonate concentration is approximately 22 mEq/L, sodium bicarbonate is not necessary.

Hypokalemia is generally improved by sodium bicarbonate supplementation; but in some patients potassium supplementation in the form of potassium citrate or bicarbonate is necessary.

Shohl's solution (page 208) can be used in place of sodium bicarbonate. Each 1 ml contains approximately 1 mEq bicarbonate ions. Therefore, a daily dose of approximately 50 to 75 ml can be used.

Patients with proximal renal tubular acidosis will need larger doses of sodium bicarbonate or other alkaline salts and often require substantial potassium supplements.

Osteomalacia or rickets can be treated with a high calcium diet and larger doses of vitamin D—20,000 to 100,000 units daily or 0.125–1.0 microgram of 1.25 vitamin D_3—may be necessary. However, these doses may cause severe hypercalcemia with secondary renal failure. The serum calcium concentration should be checked every several weeks. If it rises above 10.5 mg/dl, the vitamin D therapy should be stopped.

Richards and his associates have recently reported the use of sodium bicarbonte alone in the treatment of osteomalacia of renal tubular acidosis.

In those patients who have RTA associated with hyperkalemia, potassium-binding resins. thiazide diuretics, furosemide and sodium bicarbonate may help to correct the hyperkalemia and acidosis. Fludrocortisone is also useful in selected cases.

REFERENCES

Albright, F., Burnett, C.H., Parson, W., Reifenstein, E.C., Jr., and Roos, A.: Osteomalacia and late rickets: various etiologies met in United States with emphasis on that resulting from specific form of renal acidosis: therapeutic indications for each etiological group and relationship between osteomalacia and Milkman's syndrome. Medicine, 25:399, 1946.

Arruda, J., and Kurtzman, N.: Metabolic acidosis and alkalosis. Clin Nephrol, 7:201, 1977.

Carroll, H.J., and Farber, S.J.: Hyperkalemia and hyperchloremic acidosis in chronic pyelonephritis. Metabolism, 13:808, 1964.

Courney, W.R., and Pfister, R.C.: The radiographic findings in renal tubular acidosis. Radiology, 105:497, 1972.

DeFronzo, R.A.: Hyperkalemia and hyporeninemic hypoaldosteronism. Kidney Int., 17:118, 1980.

Elkinton, J.R., Huth, E.J., Webster, G.D., and McCance, R.A.: The renal excretion of hydrogen ion in renal tubular acidosis. Am J Med, 29:554, 576, 586, 1960.

Gennari, F.J., and Cohen, J.J.: Renal tubular acidosis. Ann Rev Med, 29:521, 1978.

Gouttas, A., et al.: Adult Fanconi syndrome. New York State J Med, 65:295, 1965.

Harrington, T.M., et al.: Renal tubular acidosis. A new look at treatment of musculoskeletal and renal disease. Mayo Clin Proc, 58:354, 1983.

Lathem, W.: Hyperchloremic acidosis in chronic pyelonephritis. N Engl J Med, 258:1031, 1958.

Lew, H.T., and French, S.W.: Tetracycline nephrotoxicity and nonoliguric acute renal failure. Arch Intern Med, 118:123, 1966.

Mason, A.M.S., and Golding, P.L.: Hyperglobulinemic renal tubular acidosis. Br Med J, *3*:143, 1970.

Morris, R.C., Jr.: Renal tubular acidosis. Mechanisms, classification and implications. N Engl J Med, *281*:1405, 1969.

Morris, R.C., Jr.: Renal tubular acidosis, editorial. N Engl J Med, *304*:418, 1981.

Morris, R.C., Jr., and Sebastian, A.: Disorders of the renal tubule that cause disorders of fluid, acid-base, and electrolyte metabolism. In *Clinical Disorders of Fluid and Electrolyte Metabolism.* 3rd ed. (Maxwell, M.H., and Kleeman, C.R., (Eds.). New York, McGraw-Hill Book Co., 1980.

Owen, E.E., and Verner, J.V.: Renal tubular disease with muscle paralysis and hypokalemia. Am J Med, *28*:8, 1960.

Patterson, R.M., and Ackerman, G.L.: Renal tubular acidosis due to amphotericin B nephrotoxicity. Arch Intern Med, *127*:241, 1971.

Pines, K.I., and Mudge, G.H.: Renal tubular acidosis with osteomalacia. Am J Med, *11*:302, 1951.

Reynolds, T.R.: Renal tubular disorders. In *Clinical Disorders of Fluid and Electrolyte Metabolism.* 2nd ed. (Maxwell, M.H., and Kleeman, C.R., Eds.). New York, McGraw-Hill Book Co., 1972.

Richards, P., et al.: Treatment of osteomalacia of renal tubular acidosis by sodium bicarbonate alone. Lancet, *2*:994, 1972.

Sebastian, A., and Morris, R.: Renal tubular acidosis. Clin Nephrol, *7*:216, 1977.

Sebastian, A., Schambelan, M., Lindenfeld, S., et al.: Amelioration of metabolic acidosis with fludrocortisone therapy in hyporeninemic hypoaldosteronism. N Engl J Med, *297*:576, 1977.

Shear, L., Bonkowsky, H.L., and Gabuzda, G.J.: Renal tubular acidosis in cirrhosis. N Engl J Med, *280*:1, 1969.

Vander, A.J.: *Renal Physiology,* 3rd ed. New York, McGraw-Hill Book Co., 1985.

Wilson, D.R., and Siddiqui, A.A.: Renal tubular acidosis after kidney transplantation. Ann Intern Med, *79*:352, 1973.

Wrong, O.M.: Renal tubular acidosis. Letter. New Engl J Med, *304*:1548, 1981.

Wrong, O.M., and Davies, H.E.F.: The excretion of acid in renal disease. Quart J Med, N.S. *28*:258, 1959.

CHAPTER 19

METABOLIC ACIDOSIS SYNDROMES (Continued)

LACTIC ACIDOSIS

Lactic acidosis is a metabolic acidosis due to the accumulation of lactate ions above a concentration of 2 mEq/L, in association with a decreased arterial pH.

Lactic acid is the end-product of the anaerobic metabolism of glucose (dextrose). It is formed in nearly all tissues in the body, particularly in skeletal muscles and red blood cells. Glycogen is normally metabolized to pyruvic acid in the first stage of carbohydrate metabolism. If adequate oxygen is present, little lactic acid is formed, because the pyruvic acid is metabolized to carbon dioxide. However, under anaerobic conditions, pyruvic acid is metabolized (reduced) to lactic acid in the cells. (This reaction occurs mainly in the liver.) Although this chemical reaction is reversible, so that pyruvic acid can be formed from lactic acid, the kinetics of the reaction normally produces a lactate-pyruvate ratio of 10:1.

Lactic acid can accumulate in two ways:

1. By increased production of lactic acid. This occurs in lactic acidosis because there is an increased breakdown of glycogen in the liver. (An increased production of lactic acid also occurs with muscular exercise or hyperventilation, or when epinephrine, fructose, or glucagon is administered. However, these latter conditions do *not* produce a significant lactic acidosis.)
2. By decreased metabolism of lactic acid. Shock and hypoxia are the most common causes of this decreased metabolism of lactic acid.

ETIOLOGY

Lactic acidosis can occur from the following causes.

1. Shock. This is the most frequent cause of lactic acidosis, for reasons just mentioned. In addition, the arterial lactate concentration is a good prognosticator in shock. When the lactic acid concentration is below 4.3 mEq/L, almost all patients recover; when the concentration is between 4.4 and

8 mEq/L, there is only approximately a 33% chance of survivial; when the lactic acid concentration rises above 8 mEq/L, there is only approximately a 10% chance of survival. However, when shock is treated with a vasodilating drug, such as phentolamine (Regitine), or isoproterenol (Isuprel), etc., and tissue perfusion improves, lactic acid will be flushed into the general circulation and its concentration in the blood will rise temporarily, as the patient's condition improves.

2. Metabolic acidosis. Lactic acidosis also occurs when the pH falls to approximately 7.10 or less.
3. Diabetes mellitus. Lactic acidosis can occur in one of three ways in diabetic patients:
   a. If renal insufficiency, due to shock, sepsis, pancreatitis, or any other cause, occurs, the diabetic patient is particularly susceptible to the development of lactic acidosis.
   b. Lactic acidosis can occur simultaneously with diabetic ketoacidosis. This combination can be suspected when a weakly positive Acetest (nitroprusside) reaction is found on the serum of a patient in diabetic ketoacidosis. The reason for this is that the Acetest is specific for aceto-acetate ketones, but does not measure beta-hydroxybutyrate and other ketones. (Measurement of beta-hydroxybutyrates and lactic acid should be made on such patients.)
   c. Phenformin (DBI) therapy of diabetes mellitus. (Phenformin has been withdrawn from general use, although it is still available as an investigational drug.)
4. Acute pulmonary edema due to left-sided congestive heart failure.
5. Generalized (grand mal) convulsive seizures.
6. Severe hypoxemia (PaO_2 below 35 mm Hg), or severe anemia (hemoglobin below 6 g/dl).
7. During cardiopulmonary bypass operations, especially if hypothermia is used during the bypass surgery.
8. Acute leukemia. An excessive amount of lactic acid is produced by the excessive numbers of white blood cells. In addition, tissue hypoxia occurs from sludging in small blood vessels. The situation is aggravated if leukemia infiltration of the liver occurs, producing impaired liver function.
9. Excessive ethanol intake.
10. Spontaneous (idiopathic) causes. Lactic acidosis has been described in association with numerous infectious or inflammatory conditions such as acute pyelonephritis, acute peritonitis, acute pancreatitis, subacute bacterial endocarditis, acute poliomyelitis, and in noninfectious conditions such as gastrointestinal hemorrhage, acute myocardial infarction, and postoperatively. The mechanisms of lactic acidosis in these cases are not known. Shock or severe tissue hypoxia is usually present, due to other causes, and is probably the precipitating factor producing the lactic acidosis.

SYMPTOMS AND SIGNS

Lactic acidosis usually develops acutely. Symptoms include weakness, fatigue, or moderate to marked dyspnea. Hyperventilation is a common finding. This may be slight cyanosis. Changes in consciousness may vary from mild lethargy to stupor and eventually to coma. Death usually occurs in hours or days.

These symptoms and signs are not specific for lactic acidosis and can occur with metabolic acidosis due to any cause.

LABORATORY FINDINGS

The normal arterial concentration of lactate is less than 1.5 mEq/L (approximately 10 mg/dl). A concentration greater than 2 mEq/L is abnormal. However, a rise in arterial lactate concentration to 2 to 3 mEq/L is usually associated with no change in pH, because buffers in the extracellular fluid can neutralize this increase in lactate ions. However, when the arterial lactate concentration rises above this, the pH begins to fall. When lactic acidosis is present, the arterial lactate concentration is usually higher than 7 mEq/L, and may rise as high as 30 mEq/L.

(*Lactate concentration in mEq/L can be converted to its concentration in mg/dl by* multiplying *by the factor 9. To convert lactate concentration in mg/dl to mEq/L,* divide *by this factor.*)

The normal arterial concentration of pyruvate is less than 0.15 mEq/L.

(*Pyruvate concentration in mEq/L can be converted to its concentration in mg/dl by* multiplying *by the factor 8.8. To convert pyruvate concentration in mg/dl to mEq/L,* divide *by this factor.*)

The Arterial Lactate-Pyruvate Ratio

Since the normal arterial lactate concentration is approximately 1.5 mEq/L, and the normal arterial pyruvate concentration is approximately 0.15 mEq/L or less, the arterial lactate-pyruvate ratio is normally approximately 10:1. When lactic acidosis is present, the lactate concentration rises much higher than the pyruvate concentration, so that the arterial lactate-pyruvate ratio may rise to 60:1.

Arterial blood should be used to determine lactate and pyruvate concentrations because contractions of the muscles of the arm occluded with a tourniquet will raise the lactate concentration in venous blood. (If venous blood is used, it should be drawn without stasis from a resting extremity. The venous lactate concentration exceeds the arterial lactate concentration by approximately 3 mEq/L.)

The pH is low and the anion gap is usually greater than 22 mEq/L.

Other Findings

Other laboratory findings include: leukocytosis and increased SGOT value, probably due to decreased blood flow through the liver. An increased serum phosphate concentration commonly occurs. Hypoglycemia in association with lactic acidosis has also been noted in some patients.

Example: Patient with lactic acidosis
pH 7.30 CO_2 content 9.0 mEq/L

Cation-anion balance
Na 131   K 5   Cl 86 HCO_3 9 mEq/L
Anion Gap = (Na + K) − $(HCO_2$ + Cl)
$$= (131 + 5) - (9 + 86)$$
$$= 136 - 95$$
$$= 41 \text{ mEq/L. This is markedly abnormal.}$$

DIAGNOSIS

Lactate acidosis can be suspected when a metabolic acidosis occurs with an abnormal anion gap and diabetic ketoacidosis, azotemic acidosis, salicylate intoxication, ethylene glycol poisoning, paraldehyde or methanol intoxication can be ruled out. The presence of shock or severe hypoxia further suggests lactic acidosis. However, the diagnosis should be confirmed by measuring arterial lactate and pyruvate concentrations.

TREATMENT

1. Eliminate the source or sources of excessive lactate acid production. For example, if it is ethanol, stop it immediately.
2. Maintain an adequate peripheral perfusion of tissues and an adequate cardiac output. Correct hypoxia, if possible. If shock is present, vasoconstrictors such as dopamine (Intropin), or levarterenol (Levophed) should *not* be used, because they cause further vasoconstriction and may worsen the lactic acidosis. Instead, it is preferable to treat the patient with intravenous fluids, monitoring with CVP or with pulmonary-wedge pressure measurements. Vasodilating drugs, such as phentolamine (Regitine) or intravenous corticosteroids, may also be helpful in association with intravenous fluids. Sodium nitroprusside has also been used because it is an excellent vasodilator. However, when large doses are used for a long time, it may produce lactic acidosis.
3. Correct the metabolic acidosis. Sodium bicarbonate is the drug of choice. It is given intravenously to raise the pH to approximately 7.30 (see Chap 35).
   An alkalinizing solution such as lactated Ringer's solution (which contains lactate ions) should not be used. However, if a patient with unrecognized lactic acidosis is given sodium lactate, no harm will occur.
   When a patient in shock develops acute renal insufficiency and requires peritoneal dialysis, one should also remember that the commercially available peritoneal dialysis solutions contain 35 mEq/L lactate ions. Here again the lactate ions will not harm the patient, but they will not produce an alkalinizing effect until the peripheral perfusion of tissues improves and the lactate can be oxidized and bicarbonate ions formed.
4. If diabetic acidosis is also present, insulin and dextrose may also be of value (Freeman and Campbell).
5. Methylene blue in a single intravenous dose of 1 to 5 mg per kg body weight has been used to increase the conversion of lactic acid to pyruvic

acid. However, there are no conclusive studies to indicate that it is effective clinically.

6. Treat pulmonary edema due to left-sided congestive heart failure in the usual ways. (These patients do not need sodium bicarbonate to correct the lactic acidosis. This spontaneously disappears when the pulmonary edema disappears.)

REFERENCES

Anderson, C.T., et al.: Contribution of arterial blood lactate measurements to the care of critically ill patients. Am J Clin Path, *68*:63, 1977.

Buehler, J.H., et al.: lactic acidosis from carboxyhemoglobinemia after smoke inhalation. Ann Intern Med, *82*:803, 1975.

Cohen, R.D.: Lactic acidosis. Clinical considerations. Practical Cardiol, *8*:83, 1982.

Cohen, R.D., and Woods, H.F.: *Clinical and Biochemical Aspects of Lactic Acidosis.* London, Blackwell Scientific Publications, and Baltimore, Williams & Wilkins, 1976.

Dahlquist, N.R., et al.: D-lactic acidosis and encephalopathy after jejunoileostomy. Mayo Clin Proc, *59*:141, 1984.

Freeman, H., and Campbell, D.: Therapy of lactic acidosis. N Engl J Med, *292*:263, 1975.

Fulop, M., et al.: Lactic acidosis in pulmonary edema due to left ventricular failure. Ann Intern Med, *79*:180, 1973.

Fulop, M., and Hoberman, H.D.: Is lactic acidosis "spontaneous"? New York State J Med, *77*:24, 1977.

Goldberger, E.: Cardiogenic shock. In *The Treatment of Cardiac Emergencies,* 4th Ed. St. Louis, C.V. Mosby Co., 1984.

Huckabee, W.E.: Abnormal resting blood lactate. I. Significance of hyperlactatemia in hospitalized patients. Am J Med, *30*:833, 1961. II. Lactic acidosis. Am J Med, *30*:840, 1961.

Humphrey, S.H., and Nash, D.A., Jr.: Lactic acidosis complicating sodium nitroprusside therapy. Letter. Ann Intern Med, *88*:58, 1978.

Medalle, R., Webb, R., and Waterhouse, C.: Lactic acidosis and associated hypoglycemia. Arch Intern Med, *128*:273, 1971.

Misbin, R.I.: Phenformin-associated lactic acidosis. Pathogenesis and treatment. Ann Intern Med, *87*:591, 1977.

O''Connor, L.R., Klein, K.L., and Bethune, J.E.: Hyperphosphatemia in lactic acidosis. N Engl J Med, *297*:707, 1977.

Oliva, P.B.: Lactic acidosis. Am J Med, *48*:209, 1970.

Orringer, C.E., et al.: Natural history of lactic acidosis after grand-mal seizures. N Engl J Med, *297*:796, 1977.

Schweizer, O., and Howland, W.S.: Prognostic significance of high lactate levels. Anesth Analg, *47*:383, 1968.

Stackpoole, P.W., et al.: Treatment of lactic acidosis with dichloroacetate. N Engl J Med, *309*:390, 1983.

Stolberg, L., et al.: d-lactic acidosis due to abnormal gut flora. N Engl J Med, *306*:1344, 1982.

Taradash, M.R., and Jacobson, L.B.: Vasodilator therapy of idiopathic lactic acidosis. N Engl J Med, *293*:468, 1975.

Tranquada, R.E., Bernstein, S., and Grant, W.J.: Methylene blue in the treatment of lactic acidosis. Clin Res, *11*:230, 1963.

CHAPTER 20

METABOLIC ACIDOSIS SYNDROMES (Continued)

AZOTEMIA AND ACIDOSIS

Azotemia (uremia) is the accumulation in the blood and extracellular water of nonprotein nitrogenous substances, caused by acute or chronic renal failure.

ETIOLOGY

Azotemia may result from any pathological process that produces significant acute or chronic impairment of renal function—for example, disturbances of glomerular function, disturbances of tubular function, renal vascular disturbances, renal infections, obstruction of the upper or lower urinary tract, collagen diseases, hypercalcemia, hyperuricemia, and so on.

PATHOPHYSIOLOGY

Normally, the glomerular filtrate rate (GFR), or the creatinine clearance, is 100 ml or more per minute. When either of these values decreases to approximately 10 to 15% of normal, overt signs of azotemia appear.

Creatinine clearance can be measured by using the following formula:

$$\text{Creatinine clearance (ml/min)} = \frac{\text{total creatinine in 24-hour urine sample} \times 0.07^*}{\text{serum creatinine concentration (mg/dl)}}$$

The creatinine clearance varies with the surface area of a person. The

---

*The constant 0.07 is obtained by dividing the constant 100 (which converts mg/dl into mg/1 ml, by the constant 1440, the number of minutes in 24 hours.

normal range is from 91 to 131 ml per min, expressed per 1.73 m²
surface area.

A complete 24-hour urine sample must be obtained. If this is not
done, the calculated creatinine clearance will be underestimated.

Since creatinine is produced at a stable rate by the body, the serum
creatinine concentration is a useful index of the creatinine clearance.
The following simple rule can be used to approximate the creatinine
clearance, or the glomerular filtrate rate: *Divide the constant 100 by
the serum creatinine concentration (in mg/dl). The result is the creatinine clearance (or the glomerular filtration rate) in ml per min.* It must
be recognized that the use of this approximation is valid only for patients of relatively normal size and muscle mass (60 to 80 kg). Exceedingly small, frail patients may produce unusually small amounts of
creatinine per day so that the above formula will overestimate actual
clearance. In such patients, 24-hour urine measurement is required.
Furthermore, the above approximation is useful only when renal function is relatively stable.

As glomerular filtration (GFR) decreases, retention of nitrogenous
substances, uric acid, phosphates, and metabolic acids occurs. In addition, as GFR is reduced, tubular function is compromised, and deficits
in sodium, H_2O, and acid handling become evident. In some diseases,
such as chronic interstitial nephritis, tubular dysfunction may be impaired out of relation to GFR. Finally, endocrine functions of the kidneys, such as the 1 position hydroxylation, 25 hydroxyvitamin D3, and
the secretion of erythropoietin also become impaired.

One of the most important physiological functions of the kidneys is
to maintain a balance of fixed (nonrespiratory) acids. The kidneys do
this by excreting in the urine an amount of hydrogen ions that is approximately equal to the amount of hydrogen ions produced by metabolism, or ingested. The major source of hydrogen and sulfate ions
is the metabolic oxidation of organic sulfur-containing amino acids.
Phosphate and other ions are mostly derived from dietary sources. Uric
and other acids are also excreted by the kidneys.

When renal failure occurs, the primary disturbance is a decreased
glomerular filtration. This causes retention of urea, creatinine, uric acid,
other nonprotein nitrogenous products and organic metabolic acids. In
addition, there is an accumulation of sulfuric and particularly phosphoric acids. These acids react with sodium bicarbonate to form carbonic acid. This dissociates into water and carbon dioxide, which is
eliminated by the lungs. As a result of the loss of bicarbonate ions, the
bicarbonate-carbon dioxide ratio and the pH fall, resulting in a metabolic acidosis.

The acid-base abnormalities of azotemia result from retention of metabolic acids (such as sulfuric and phosphoric acid), and from the inability of tubular function to excrete the daily H^+ load as ammonium

ions and titratable acids. The result is an increased anion gap acidosis. However, when tubular disease is disproportionately severe, the acidosis results more from the tubular disease, and may be associated with a normal or minimally elevated anion gap. Some patients may also lose bicarbonate ions in the urine, which may further contribute to the acidosis. Respiratory compensation will occur as described in Chap 16.

There is also progressive loss of concentrating ability, so that urine osmolality becomes fixed at approximately 300 mOsm/kg H_2O). With severely reduced GFR, sodium loads may not be excreted, so that salt and H_2O overload may develop. Conversely, some patients may be unable to conserve sodium ions, so that when they eat a salt restricted diet, a sodium loss syndrome (Chap 8) may develop. Recent studies suggest that such an inability to conserve sodium ions is rare and reversible.

The disturbances in calcium metabolism result from 2 basic pathophysiologic mechanisms: inability to excrete phosphate ions and inability to 1-hydroxylate 25-vitamin D_3, so that a decreased blood level of 1,25 dihydroxyvitamin D_3 develops (see Chap 32).

The retention of phosphate ions which results from diminished GFR, causes hyperphosphatemia, which may in fact be quite subtle and may occur early in the course of chronic renal disease. The hyperphosphatemia causes reciprocal depression of serum calcium which, in turn, stimulates the parathyroid glands. The resultant hyperparathyroidism produces a variety of signs and symptoms (see Chap 33).

The inability to activate vitamin D causes reduced calcium absorption, which further promotes hypocalcemia and hyperparathyroidism. In addition, this hydroxylation deficiency results directly in defective bone mineralization. Poorly mineralized bone may, in addition, be resistant to the effects of parathyroid hormone, which further worsens the severity of the hyperparathyroidism.

DIAGNOSIS

The diagnosis of chronic renal failure is not difficult if the patient shows an increased blood urea nitrogen concentration, a fixed urinary specific gravity, albuminuria, and granular casts. Small renal size (<8 cm) by ultrasound or x-ray examination is confirmatory. However, any factor which causes a decreased renal blood flow, such as severe congestive heart failure, sodium loss, shock, or severe water loss, can cause decreased renal function which simulates primary renal failure. The diagnosis of such patients is important. Unfortunately, there is no simple way in which this can be done. If the patient does not give a history of pyelonephritis, or if previous examinations of the urine and blood have shown normal values, and if there is a history of an acute loss of sodium, water, or blood, the patient should be treated as quickly as possible with the electrolytes or fluids which have been lost.

In some diseases, such as chronic interstitial nephritis, tubular dysfunction may be impaired more proportionately than the glomerular filtration rate.

A typical partially compensatory respiratory alkalosis, described in Chapter 17, develops as a result of the metabolic acidosis. However, patients with chronic renal disease and metabolic acidosis and azotemia may develop a metabolic alkalosis, if severe vomiting occurs or if prolonged gastric suction is used. The metabolic acidosis is due not only to the retention of sulfuric and phosphoric acids but also to the reduced capacity of the tubules to produce ammonium ions and to excrete acid phosphate salts. However, the ability to acidify the urine and to excrete a urine with a low pH often remains. (Some patients also show excessive secretion of bicarbonate ions in the urine. This also produces a metabolic acidosis.)

There is also a progressive decrease in the ability of the kidney tubules to concentrate water. Normally, a concentrated urine (even 1100 mOsm/kg or more) can be excreted. When severe azotemia is present, the urine osmolality decreases to approximately 300 mOsm/kg (slightly higher than the normal serum osmolality).

When azotemia is present, the kidneys are unable to excrete as much sodium ions as a normal person (unless a salt-losing nephritis is present). Therefore, if too many sodium ions are ingested (or infused), sodium and water retention occurs and signs of congestive heart failure will develop. Conversely, if the patient is given a diet containing less than approximately 2 g of salt a day, the kidneys will continue to excrete sodium ions in the urine, unlike a normal person, so that a sodium loss syndrome (Chap 8) may develop.

Azotemia is also associated with a marked disturbance in calcium metabolism. The hypocalcemia associated with the retention of phosphate ions has already been mentioned. In addition, a defective absorption of calcium ions from the intestines occurs. This is due to vitamin D resistance (which probably results from the inability to 1-hydroxylate 25-vitamin D_3 to 1,25 dihydroxyvitamin D_3, which promotes the absorption of calcium ions in the intestines and mobilizes calcium ions from the bones. As a result, hypocalcemia often (but not always) develops. The hypocalcemia also causes stimulation of the parathyroid glands, so that secondary hyperparathyroidism develops, and the serum calcium concentration tends to rise toward normal.

The impaired activation of vitamin D results directly in defective bone mineralization. Poorly mineralized bone may be resistant to the effects of parathyroid hormone. This further worsens the severity of the hyperparathyroidism.

The secondary hyperparathyroidism may become severe, so that actual hypercalcemia may occur in association with osteodystrophy and metastatic calcification (see below). (Hypercalcemia can also be produced if the azotemic patient is given thiazides.) In some patients, the hyperparathyroidism may persist even after maintenance hemodialysis or renal transplantation. This is known as irreversible secondary (tertiary) (autonomous) hyperparathyroidism.

Calcium is present in the plasma in two forms: as ionized calcium, and as calcium bound to protein. When the ionized calcium concentration decreases, muscle irritability increases and muscle twitching may occur. In acidosis, the ionized calcium concentration is increased, even though the total calcium concentration is decreased. This is the reason that tetany does not occur in acidosis, even though muscle twitching may occur. However, if the acidosis is treated with an alkalinizing salt, such as sodium bicarbonate or sodium lactate, tetany may result, because the alkalinizing salt decreases the ionized calcium concentration. The tetany can be prevented by giving the patient calcium along with the alkalinizing salt.

Normally, the secretion of parathyroid hormone is associated with an increased excretion of phosphate ions in the urine and the development of hypophosphatemia. However, when azotemia develops, this effect decreases, so that phosphate ions are retained in the body and hyperphosphatemia develops. In addition, parathyroid hormone mobilizes calcium and phosphate ions from the skeleton. This further increases the serum concentration of phosphates.

The hyperphosphatemia causes the serum calcium concentration to fall still further, because there is an inverse relationship between the serum concentrations of these two ions. However, the degree of hyperphosphatemia is not exactly related to the degree of hyper- or hypocalcemia.

The hyperphosphatemia tends to become higher as the severity of the azotemia worsens and when the dietary phosphate intake is high. Conversely, the serum phosphate concentration tends to decrease with a high dietary *calcium* intake, or when phosphate-binding antacids (page 209) are ingested.

Disturbances in intermediary metabolism may also occur. Carbohydrate tolerance may become impaired, producing mild to moderate hyperglycemia. Conversely, diabetic patients who become azotemic may need less insulin, because insulin has a longer half-life when azotemia is present. Fat wasting may also occur.

SYMPTOMS AND SIGNS

The general signs of metabolic acidosis may be present (Chap 17). Hyperventilation of the Kussmaul type usually does not occur until the serum bicarbonate concentration falls below 10 mEq/L.

The usual symptoms and signs can be described in three categories: the uremic syndrome, secondary hyperparathyroidism, and renal osteodystrophy.

The Uremic Syndrome

Symptoms and signs are caused by the retention of urea, guanidine compounds, and other unknown substances. Any of the following may be present:

1. Central nervous symptoms. Mental depression or confusion, decreased libido, convulsive seizures (which may be due to hypertensive encephalopathy), coma, muscle cramps (which may be due to sodium loss), muscle fasciculations, or peripheral neuropathy.

   The neuropathy begins in the distal legs. The arms are usually spared and the cranial nerves are not involved. The first symptom is often a complaint of *restless legs,* relieved by moving the legs or walking. Paresthesias of the feet develop and loss of vibratory sense occurs early. Motor changes may also occur, including foot drop or even paraplegia. Peroneal nerve conduction velocity decreases (normal, 45 meters/sec); a value less than 40 meters/sec is abnormal.

   The electroencephalogram may show diffuse slowing, and a tendency to paroxysmal bursts of slow waves. The cerebrospinal fluid may show an increased lymphocyte count, and a slightly increased protein content.
2. Skin. Dry scaly skin, pruritis, nail changes, purpura, a grayish-brown discoloration (due to anemia and the deposition of urochrome pigment), or uremic "frost" (due to the precipitation of urea microcrystals in the skin).
3. Cardiovascular system. High- (or low-) output right- or left-side congestive heart failure, fibrinous pericarditis, pericarditis with effusion, occasionally constrictive pericarditis, essential or accelerated (malignant) hypertension (with or without increased renin activity in the blood), pulmonary edema, which may produce a characteristic "bat wing" exudate in the hilar areas, due partly to increased capillary permeability and to overhydration.
4. Gastrointestinal system. Nausea, vomiting, diarrhea, hiccups, stomatitis, parotitis, pancreatitis, gastrointestinal bleeding due to ulcerations. The patient may complain of an unpleasant metallic taste. The breath may show a characteristic "uremic" odor.
5. Musculoskeletal system. Muscle weakness, bone pain, fractures, pseudofractures, tendinitis, osteodystrophy (see below).
6. Genitourinary system. Nocturia, or paradoxical polyuria (during the day).
7. Hematological signs. Anemia (due partly to decreased erythropoietin), bleeding, particularly from the gums, nasal mucosa, or gastrointestinal tract, bleeding tendencies (partly due to abnormal platelet function), hemolysis.
8. Ophthalmic signs. Severe loss of vision (uremic amaurosis), nystagmus, miosis and pupillary asymmetry, decreased intraocular pressure. Ocular muscle paralysis is rare.
9. Auditory signs. Decreased hearing.

Secondary Hyperparathyroidism

This develops early in azotemia because of the continual stimulation of the parathyroid glands by the hypocalcemia. It may or may not produce symptoms or signs. However, the following signs suggest that it is present (Massry and Coburn):

1. Soft-tissue calcification, for example, calcium deposits in the conjunctive and/or cornea. The conjunctival deposits are irritating and produce the painful *red eyes* of uremic patients. Corneal deposits are asymptomatic. They are small and punctate and may show the characteristics of band keratopathy (Chap 31). In other patients, they can be observed only on slit-lamp examination.

   Other soft-tissue calcifications include vascular calcifications of the media of medium and large arteries, which may produce gangrene; visceral calcification in the heart, lungs, kidneys; calcification affecting joints, capsules, bursae, or tendons; tumor-like calcium masses around joints; pseudogout (due to the precipitation of calcium phosphate) or typical gout; or small macular or papular calcifications in the skin (particularly in patients on maintenance dialysis).

   These calcium deposits tend to appear when the product of the serum calcium and phosphate concentrations (Ca × P) reaches and exceeds 75, or if alkalosis develops. (The ionization and solubility of calcium salts is *decreased* when alkalosis is present.)

2. Osteitis fibrosa (with bone cysts), or subperiosteal bone resorption. The x-ray signs include subperiosteal resorption of the small bones of the hands (especially in the phalanges), feet, medial margin of the upper end of the tibia or distal end of the ulna, outer ends of the clavicle, skull (which develops a granular, moth-eaten appearance), and other bones.

3. Spontaneous hypercalcemia, or hypercalcemia which develops following phosphate restriction.

4. Pruritis which does not respond to adequate dialysis.

5. An elevated alkaline phosphatase level. (However, this can occur when secondary hyperparathyroidism is absent.) Hyperparathyroidism may persist even after the azotemia has been alleviated by dialysis or transplantation of a kidney (irreversible secondary [tertiary] [autonomous] hyperparathyroidism).

Renal Osteodystrophy

The term *renal osteodystrophy* includes osteitis fibrosa, osteoporosis, osteomalacia, and osteosclerosis. These changes are present in many azotemic patients, especially those maintained on chronic dialysis.

Chronic azotemia is associated with vitamin D resistance (possibly due to abnormal metabolism of vitamin D_3, associated with decreased production of 1,25-dihydroxycholecalciferol). Decreased absorption of calcium ions from the gastrointestinal tract, a secondary decreased absorption of phosphate ions, and a decreased ability of the skeleton to respond to parathyroid hormone result.

The hypocalcemia that develops is often associated with a defective mineralization of cartilage and organic bone matrix, so that (renal) rickets in children or (renal) osteomalacia in adults may develop. The metabolic acidosis also contributes to the loss of calcium ions from bone. Other factors include the loss of calcium ions from repeated hemodialyses, toxic effects of heparin which is used in the dialysate solution, or the use of fluorinated water in the solution. In addition, because of the hypocalcemia, there is continual stimulation of the parathyroid glands, so that secondary hyperparathyroidism develops. This produces osteitis fibrosa. Areas of osteitis fibrosa and osteomalacia may coexist in the same patient. These bone changes can be associated with bone pain, pseudofractures, and even fractures.

Osteosclerosis is most often localized in the vertebrae, which show a characteristic band-like increased density in the upper and lower margins separated by a central horizontal band of decreased density. The mechanism producing osteosclerosis is obscure.

LABORATORY FINDINGS

A typical example of a patient with partially compensated metabolic acidosis due to chronic renal failure is shown on page 178.

Blood Values

The blood urea nitrogen concentration is elevated and may be above 100 mg/dl (normal 10 to 20 mg/dl). The serum creatinine is also elevated above its normal concentration of 0.7 to 1.5 mg/dl.

The BUN concentration is affected by both renal and prerenal factors. The major prerenal determinant is dietary protein content. Other factors include the effective circulating blood volume (and renal blood flow). For example, the BUN concentration will rise with sodium loss and hypovolemia due to any cause. Upper gastrointestinal bleeding with resorption of blood will also elevate the BUN concentration. Glucocorticoid therapy or administration of tetracycline can also elevate the BUN concentration, by catabolic effects.

The serum creatinine concentration is determined primarily by glomerular filtration rate (and body muscle mass). Therefore, it is a more reliable indicator of renal function than the BUN concentration.

The BUN-creatinine ratio is also helpful in clinical diagnosis. Normally, and in most azotemic patients, the BUN-creatinine ratio is 10:1. The ratio may exceed 10:1 with ingestion of excessive protein, with upper gastrointestinal bleeding, with excessive tissue catabolism (for example, after burns, high corticosteroid dosage, tetracycline, acute muscle wasting), or with increased resorption of urea from the renal tubules. (This latter occurs in patients with glomerulonephritis, severe congestive heart failure, urinary tract obstruction, or in whom the urine is diverted into the ileum.)

The BUN-creatinine ratio is lower than 10:1 if the patient has a low protein intake, after repeated hemodialyses or peritoneal dialyses, if there is severe hepatic insufficiency or extreme muscle wasting.

The blood uric acid concentration may be elevated. The serum magnesium concentration is either normal or slightly elevated.

Hypertriglyceridemia (Type IV) may develop.

Urine

The urine shows a low specific gravity and may be fixed at about 1.008 to 1.012. Albumin, red and white blood cells, and short, broad, dark (renal failure) casts may be present, depending on the cause of renal insufficiency.

COURSE AND PROGNOSIS

No detailed statement can be made because each patient must be considered individually. However, nonspecific factors such as respiratory, urinary, or systemic infection, congestive heart failure, water loss, or sudden sodium loss can cause a marked decrease of renal function and an exacerbation of the acidosis.

TREATMENT

Developments in the past decade of maintenance dialysis and renal transplantation have caused marked improvement in the treatment and prognosis of chronic renal failure. However, medical treatment is still valuable for most patients.

Recognition of Potentially Reversible Azotemia

The first priority in treatment is to determine if the azotemia is due to a reversible condition, for example, obstruction (congenital or acquired) of the upper or lower urinary tract; poor renal perfusion and decreased renal blood flow due to sodium or water loss, gastrointestinal bleeding, anemia, diuretics, and so on; pyelonephritis; hypercalcemia or kidney failure due to gout; cardiovascular disturbances such as congestive heart failure, pericardial effusion, constrictive pericarditis, accelerated (malignant) hypertension; infection; renal vascular disturbances such as renal artery stenosis or thrombosis, (infectious subacute bacterial) endocarditis; chronic use of phenacetin or other nephrotoxins, lupus nephritis, periarteritis or other treatable diseases affecting the kidneys, such as multiple myeloma or lymphoma.

Diet

The diet should be low in urea-producing (protein) foods (Table 20–1) (4 g of protein produce 1 g of urea), and should be high in carbohydrates

Table 20–1. Basic Protein Foods

Food	Portion
Milk (whole or skimmed)	1 cup (200 ml)
Egg	1
Fresh meat or fish (lean or fatty)	1 oz (30 g)
Cheese (cottage)	1 rounded tblsp
Cheese (processed)	1 slice (1 oz)
Soybeans (fresh)	1/4 cup
Other legumes	1/2 cup
Nuts	1 oz
Bread	2/3 of a 1/2″ slice

*Each portion contains about 6 g of protein (24 calories).

(which have a protein-sparing effect) (Fig. 3–1, page 42). Many proteins do not provide the essential amino acids. Therefore, it is important that foods such as egg white, beef, lamb, veal, fish, and pork, which provide the essential amino acids and therefore have a high biological value, should be eaten. (Milk is used in the Giordano-Giovannetti diet [see below] but has a high phosphate concentration.) Vegetables generally have a protein content poor in essential amino acids.

Protein restriction is not indicated until the BUN concentration rises to approximately 70 mg/dl, or when uremic symptoms develop. Then, the daily protein intake should be maintained below 0.38 g per kg body weight. Therefore, a 70-kg (154-lb) patient would receive approximately 25 g protein a day. If the patient is on maintenance dialysis, the daily protein intake should be increased to 0.75 to 1.0 g per kg body weight. If the patient has severe proteinuria, daily protein needs will also be higher. After renal transplantation, protein restriction is not necessary.

At least 100 g of carbohydrate should be eaten daily. A multivitamin capsule and 1 mg folic acid daily should also be prescribed. (Patients on maintenance dialysis may require more water-soluble vitamins because they are removed during dialysis.)

The Giordano-Giovannetti Diet. In the patient with severely reduced GFR, the need for dialysis may be postponed by rigid dietary control. The key goals in such a diet are achieving a reduction in BUN concentration while avoiding net negative nitrogen balance (i.e., avoiding breakdown of endogenous protein). These goals are best achieved: (1) when the diet includes an adequate amount of calories (approximately 30 to 40 calories per kg a day); (2) when the diet has a basic minimum nitrogen content, derived from eggs and milk, rather than from meat, vegetables, or grain (vegetable and grain protein have less of the essential amino acids, and meat has too many unessential amino acids); (3) when the diet includes all the essential amino acids. This diet provides enough calories and essential amino acids in approximately 20 g of protein to lower the BUN and avoid tissue catabolism. Actual reuse of urea in synthesizing nonessential amino acids may contribute to the effectiveness of the diet, although the magnitude of this effect is probably small. Shaw has described a modified Giordano-Giovannetti diet, providing 20 g of protein daily, which is suitable for American tastes.

This diet has been successful in controlling the BUN concentration and uremic symptoms in patients with initial BUN's as high as 200 mg/dl. However, when creatinine clearance is less than 3.5 ml/min, the diet is unlikely to have long term value.

Water Balance

Renal failure is associated with a diminished ability to concentrate the urine. As a result many azotemic patients have a daily urine volume of 2 to 3 liters. Such patients require a liberal water intake to prevent dehydration.

Some patients with chronic renal disease become oliguric when the GFR is exceedingly low. Oliguria is, in fact, quite usual in patients who are receiving intermittent dialysis therapy (when urea load and sodium excess are controlled by the dialysis. Therefore, restriction of H_2O intake is necessary in these patients. A patient should receive the maximal amount of fluid per 24 hours that the kidneys can excrete without developing edema or congestive heart failure.

The following is a simple way to determine the daily water needs of a nonedematous patient: The body weight, fluid intake, and urine output must be measured daily. Have the patient collect the 24-hour urine output in a large measuring jar. The next day have him drink a volume of water equal to the previous day's volume, plus 400 to 600 ml (for water loss due to insensible evaporation).

If the weight falls, this indicates that the fluid intake is too low. If the weight rises rapidly in 2 to 3 days, this indicates excessive water intake. Other signs of excessive water intake include a rise in blood pressure, increased pulse rate, or edema or other signs of congestive heart failure.

Sodium Balance

Most azotemic patients do not lose an excessive amount of sodium ions through the kidneys. They can eat regularly prepared food, but should not use a salt shaker. If the diet contains an inadequate amount of sodium ions, a sodium loss syndrome may develop with decreased renal blood flow and worsening azotemia. Conversely, if the diet is too high in sodium ions, congestive heart failure may develop.

The following method can be used to determine if the sodium is adequate (if the patient's renal function is stable): Place the patient on a fixed sodium intake of 2 g sodium chloride (salt) (approximately 35 mEq sodium ions) a day for several days. Measure the urine sodium excretion daily. If the urinary sodium excretion is higher than the sodium intake, increase the salt intake. If the patient develops edema or other signs of congestive heart failure, decrease the sodium intake.

The patient should not use a salt substitute, because most such substances contain potassium chloride.

Some azotemic patients (particularly those with chronic pyelonephritis, polycystic disease, or medullary cystic disease) may not be able to conserve sodium ions and may develop a sodium loss syndrome (*renal salt wasting, salt-losing nephritis*) unless they are given extra salt. As much as 40 g of salt daily may be needed. The patient should be instructed to add the salt to the food, but not to use salt tablets (which dissolve poorly and may cause gastrointestinal irritation).

Danovitch, Bourgoignie and Bricker have recently demonstrated that some azotemic patients, who have been considered salt wasters, can, in fact, reduce their urinary sodium loss when dietary sodium is gradually reduced under controlled conditions. Thus, true sodium wasting is probably a rare phenomenon.

If congestive heart failure develops, a "loop" diuretic, furosemide (Lasix) can be prescribed. Massive doses (as much as 1 g or more daily) have been used in azotemic patients. However, when such large doses are used, hyponatremia, hypokalemia, hypochloremia, and metabolic alkalosis can develop, with worsening of the azotemia.

Metabolic Acidosis

No treatment is needed until the serum bicarbonate concentration decreases below 15 mEq/L. A high-protein diet aggravates the metabolic acidosis. Therefore, a low-protein diet (see above) should be used. Some phosphate-binding salts (see below) are also helpful in raising the bicarbonate concentration, by eliminating hydrogen and phosphate ions.

If a severe metabolic acidosis develops, sodium bicarbonate can be given orally in a dose of 5 g or more, or parenterally, to raise the serum bicarbonate concentration to 18 to 20 mEq/L, but not higher. If the serum bicarbonate concentration is raised too high, a metabolic alkalosis may develop, as may hypocalcemic tetany. If an excessive amount of sodium bicarbonate is given, the excessive sodium ions may precipitate congestive heart failure. If a patient needs sodium bicarbonate but cannot tolerate the sodium ions, dialysis is needed.

Shohl's solution, instead of sodium bicarbonate, can be used to correct the metabolic acidosis. It has a pleasant taste, unlike the slippery taste of sodium bicarbonate. (It is prepared by dissolving 90 g crystalline sodium citrate and 140 g citric acid in water to make 1 liter of solution. Each 1 ml of this solution contains the equivalent of 1 mEq sodium ions. Therefore, 15 ml is equivalent to approximately 1.2 g of sodium bicarbonate.)

Hyperphosphatemia

The serum phosphate concentration can be lowered by avoiding foods high in phosphates (see below) and by decreasing the dietary protein intake (see above). In addition, a phosphate-binding gel such as aluminum hydroxide gel (Amphogel) or aluminum carbonate gel (Basalgel) can be given in a dose of approximately 45 ml 1 hour after meals and at bedtime. It has a constipating effect and can cause fecal impaction. Because of the possible contribution of oral aluminum intake to aluminum overload syndromes (dementia, osteomalacia), calcium carbonate has recently been used as an effective phosphate binder, which also provides some calcium supplement. Gastrointestinal upset and hypercalcemia may limit its usefulness.

LOW PHOSPHORUS DIET

EAT:
1. Meat, fish, chicken
2. Vegetables
3. White bread with butter or oleomargarine
4. Sugar, jam, jelly, hard candy
5. Coffee, tea, carbonated drinks
6. Fruits
7. Milk, 1 cup a day
8. Eggs, 1 a day
9. Cereals, such as cream of wheat, corn flakes, rice krispies

DO NOT EAT:
1. Hard cheese or cream
2. Whole grain cereals, such as bran, oatmeal
3. Nuts and nut products
4. Dried fruits
5. Dried vegetables, such as peas, beans, lentils
6. Special meats, such as brain, sweetbreads, kidneys, sardines
7. Desserts made with milk, such as puddings, ice cream

Hypocalcemia and Osteomalacia

Vitamin D is definitely indicated if osteomalacia is present with a low serum calcium concentration and minimal hyperphosphatemia. In addition, since there is good evidence that virtually all azotemic patients have reduced levels of 1,25 dihydroxyvitamin D_3, many nephrologists empirically treat all azotemic patients with vitamin D compounds (unless hypercalcemia is present). Because vitamin D resistance is present, the patient needs large doses. Calciferol (vitamin D_2) can be given in a daily dose of 50,000 to 400,000 units. When the serum calcium concentration rises to normal, the patient can be maintained on a small dose, such as 10,000 units daily. The serum calcium concentration must be checked weekly to prevent hypercalcemia. If hypercalcemia occurs, or if the serum Ca × P product rises higher than 75, the calciferol must be stopped.

Dihydrotachysterol (Hytakerol), an analog of vitamin D_3, or 25-hydrocholecalciferol, an active vitamin D_3 metabolite, has also been used to treat azotemic hypocalcemia and osteomalacia. 1,25 dihydroxyvitamin D_3 (calcitrol) is now widely used because of its potency and shorter half life.

Symptomatic improvement, such as relief of bone pain, will occur in several weeks, although x-ray signs of improvement may not appear for several months or more.

Oral calcium supplements are generally recommended in azotemic patients, especially those who are hypocalcemic. The recommended dosage is 1 g of elemental calcium daily. This is contained in 2.5 g $CaCO_3$ (which contains 40% calcium), or in 6.5 g of Ca lactate (which contains 13% calcium).

Acute hypocalcemia with muscle twitching can be treated with calcium gluconate intravenously, as needed (10 ml of a 10% solution supplies 1 g). As much as 10 g a day can be given.

Hyperkalemia

The retention of potassium ions is usually not serious until severe azotemia occurs and the creatinine clearance decreases to approximately one-tenth normal. However, foods high in potassium ions (page 256) should be avoided. If severe hyperkalemia occurs, it should be treated promptly (Chap 24).

Hypermagnesemia

The excretion of magnesium ions is impaired in azotemia even though the serum magnesium concentration may be normal. Therefore, magnesium-containing antacids (see page 345) and magnesium-containing laxatives (milk of magnesia, Epsom salts [magnesium sulfate], and others) should not be prescribed. Similarly, magnesium sulfate should not be used to treat azotemic convulsions.

Hyperuricemia

Clinical gout does not occur frequently in azotemia, unless the serum uric acid concentration rises to 10 to 12 mg/dl or higher. Colchicine can be given for symptomatic relief. Allopurinol (Zyloprim) is also beneficial. However, azotemic patients develop exfoliative dermatitis from allopurinol more frequently than patients with normal kidneys and the dosage required is generally less than 300 mg/day. Also, if the patient has had a renal transplant, allopurinol diminishes the metabolism of azathioprine so that azathioprine dosage must be reduced.

Infections

Infections must be treated promptly. Generally, if less than 15% of a drug is excreted by the kidneys, no decreased dosage is necessary. However, if a drug is toxic and is largely excreted in the urine, a marked decrease in dosage is needed (Bennett et al.).

Nitrofurantoin and methenamine mandelate are not effective if azotemia is present. Tetracycline causes a rise in BUN concentration and should not be used. Similarly, the aminoglycoside antibiotics (gentamicin, amikacin, kanamycin, neomycin, and streptomycin) are nephrotoxic and ototoxic.

Secondary Hyperparathyroidism

Virtually all patients with severely reduced GFR have some degree of secondary hyperparathyroidism. Control of hyperphosphatemia (with diet and phosphate binders), vitamin D and calcium supplementation (in patients who are not hypercalcemic) may control the severity of the hyperparathyroidism.

Indications for subtotal parathyroidectomy in renal failure patients are hypercalcemia (which is persistent and not the result of excessive calcium supplementation, or some other disorder); severe osteitis fibrosa (with pain, fractures, etc.), intractable pruritus, soft tissue calcification (particularly visceral calcification), or ischemic necrosis of skin or muscle).

Irreversible Secondary (Tertiary) (Autonomous) Hyperparathyroidism

This usually disappears spontaneously.

Indications for Maintenance Hemodialysis

Hemodialysis is not the perfect solution to the treatment of azotemia and is associated with many complications. It decreases the severity of many but not all uremic symptoms and signs. However, it does not prevent anemia; it may not control the progress of hypertensive cardiovascular disease (which may actually increase); impotence and decreased libido may persist; neuropathy (particularly motor) may progress; pericardial effusion or constrictive pericarditis may occur; osteodystrophy and metastatic calcification, pseudogout, or irreversible secondary hyperparathyroidism may occur.

Indications for Peritoneal Dialysis

Acute Renal Failure. There are no rigid criteria for the use of peritoneal dialysis in acute renal failure. Some physicians use it only when uremic symptoms are severe. Others use it when the BUN concentration rises above an arbitrary level, for example, 125 or 150 mg/dl. It can be done every 2 to 3 days, depending on the clinical condition of the patient.

Chronic Renal Failure. Dialysis is useful when acute deterioration of renal function occurs due to intercurrent infection, congestive heart failure, volume depletion, or when the patient has improved from a previous peritoneal dialysis. It is also helpful when uremic complications such as peripheral neuropathy, encephalopathy or pericarditis occur. Laboratory indications for peritoneal dialysis in chronic renal failure include: creatinine concentration more than 10 mg/dl, creatinine clearance less than 2.5 ml per minute, uncontrollable hyperkalemia. In recent years, chronic peritoneal dialysis has been utilized for selected patients, using a specially designed reusable indwelling catheter. Patients with severe angina, bleeding problems, hemodialysis, vascular access problems, and children are all good candidates for this approach. In addition, patients who wish to dialyze themselves at home, but do not have a partner for assistance may be trained to perform home peritoneal dialysis, using an automated device for preparation and instillation of dialysate. The patients usually require three or four 12-hour dialysis sessions per week.

A technic known as chronic ambulatory peritoneal dialysis has also recently been attempted. Here, the patient performs only four 2 liter exchanges daily; but the patient does this continually. Results so far have been impressive, but a high incidence of peritonitis has been a serious problem.

Hyperkalemia. With hyperkalemia which has not responded to medical treatment, or which is life threatening, dialysis is advisable.

Intoxication from a Dialyzable Poison or Drug. If the blood level is potentially fatal, or the patient's condition is critical, peritoneal dialysis may be used to reduce the concentration of the drug or poison to a safe level; complete removal is not attempted.

Generally, however, peritoneal dialysis is remarkably less efficient than hemodialysis (or hemoperfusion utilizing a resin or charcoal column) and is of limited usefulness. For salicylate and methanol intoxication, peritoneal dialysis may be adequate, but for most other intoxications it is generally not valuable.

Other Indications
1. Severe congestive heart failure, when the patient is no longer responsive to digitalis and diuretics and when renal function is impaired.
2. Severe edema (nephrotic or cirrhotic), when the patient has not responded to diuretics or other medication.
3. Symptomatic hyponatremia, if water restriction would take too long, or if salt administration would be dangerous.

Contraindications to Hemodialysis or Peritoneal Dialysis

Although the choice of hemodialysis or peritoneal dialysis is often dependent on personal factors, specific contraindications to either form of therapy may exist. Relative contraindications to hemodialysis include chronic bleeding exacerbated by anticoagulation, angina or symptomatic hypotension induced by dialysis, or peripheral vascular disease which is worsened by dialysis vascular access procedures. Relative contraindications to peritoneal dialysis include extensive prior abdominal surgery with adhesions, ostomy appliances or malnutrition.

Indications for Renal Transplantation

Theoretically, any patient on maintenance hemodialysis is a candidate for renal transplantation. However, patients older than 50 to 55 years have a markedly increased morbidity and mortality, and are generally discouraged from seeking a transplant. Chronic infections, symptomatic coronary artery disease, valvular heart disease, severe pulmonary disease, liver disease, uncontrollable hypertension, severe peripheral vascular disease and a history of previous malignancy are all relative contraindications to transplantation.

Almost all transplants are elective. Rarely, progressive neuropathy despite adequate dialysis, or progressive debility (especially in children or adolescents), makes transplantation an indicated procedure.

The results of living related donor transplants depend on the degree of compatibility between donor and recipient. With the best matching, the probability of 2-year function of the kidney exceeds 80%. With less well-matched living related donor transplants the 2-year graft survival has been 60%, but donor specific transfusion has improved these results to 80 to 90%. Cadaver transplant results, although quite variable, seem to be reaching the 70% success rate with the use of cyclosporine.

Renal transplantation may arrest peripheral neuropathy or uncontrollable hypertension. However, it is also associated with complications related to the use of immunosuppressive drugs and corticosteroids. In addition, there may be a tendency for cancers of various types to develop de novo in transplant patients.

REFERENCES

Anderson, C.F., et al.: Nutritional therapy for adults with renal disease. JAMA, *223*:68, 1973.

Armbruster, K.F.W., Ing, Y.S., and Kark, R.M.: Nondialytic treatment of chronic renal insufficiency. Rational Drug Ther, *7*:5, 1973.

Avram, M.M., et al.: Uremic hypoglycemia. A preventable life-threatening complication. NY State J Med, *84*:593, 1984.

Bailey, G.L., and Sullivan, N.R.: Selected protein diet in terminal uremia. J Am Diet Assoc, *52*:125, 1968.

Bennett, W.M., Singer, I., et al.: Guides for drug therapy in renal failure. Ann Intern Med, *86*:754, 1977.

Bennett, W., et al.: Drug prescribing in renal failure. Am J Kidney Dis, *3*:155, 1983.

Berl, T., Berns, A., Hyfer, W., et al.: 1,25 Dihydroxycholecalciferol effects in chronic dialysis. Ann Intern Med, *88*:774, 1978.

Berlyne, G.M., and Shaw, A.B.: Giordano-Giovannetti diet in terminal renal failure. Lancet, *2*:7, 1965.

Berlyne, G.M.: Red eyes in renal failure. Lancet, *1*:4, 1967.

Danovitch, G., Bourgoignie, J., Bricker, N.: Sodium conservation in renal failure. N Engl J Med, *296*:14, 1977.

David, D.S., et al.: Dietary management in renal failure. Lancet, *2*:34, 1972. Also Am Heart J, *86*:1, 1973.

DeLuca, H.F.: The kidney as an endocrine organ. Production of 1,25-hydroxyvitamin D_3. N Engl J Med, *289*:359, 1973.

DeStrihou, C.V.Y., and Frans, A.: Pattern of respiratory compensation in chronic uremic acidosis. Nephron, *7*:37, 1970.

Diloy, M.M., and Givens, D.H., Jr.: Urinary salt-wasting in chronic renal disease. Grace Hosp Bull, *48*:41, 1970.

Dossetor, J.B.: Creatinemia versus uremia. The relative significance of blood urea nitrogen and serum creatinine concentrations in azotemia. Ann Intern Med, *65*:1287, 1966.

Editorial: Tertiary hyperparathyroidism after renal transplantation. JAMA, *209*:2048, 1969.

Eichenholtz, A., Mulhausen, R.O., and Blumentals, A.: Management of metabolic alkalosis in patients with azotemia. Arch Intern Med, *114*:236, 1964.

Eilert, J., et al.: Experience with subtotal parathyroidectomy for "tertiary" hyperparathyroidism. Arch Surg, *103*:303, 1971.

Eliahou, H.E., et al.: Acetate and bicarbonate in the correction of uremic acidosis. Br Med J, *4*:399, 1970.

Flamenbaum, W., and Kaufman, J.S.: Acute renal failure. The Kidney 9, no. 5, September 1976.

Gabow, P.A., Anderson, R.J., and Schrier, R.W.: Acute renal failure, Cardiovasc Med, *2*:1161, 1977.

Giovannetti, S., and Maggiore, Q.: A low nitrogen diet with proteins of high biological value for severe chronic uremia. Lancet, *1*:1000, 1964.

Johnson, W.J., et al.: Effects of urea loading in patients with far-advanced renal failure. Mayo Clin Proc, *47*:21, 1972.

Kassirer, J.P.: Clinical evaluation of kidney function-glomerular function. N Engl J Med, *285*:385, 1971.

Kim, K.E., et al.: Creatinine clearance in renal disease. A reappraisal. Br Med J, *4*:11, 1969.

Kurtin, P.: Principles of nutritional support for patients with renal disease. Bull NY Acad Med, *60*:1002, 1984.

Levin, D.M., and Cade, R.: Influence of dietary sodium on renal function in patients with chronic renal disease. Ann Intern Med, *62*:231, 1965.

Lowrie, E.G., et al.: Editorial: Cardiovascular disease in dialysis patients. N Engl J Med, *290*:737, 1974.

Luke, R.G.: Uremia and the BUN. Editorial. N Engl J Med, *305*:1213, 1981.

Mann, J.F.E., and Ritz, E.: Supplemental low-protein diet in chronic renal failure. Letter. N Engl J Med, *311*:1517, 1984.

Massry, S.G., and Coburn, J.W.: Renal osteodystrophy. In *Clinical Disorders of Fluid and Electrolyte Metabolism.* 2nd ed. (Maxwell, M.H., and Kleeman, C.R., Eds.). New York, McGraw-Hill Book Co., 1972.

Merrill, J.P., and Hampers, C.L.: *Uremia. Progress in Pathophysiology and Treatment.* New York, Grune & Stratton, 1971. Also N Engl J Med, *282*:953, 1014, 1970.

Muth, R.G.: Diuretic properties of furosemide in renal disease. Ann Intern Med, *69*:249, 1968.

Ogg, C.S.: Total parathyroidectomy in treatment of secondary (renal) hyperparathyroidism. Br Med J, *4*:331, 1967.

Popovtzer, M.M., et al.: Secondary hyperparathyroidism. Conservative management in patients with renal insufficiency. JAMA, *231*:960, 1975.

Rae, A., and Pendray, M.: Advantages of peritoneal dialysis in chronic renal failure. JAMA, *225*:937, 1973.

Relman, A.S.: The acidosis of renal disease. Am J Med, *44*:706, 1968.

Rose, W.C., and Dekker, E.E.: Urea as a source of nitrogen for the biosynthesis of amino acids. J Biol Chem, *223*:107, 1956.

Salvesen, H.A.: Alkali treatment of renal acidosis. Acta Med Scand Suppl. *259*:75, 1951.

Schoch, H.K.: Potassium deficiency in chronic renal disease. Arch Intern Med, *88*:20, 1951.

Schwartz, W.B., and Kassirer, J.P.: Medical management of chronic renal failure. Am J Med, *44*:786, 1968.

Schwartz, W.B., and Relman, A.S.: Acidosis in renal disease. N Engl J Med, *256*:1184, 1957.

Shaw, A.B., et al.: The treatment of chronic renal failure by a modified Giovannetti diet. Quart J Med, *34*:237, 1965.

Stanbury, W.S.: The treatment of renal osteodystrophy. Ann Intern Med, *65*:1133, 1966.

Teitelbaum, S.L.: Calcefediol (25-hydroxyvitamin D_3) in the treatment of uremic bone disease. Editorial. Ann Intern Med, *94*:404, 1981.

Tyler, H.R.: Neurologic disorders in renal failure. Am J Med, *44*:734, 1968.

Villazon, A., et al.: Polyuric syndromes in the critically ill patient. Critical Care Med, *4*:24, 1976.

Walser, M.: Keto acid therapy in chronic renal failure. Nephron, *21*, no 2, 57, 1978.

Walser, M., and Mitch, W.: Dietary managment of renal failure. The Kidney 10, no 3, May 1977.

Woods, J., Blythe, W., Huffines, W.: Management of malignant hypertension complicated by renal insufficiency. N Engl J Med, *291*:10, 1974.

CHAPTER 21

METABOLIC ACIDOSIS SYNDROMES (Continued)

ACUTE RENAL FAILURE

Acute renal failure (ARF) is characterized by an acute suppression of kidney function, which causes a rapidly progressive azotemia. This may occur in a previously normal person or in a patient with preexistent renal disease.

Renal function may be acutely suppressed by a great variety of prerenal, intrinsic renal or obstructive renal causes. The differential diagnosis of an acute deterioration of renal function is discussed subsequently; but in this chapter the focus will be on the entity of reversible acute renal failure.

Synonyms: acute tubular necrosis (ATN), lower nephron nephrosis, vasomotor nephropathy.

PATHOLOGY

Several types of lesions may be present in the kidneys:

1. Nephrotoxic lesions are due to drugs, solvents, heavy metals, and many chemicals which are directly toxic to the renal tubular cells. Necrosis of the proximal tubules of the nephrons occurs. Both kidneys are equally affected.
2. Renal ischemic lesions are due to a decreased circulating blood volume and hypotension. This causes severe renal vasoconstriction and anoxia. As a result, a type of tubular necrosis, called tubulorrhexis, occurs. This consists of wide-spread scattered necrosis of any portion of the renal tubules, associated with disruption of the basement membranes. It may be followed by permanent kidney damage. Nephrotoxic lesions and tubulorrhexis often coexist, and are, for the most part, reversible.
3. Occasionally, in clinical situations where hypotension is associated with disseminated intravascular coagulation, actual bilateral cortical necrosis may occur. This necrosis of the cortical areas of the kidney may be patchy and therefore compatible with life-sustaining renal function. However, when cortical necrosis is bilateral and extensive, recovery of renal function is virtually unprecedented.

ETIOLOGY

Acute renal failure associated with predominant nephrotoxic lesions can be produced by: antibiotics, such as amphotericin B, colistin, gentamicin, kanamycin, neomycin, polymycin, ristocetin; the urinary antiseptic phenazopyridine (Pyridium); iodinated radiographic contrast agents; heavy metals and their compounds (arsenic, bismuth, cadmium, mercury [including the organic mercurial diuretics]), etc.; organic compounds such as carbon tetrachloride, chloroform, glycols, methanol, tetrachloroethylene, etc.; substances such as aniline dyes, carbon monoxide, chlordane, diesel fuel, Lysol and other phenols, quinacrine (Atabrine), and many others.

Acute renal failure associated with predominant tubulorrhexis can occur as a result of: major surgical operations (particularly open-heart surgery, aortic surgery, water irrigation during transurethral prostatectomy, major abdominal surgery); severe or extensive trauma such as crush injuries or fractures; the release of hemoglobin into the circulation due to mismatched transfusions; sepsis, falciparum malaria (blackwater fever), mushroom poisoning or venomous snake bites; the release of myoglobin into the circulation, due to burns, crush injuries, excessive muscular exercise, electric shock, heat stroke, severe depletion of potassium ions, and many other conditions.

Tubulorrhexis can also occur when abnormal proteins circulate, as in patients with multiple myeloma (with Bence-Jones proteinuria), Waldenstrom's macroglobulinemia, as a result of the infusion of low-molecular-weight Dextran 40; or when renal ischemia occurs as a result of decreased circulating blood volume, due to sodium and water loss, severe burns, acute myocardial infarction, or massive bleeding.

Disseminated intravascular coagulation or bilateral cortical necrosis can occur as a result of intravascular coagulation and shock, as in burns, extensive trauma, transfusion reactions, gram-negative sepsis, acute pancreatitis, or obstetric complications such as premature separation of the placenta, pre-eclampsia, hypofibrinogenemia, septic abortion.

PATHOPHYSIOLOGY

The course of acute renal failure (ARF) is often divided into an *oliguric* and a *diuretic* phase. However, many patients are never oliguric, especially when drugs are the causative agent of the acute renal failure. Rarely, anuria may develop in the course of acute renal failure. Anuria is more common with cortical necrosis. Obviously, the degree of renal failure is quite variable. Some patients will have only transient mild reductions in GFR, while others may develop prolonged periods of severely reduced GFR.

Three basic pathophysiologic processes seem to contribute to ARF.

1. Intrarenal vasomotor abnormalities resulting in a transient marked reduction in renal cortical blood flow play a variable role. Vasoconstriction
   may be the major mechanism of tubulorrhexis as seen in shock syndromes.
2. Tubular obstruction secondary to occlusion by sloughed necrotic tubular
   cells may also be a contributing factor.
3. Back leak of the filtered urine through a damaged tubular epithelium may
   also contribute to the reductions in GFR and to oliguria.

These latter two mechanisms may be of most significance in nephrotoxic ARF.

The serum creatinine concentration rises approximately 2 to 3 mg/
dl per day when there is a severe reduction in renal function. The rate
of rise of the BUN concentration depends on the degree of tissue catabolism and on the protein intake. A daily rise of less than 10 mg/dl
indicates a mild catabolic reaction. A daily rise between 10 to 30 mg/
dl indicates a moderate catabolic reaction. A daily rise of the BUN
concentration above 30 mg/dl is severe, or may suggest gastrointestinal
hemorrhage.

A metabolic acidosis develops because the kidneys are unable to
excrete the metabolic acids. As a result, the serum bicarbonate concentration and the pH fall. The serum bicarbonate concentration decreases approximately 1 to 3 mEq/L daily, but may not fall below 15
mEq/L. The serum sodium and chloride concentrations also tend to fall.
However, these changes are usually due to dilution from excessive
administration of water.

Hyperkalemia results from the inability to excrete potassium ions in
the presence of daily tissue breakdown with potassium release into the
extracellular fluid. Acidosis may worsen the hyperkalemia.

Other laboratory findings include an elevated serum magnesium concentration, elevated blood cholesterol, triglyceride, and total lipid concentrations, and hyperglycemia (uremic pseudodiabetes). High serum
amylase and lipase values may be present, without pancreatitis (due
to decreased renal clearance of these enzymes).

The white cell count may be high, without infection. A severe anemia
may develop in the first week of the oliguric phase, and the hemoglobin
level may fall to 7 or 8 g/dl.

The urinalysis reflects the tubular damage which has occurred. Renal
tubular epithelial cells, blood, tubular cell casts and coarsely granular
casts are usually present. Proteinuria is variable. Other urinary findings
are discussed subsequently.

Clinical Signs. Symptoms at first are minimal and include anorexia
and tiredness. However, a severe uremic syndrome (page 202) may
develop. The oliguric phase usually lasts 6 to 12 days, but may last 1
day to 6 weeks.

Polyuric renal failure is a variant of the oligemic phase of acute renal failure. Acute and progressive azotemia occur in association with hemo-globinuria. However, instead of oliguria, the daily urine volume exceeds 500 ml per 24 hours. Polyuric renal failure has been noted following burns, trauma, distilled water instillation during transurethral prostate surgery, falciparum malaria (blackwater fever), and other conditions.

The prognosis of patients with polyuric renal failure seems to be better than that of oliguric patients. Certainly, they tend to have a lesser need for dialysis.

Diagnosis of the Oliguric Phase of Acute Renal Failure

The differential diagnosis of an acute reduction in renal function includes a great variety of possibilities. An anatomic approach can be presented as follows:

1. Prerenal—Intravascular volume depletion
   Profoundly low cardiac output
   Aortic or renal vascular occlusion
2. Intrinsic renal—small renal vascular disease (i.e. hypertensive nephro-sclerosis, scleroderma, vasculitis)
   Atheroembolism
   Hepatorenal syndrome
   Glomerulonephritis
   Tubulointerstitial disease (i.e. pyelonephritis,
      allergic interstitial nephritis, papillary necrosis)
   Cortical necrosis
   Acute renal failure
   Tubular obstruction secondary to hyperuricemia.
3. Postrenal—obstruction

It is beyond the scope of this chapter to discuss each of these entities. However, the distinction between acute renal failure and prerenal azotemia is a frequent clinical problem, which will be discussed.

Prerenal azotemia refers to patients who develop oliguria and rising BUN and creatinine concentrations due to inadequate renal perfusion. Most commonly, the inadequate renal perfusion is due to a sodium loss syndrome and there are often signs of sodium loss and volume depletion, such as orthostatic hypotension and poor skin turgor.

The BUN concentration is often increased out of proportion to the serum creatinine concentration, and the BUN/creatinine ratio exceeds 10. The urine tends to have a high specific gravity (greater than 1.020) with high osmolality (450 or more mOsm/kg). There is also high urinary urea and creatinine concentrations, and a low urinary sodium concentration (less than 15 to 20 mEq/L).

The fractional excretion of sodium ions in the urine (Fe sodium) is an index that combines the blood and urine findings, described above, into a term that objectively helps distinguish prerenal azotemia from acute renal failure:

$$\text{Fe sodium} = \frac{\text{U/P sodium ratio}}{\text{U/P creatinine ratio}} \times 100, \text{ expressed as a percentage}$$

Example: If the urine (U) sodium concentration is 20 mEq/L, and the plasma (P) sodium concentration is 140 mEq/L, the U/P sodium ratio is 20/140 = 1/7.

If the urine (U) creatinine concentration is 50 mg/100 ml, and the plasma (P) creatinine concentration is 2.0 mg/dl, the U/P creatinine concentration is 50/2 = 25.

$$\text{Therefore, the Fe sodium} = \frac{1/7}{25} \times 100 = \frac{0.14}{25} \times 100 = 0.56\%.$$

If the Fe sodium is less than 1%, prerenal azotemia is highly likely. (The hepatorenal syndrome and acute glomerulonephritis may have similar values.) If the Fe sodium is greater than 3%, acute renal failure is highly likely. Intermediate values are not diagnostic and further information is necessary for diagnosis, for example, clinical findings, urine sediment, response to cautious volume repletion.

Clinically, it is important to differentiate prerenal azotemia from acute renal failure, because if prerenal azotemia is treated promptly, acute renal failure, which is serious and may be fatal, can be prevented.

Prerenal azotemia can be differentiated clinically from acute renal failure in the following ways:

1. Intravenous fluid tolerance test. This must be done in association with constant CVP or pulmonary artery wedge monitoring. If the CVP is less than 15 cm water, give the patient an initial test volume of 200 to 300 ml IV fluid in a period of 5 to 10 minutes. Note the changes in CVP, blood pressure, and auscultatory signs in the lungs.

    If the CVP remains unchanged or does not rise more than 2 to 3 cm water above the initial level, and the blood pressure remains stable (or rises if hypotension had been present), and if signs of pulmonary congestion do not appear or worsen, give an additional infusion of 200 ml fluid in a period of 10 minutes.

    If the CVP continues below 15 cm water, and if vital signs remain unchanged, continue the IV infusion at a rate of 500 ml per hour (approximately 125 drops per minute, using a regular drip bulb), until the urinary output improves and the hypotension or signs of shock disappear, and the CVP reaches a normal level. Check the CVP, the blood pressure, and the lungs every 15 minutes.

    The type of fluid used for the IV fluid tolerance test depends on the clinical situation. If the patient has an abnormally low CVP and there are also signs of sodium loss, isotonic saline, equal amounts of isotonic saline solution and 5% dextrose in water, half-isotonic saline, or plasma, can be infused. If there is acute blood loss, a transfusion of fresh blood should be given.

    If the oligemia is prerenal, the urinary output will increase to more than 20 ml per hour within a few hours. A lack of response usually indicates the presence of acute renal failure or urinary tract obstruction. (A Foley catheter can be inserted to measure the urinary volume accurately.)

If the patient remains oliguric after the intravenous infusion has been given and if the CVP and the blood pressure have returned to normal, it is then necessary to determine if the oliguria is still prerenal and will respond to further expansion of the circulating blood volume, or whether the volume depletion has led to acute renal failure. If renal failure has occurred, the abministration of further intravenous fluids can be dangerous. The mannitol infusion test, or the intravenous injection of furosemide (or ethacrynic acid), can be used to determine this. These drugs increase blood flow through the kidney cortices and increase glomerular filtration rate and can produce a diuresis in this way.

2. The mannitol infusion test. Mannitol is given rapidly intravenously in a dose of 0.2 g per kg body weight in a period of 3 to 5 minutes. (A 70-kg [154-lb] patient would receive 14 g—70 ml—of a 20% solution.)

   An adequate response is a urine flow of 30 to 50 ml per hour (measured over a period of 2 to 3 hours). If this occurs, intravenous hydration with an appropriate fluid should be continued, and up to 100 g of mannitol (as a 10, 15, or 20% solution) can be given in divided doses every 24 hours, to maintain a urine flow of approximately 100 ml per hour.

   If the kidneys do not respond to the test dose, another test dose can be given. If there is still no response, further mannitol should not be given.

3. Intravenous furosemide or ethacrynic acid. Either of these diuretics may cause a diuresis when mannitol is not effective, and either can be used in conjunction with mannitol.

   Bullock and Shapiro use the following regimen: An initial dose of 40 mg furosemide (Lasix) is given intravenously over a period of 5 minutes. If the urine flow increases to 40 ml or more per hour in the next hour, intravenous fluids are continued and mannitol is given as needed, in a dose of 12.5 to 20 g, to maintain the urine flow at 100 ml per hour. If the urine flow increases, but remains below 40 ml per hour, the patient should receive an infusion of 500 ml isotonic saline solution, followed by a dose of mannitol, provided the condition permits. If the urine flow is still inadequate, furosemide is infused in a progressive dose schedule, starting with 80 mg and doubling the dose every 2 hours, until either diuresis occurs or a total dose of 1200 mg furosemide has been given.

   A diuretic response to furosemide should occur within 5 minutes, with a peak effect in approximately 30 minutes. When large doses of furosemide are given, as described above, serum (and urine) electrolyte concentrations must be checked, to avoid serious losses of potassium, chloride, and sodium ions.

   Ethacrynic acid (Edecrin) can be given intravenously in a dose of 50 to 100 mg instead of furosemide. However, the thiazide diuretics must *not* be used for this purpose.

The etiologic factors that can produce acute renal failure have been described above.

Acute glomerulonephritis can produce oliguria. Differentiation from acute renal failure may be difficult because the urinary findings may be similar to those of prerenal azotemia (see above).

Acute interstitial nephritis (usually due to methicillin) may also cause oliguria. The clinical findings include dermatitis, eosinophilia, and hematuria.

Bilateral renal vein thombosis, or bilateral renal arterial occlusion, may be associated with oliguria, hematuria, severe lumbar pain and marked proteinuria. X-ray examination shows increased size of the kidneys (which is not distinctive), but the IVP shows no opacification.

If urinary tract obstruction is present, with oliguria instead of anuria, abdominal x-ray examination may reveal kidneys of unequal size, or calculi.

Necrotizing papillitis, which occurs in patients with chronic pyelonephritis, diabetes, partial urinary tract obstruction, or as a result of chronic phenacetin ingestion, may be suspected by the development of chills and fever in association with the oliguria. Shreds of necrotic papillary tissue may be present in the urine.

Disseminated intravascular coagulation (DIC) may show many varied clinical signs, including hypotension and shock; overt hemolysis and abnormal bleeding, which may vary from petechiae in the skin and mucous membranes to massive bleeding into the brain, lungs, and other organs; capillary, arteriolar, or venous emboli in many organs, such as the lungs, kidneys, brain (producing signs such as acute cor pulmonale, oliguria or anuria, convulsions or coma, and so on); decrease or absence of blood clotting elements, such as fibrinogen, Factors II, V, and VIII, and platelets; and abnormal fragmented red blood cells.

Hepatorenal Syndrome. The term hepatorenal syndrome describes patients with cirrhosis of the liver who show renal failure with oliguria. In addition, there are signs of advanced cirrhosis with jaundice, portal hypertension, and hypoalbuminemia. Ascites is almost invariably present. Oliguria develops and the urine shows a characteristically low sodium concentration in contrast to the increased urine sodium concentration in the usual patient with acute renal failure (see above). BUN and serum creatinine concentrations become elevated. Prognosis is poor.

The etiology of the hepatorenal syndrome is not known. However, the kidneys are functionally normal, because if kidneys from a patient with the hepatorenal syndrome are transplanted they typically resume normal function immediately. This suggests that extrarenal or vascular factors (such as decreased effective plasma volume, renal vasoconstriction, intrarenal shunting of blood from the kidney cortices to the medullary regions and so on) may occur, producing glomerular-tubular imbalance, circulating toxins, and so on. Other factors that may predispose patients with cirrhosis of the liver to renal failure include the metabolic abnormalities that frequently occur (hyponatremia, hypokalemia, loss of extracellular fluids due to diarrhea, or excessive diuretics).

Treatment During the Oliguric Phase. In spite of advances in treatment the mortality is still approximately 50%. Two-thirds of the patients die during the oliguric phase. (Infection, hyperkalemia, bleeding [especially gastrointestinal], and jaundice are the major causes of death.)

1. The first priority is to treat the underlying disease, if it can be ascertained. The use of intravenous fluids to prevent acute renal failure from developing from prerenal azotemia has already been discussed. Alkalinization of the urine has also been recommended when acute renal failure is due to the precipitation of sulfonamide or uric acid crystals. If the acute renal failure is due to heavy metal poisoning, dimercaprol (BAL) can be used. If anuria is present, one must be certain that genitourinary obstruction is not present.

2. Stop all nephrotoxic antibiotics and drugs. In addition, do not use methicillin, sulfonamides, or tetracyclines.

3. Restrict water intake. Insensible water loss by evaporation from the skin and lungs is approximately 12 ml per kg body weight (840 ml for a 70-kg [154-lb] patient). In addition, if the patient is not eating, the catabolism of body fat and protein will provide approximately 460 ml water a day (see page 42). There is therefore a negative water balance of 840–460 = 380 ml. This amount of water should be given daily (by mouth or intravenously). (However, if there are water losses from vomiting, diarrhea, fever, or severe sweating, more water will be needed.) A simple guide to water intake is that the patient should lost 0.2 to 0.5 kg weight per day.

4. Plan the diet to decrease or prevent protein catabolism. At least 100 g of carbohydrate (or more) daily can be given. The diet should also be low in potassium salts (page 256), and absent (or low) in protein. For example, the following foods can be used: butter (or frozen butter balls), carbonated beverages (ginger ale and others), cereals (such as oatmeal, farina, cream of wheat, corn meal), sugar, Karo and other syrups, hard candy. A palatable high-carbohydrate drink can be prepared by mixing equal amounts of Karo syrup and ginger ale, flavored with lemon juice. It is served chilled (Franklin and Maxwell).

   If the patient cannot eat, a solution of dextrose in water can be infused. Since it is necessary to limit the patient's daily water intake to approximately 400 ml, an infusion of 400 ml of 10% dextrose in water will provide only 40 g of carbohydrate daily.

   Total avoidance of protein may not be necessary, and Berlyne and others have given 14 g of animal protein (high in essential amino acids [page 206]) daily. If too much protein is ingested, the BUN concentration will rise excessively daily (see above).

5. Recently, administration of essential amino acids (usually by the intravenous route) has been advocated in the management of ARF. Provision of 20 to 30 g of amino acids daily in addition to adequate calories may improve survival (and possibly hasten renal recovery). This increased nitrogen and fluid input may also increase the requirement for dialysis.

6. Hyponatremia ordinarily does not require treatment. The serum sodium concentration is usually low because of the administration of sodium-free fluids. However, if there has been a loss of sodium ions because of vomiting, diuretics, and so on, and if the serum sodium concentration is 120 mEq/L or less, salt can be added to the food, or if necessary, small volumes of sodium chloride solution can be infused.

7. Hyperkalemia does not require treatment if the serum potassium concentration does not rise above 6.5 mEq/L. However, the diet should be

low in potassium salts (see page 256). If the serum potassium concentration rises to 7.0 mEq/L or higher, active treatment is indicated. Conversely, if the serum concentration falls below 3.5 mEq/L, the potassium content of the diet can be increased.

8. Hypocalcemic symptoms can be treated with intravenous calcium salts.
9. Acidosis does not require treatment if the serum bicarbonate concentration does not fall below 15 mEq/L. Sodium bicarbonate can be used if severe acidosis develops.
10. Infections must be treated promptly. It may be difficult to determine if an infection is present, because fever may be absent and a high white blood count may be present without infection. However, unexplained hypotension or an unexplained excessive daily rise in the BUN concentration may suggest an infection. Antibiotics should not be used prophylactically. In addition, nephrotoxic antibiotics must be avoided.
11. Uremic symptoms are treated as indicated. Coma or convulsions are common neurological complications. Diastolic hypertension may develop in the second week of the oligemic phase, and may require an antihypertensive drug such as methyldopa.
12. Indications for dialysis include (after Elwood):
    a. A toxic concentration of a dialyzable nephrotoxic antibiotic or chemical.
    b. Hyperkalemia (more than 7 mEq/L) that cannot be controlled medically.
    c. Severe metabolic acidosis (pH less than 7.1, or serum bicarbonate concentration less than 5 mEq/L) that does not respond to treatment with sodium bicarbonate.
    d. A BUN concentration 200 mg/dl or higher, or a daily rise of the BUN concentration of 30 mg/dl or more, beyond a concentration of 100 mg/dl.
    e. Development of the uremic syndrome.
    f. Development of edema or congestive heart failure.
    g. Development of a pericardial rub.
    h. Encephalopathy or uremic seizures.
    i. Gastrointestinal hemorrhage.
        Hemodialysis or peritoneal dialysis can be used. Hemodialysis is indicated for the rapid correction of severe azotemia, metabolic acidosis, or hyperkalemia. In addition, toxins are more rapidly removed by hemodialysis.
13. As soon as a diagnosis of acute renal failure has been made, remove the Foley urinary catheter to avoid infection.
14. Treatment of the *hepatorenal syndrome* is mostly empirical. Papper has pointed out that measures to improve the circulation directly, using volume expansion, paracentesis, or paracentesis with reinfusion of ascitic fluid, or vasopressor drugs have not been successful. Acute dialysis to allow time to assess an individual patient is sometimes helpful. However, chronic intermittent dialysis does not appear to be helpful. A peritoneojugular venous shunt may be helpful. However, the data are still preliminary.
    Prophylactically, patients with cirrhosis of the liver must be given diuretics cautiously, ascitic or pleural effusions must be cautiously removed, and even a slight decrease in renal function or decreasing urine volume must be treated promptly.
15. The treatment of acute renal failure associated with disseminated intra-

vascular coagulation, or with complications of pregnancy is outside the scope of this book.

The Diuretic Phase

The *early* diuretic phase occurs when the daily urine volume is consistently more than 400 ml. Massive urine volumes, even 5 to 10 liters daily, may be present, if the patient is receiving too much fluid. However, the daily urine volume should not be allowed to exceed 4 liters. The early diuretic phase lasts approximately 4 to 7 days. During this time, the BUN concentration may continue to rise, and uremic symptoms and signs may temporarily increase.

The *late* diuretic phase occurs when the BUN concentration starts to decrease. The BUN concentration becomes normal approximately 15 to 20 days after the start of the diuretic phase. The fall in BUN concentration is associated with marked improvement of uremic symptoms and signs. However, the patient may not feel normal for another 2 to 3 months. In addition, anemia may persist for months and decreased kidney function may continue for a year or more.

Treatment During the Diuretic Phase. Treatment depends on the amount of water and electrolytes excreted daily. There are no rigid rules for therapy. If the patient has received an excessive amount of water, sodium or other ions during the oliguric phase, an excessive amount of water and electrolytes will be excreted in the urine during the diuretic phase.

The patient should receive both water and electrolytes. Water intake should be maintained at 400 to 500 ml a day, plus approximately two-thirds the volume of urine that had been excreted the previous day. (However, the daily fluid intake should not exceed 3500 ml because the diuretic phase may be prolonged by replacing the *total* volume of urine lost daily.) In addition, an excessive amount of electrolytes may be excreted and lost by this marked diuresis. The patient should continue to lose approximately one-half pound daily. However, care should be taken to prevent shock due to sodium loss or desiccation due to water loss.

There are several methods of replacing the electrolytes that are lost in the urine. The urine can be collected daily and its electrolyte content determined. This may be difficult to do.

Use of the following solution is based on the observation that the urine in the diuretic phase contains sodium ions in a concentration of approximately 50 mEq/L (approximately one-third that of plasma). In addition, a large amount of potassium and magnesium ions may be excreted in the urine.

Isotonic sodium chloride solution	225 ml
⅙ molar sodium lactate solution	110 ml
Potassium chloride, 35 to 40 mEq if the serum potassium concentration is less than 5 mEq/L	
10% dextrose in distilled water	665 ml
Total	1000 ml

If the sodium concentration of this solution is less than or more than the daily loss of sodium ions, changes in the serum sodium concentration will occur. (However, these changes may be difficult to analyze because the BUN concentration may vary from day to day.) In addition, the serum potassium concentration should not be allowed to rise higher than 5.5 mEq/L, or to fall below 3.5 mEq/L.

The patient should be encouraged to eat and drink as soon as possible. When the BUN concentration is less than 100 mg/dl, the patient can be placed on a 40-g protein diet, high in essential amino acids (page 206). As soon as the azotemia subsides, the patient can be placed on a high-protein, high-carbohydrate intake, to promote weight gain.

PROPHYLAXIS OF ACUTE RENAL FAILURE

During major surgery, the anesthetist should make certain that the patient has a urine output of at least 50 ml (or even 75 to 100 ml) per hour (also see Chap. 34). In addition, patients with the nephrotic syndrome, multiple myeloma, obstructive jaundice, undergoing open-heart surgery, biliary and gastrointestinal surgery, are prone to acute renal failure. Low-molecular-weight Dextran 40 must be used cautiously in elderly patients. Diagnostic radiography with a triiodinated dye also increases the likelihood of acute renal failure.

REFERENCES

Abel, R., Beck, G., and Abbott, W.: Improved survival of acute renal failure after therapy with intravenous essential L-amino acids and glucose. N Engl J Med, *288*:695, 1973.

Auger, R.C., et al.: Use of ethacrynic acid in mannitol-resistant oliguric renal failure. JAMA, *206*:891, 1968.

Barry, K.G., and Berman, A.R.: Mannitol infusion. N Engl J Med, *264*:1085, 1961.

Berlyne, G.M., et al.: The dietary treatment of acute renal failure. Quart J Med, *36*:59, 1967.

Brown, J.J., et al.: Renin and acute renal failure. Br Med J, *1*:253, 1970.

Bullock, M.L., and Shapiro, F.L.: Acute renal failure. Part 2. Hydration: first principle of prevention. Mod Med, April 29, 56, 1974.

Burton, J.R., et al.: Acute renal failure during cephalothin therapy. JAMA, *229*:679, 1974.

Butkus, D.E.: Persistent high mortality in acute renal failure. Editorial, Arch Intern Med, *143*:209, 1983.

Cantarovich, R., et al.: High dose frusemide in established acute renal failure. Br. Med J, *4*:449, 1973.

Conn, H.F.: Rational approach to the hepatorenal syndrome. Gastroenterology, *65*:321, 1973.

Diamond, J.R., and Yoburn, D.C.: Nonoliguric acute renal failure. Arch Intern Med, *142*:1882, 1982.

Eliahou, H.E.: Mannitol therapy of oliguria of acute onset. Br Med J, *1*:807, 1964.

Eliahou, H.E., and Bota, A.: The diagnosis of acute renal failure. Nephron, 2:287, 1965.

Franklin, S.S., and Maxwell, M.H.: Acute renal failure. In *Clinical Disorders of Fluid and Electrolyte Metabolism* (Maxwell, M.H., and Kleeman, C.R., Eds.). New York, McGraw-Hill Book Co., 1972.

Goggin, M.J., and Joekes, A.M.: Gas exchange in renal failure. I. Dangers of hyperkalemia during anesthesia. Br Med J, 2:244, 1971.

Hilton, P.J., et al.: Urinary osmolality in acute renal failure due to glomerulonephritis. Lancet, 2:655, 1969.

Hollengang, N.K., et al.: Acute renal failure in man. Evidence for preferential renal cortical ischemia. Medicine, 47:455, 1968.

Kleinknecht, D., et al.: Uremic and non-uremic complications in acute renal failure. Evaluation of early and frequent dialysis on prognosis. Kidney, 1:190, 1972.

Lauler, D.P., and Schreiner, G.E.: Bilateral renal cortical necrosis. Am J Med, 24:519, 1958.

Lauler, D.P., Schreiner, G.E., and David, A.: Renal medullary necrosis. Am J Med, 29:132, 1960.

Levinsky, N.G.: Management of emergencies. Acute renal failure. N Engl J Med, 274:1016, 1966.

Levinsky, N.: The interpretation of proteinuria and the urinary sediment. Disease-a-Month, March, 1967.

Levinsky, N.: Pathophysiology of acute renal failure. N Engl J Med, 296:1453, 1977.

Levitt, M.F.: Therapy for acute renal failure. Mod Med, Jan 1, 71, 1958.

Luke, R.G., et al.: Mannitol therapy in acute renal failure. Lancet, 1:980, 1965.

Maher, J.F.: Nephrotoxicity of drugs and chemicals. Pharmacol. Physicians, 4:1, 1970.

Miller, F.C. et al.: Zomepirac-induced renal failure. Arch Intern Med, 143:1171, 1983.

Merrill, J.P.: Acute renal failure. JAMA, 211:289, 1970.

Miller, T., Anderson, R., and Linas, S.: Urinary diagnostic indices in acute renal failure. Ann Intern Med, 89:47, 1978.

Moncrief, J.W.: Acute renal failure. Hints on how to avoid it. Consultant, 13:76, 1973.

Montoreano, R., et al.: Prevention of the initial oliguria of acute renal failure by the administration of furosemide. Postgrad Med, 47:7, 1971.

Papper, S.: The hepatorenal syndrome. The Kidney 10: No. 1, January 1978.

Perlmutter, M., et al.: Urine-serum urea nitrogen ratio. JAMA, 170:1533, 1959.

Siegler, R.L., and Bloomer, A.: Acute renal failure with prolonged oliguria. JAMA, 225:133, 1973.

Smolens, P., and Stein, J.H.: Pathophysiology of acute renal failure. Am J Med 70:479, 1981.

CHAPTER 22

METABOLIC ACIDOSIS SYNDROMES (Continued)

DIABETIC ACIDOSIS

INTRODUCTION

The National Diabetic Data Group in 1979 described the following clinical classification of diabetes mellitus:

Type I—insulin-dependent (formerly called juvenile-onset, or ketosis-prone) diabetes mellitus. The fasting plasma glucose concentration is more than 140 mg/dl. Insulin is needed to prevent ketosis.

Type II—noninsulin-dependent (formerly called maturity-onset or ketosis-resistant) diabetes mellitus. The fasting plasma glucose concentration is more than 140 mg/dl. Insulin may be needed to control hyperglycemia. Ketosis does not develop unless the patient is subjected to stress of various kinds.

Impaired glucose tolerance. The fasting plasma glucose concentration is less than 140 mg/dl.

Gestational diabetes mellitus.

Secondary diabetes mellitus, associated with certain conditions and syndromes, such as pancreatic disease, excessive glucocorticoid hormones (Cushing's syndrome), drug or chemically induced, and so on.

PATHOPHYSIOLOGY

The major sources of glucose (dextrose) in the body are food, liver glycogen, and glycogenesis from the metabolism of protein and fat. In the presence of insulin, a portion of the glucose is converted into glycogen in the liver. Part is oxidized to lactate and pyruvate, and then to carbon dioxide and water. A part of the glucose is also converted into acetate and then to amino acids and protein, or to fatty acids. Insulin also has a fat-sparing and protein-sparing effect, because it helps prevent the oxidation of fat and protein for energy.

The primary metabolic defect of a diabetic patient is a decreased ability to utilize glucose. This in turn is due either to a decreased secretion or a decreased effectiveness of insulin. The exact way in which insulin acts is not completely understood. It probably increases the passage of glucose into the cells through the cell membrane and stimulates carbohydrate metabolism in skeletal and cardiac muscles and in adipose tissues. It may also increase the conversion of glucose to glucose-6-phosphate. The glucose-6-phosphate can then be converted into glycogen or is further metabolized.

Diabetic ketoacidosis is characterized by the overproduction of glucose and ketone bodies in the liver, and by excessive mobilization of free fatty acids from adipose tissue. Recent studies by Unger and others indicate the pancreatic hormone, glucagon, is important in the pathogenesis of both diabetes mellitus and of diabetic ketoacidosis. For example, when a defect of insulin secretion is present, either an absolute excess or an excess of glucagon relative to the amount of available insulin, can cause the liver to form glucose at a rate that exceeds the limited capacity of the diabetic patient to clear it from the blood stream. McGarry and Foster have shown that insulin lack by itself will increase the supply of free fatty acids, but that glucagon is essential for the liver to produce ketone bodies in massive quantities. When the hyperglucagonemia of the diabetic patient is blocked, as by the administration of the hormone, somatostatin, a lack of insulin results in a rise in the level of free fatty acids, but ketone production does not increase unless an excessive amount of glucagon is present.

When insulin is not secreted nor utilized, the following physiological and chemical disturbances occur:

1. Hyperglycemia develops because the insulin supply is inadequate. The concentration of glucose in the extracellular water and blood rises because glucose is not being utilized. When the renal circulation is normal, the plasma glucose concentration rarely rises higher than 400 mg/dl. However, when renal circulation is inadequate and water loss occurs, much higher blood glucose concentrations occur.

   The renal threshold for glucose is approximately 170 mg/dl. When this threshold is exceeded, glycosuria occurs. As a result large amounts of water and electrolytes are lost (osmotic diuresis) as well as glucose. And severe water loss can occur.

2. When the insulin supply is inadequate, the action of lipase is no longer inhibited. As a result, uncontrolled lipolysis occurs and the concentration of free fatty acids exceeds the capacity of the body to metabolize them. They are partially metabolized by the liver into ketones. The increased lipolysis also causes the fat content of the blood to rise greatly.

3. Hyperosmolality occurs because the high concentrations of glucose and fat in the blood increase the osmotic pressure of the extracellular water. This lowers the serum sodium concentration (Appendix 4).

   When the plasma glucose concentration is more than 500 mg/dl, this suggests that significant hyperosmolality is present.

4. Metabolic acidosis and ketosis occur. Fat is metabolized at an excessive

rate to supply energy. As a result large amounts of ketone acids (b-hy-droxybutyric acid and aceto-acetic acid) are formed. (This produces the metabolic acidosis with an abnormal large anion gap.)

Acetone (formed from the aceto-acetic acid) also accumulates in the blood. It produces a characteristic fruity odor on the patient's breath, but it does not lower the pH.

These metabolic and ketone acids react with the sodium bicarbonate of the blood forming sodium ketone and metabolic acid salts, water, and carbon dioxide. The carbon dioxide is eliminated through the lungs. As a result, the bicarbonate-carbonic acid ratio and the pH fall, producing a metabolic acidosis.

5. Sodium and water loss occurs. This may be severe. This may be due to the osmotic diuresis. It may also be due to vomiting. One must remember that the low serum sodium concentration in patients with hyperglycemia may be more apparent than real (Appendix IV).

    The sodium and water loss is associated with hypotension and even with shock.

6. Hyperkalemia may occur because the metabolic acidosis causes a shift of potassium ions from the cells into the extracellular water in exchange for hydrogen ions, which enter the cells and are buffered there. This movement of potassium ions out of the cells tends to produce an increased serum potassium concentration. However, potassium ions are continually lost with the osmotic diuresis so that the serum potassium concentration may be high, normal or low.

7. The cholesterol concentration of the blood increases. This is due to an increased synthesis of cholesterol in the absence of insulin.

8. Protein is metabolized at an excessive rate to supply glucose and energy. This increases the amount of nitrogenous wastes and acid metabolites in the blood.

9. The acidosis may cause a compensatory respiratory alkalosis, which may persist even after the pH has returned to normal. This is not unique to patients with diabetic acidosis, and occurs in all types of metabolic acidosis.

10. An acidosis associated with an excessive amount of lactic acid in the blood may develop with phenformin (DBI) treatment. (DBI is no longer marketed for general use, although it is still available as an investigational drug.) One should also remember that diabetic ketoacidosis and lactic acidosis may be present simultaneously.

11. A precipitating factor (or factors) must be sought in every patient who develops diabetic acidosis. Common precipitating factors include failure to take insulin and infections of any type. Other underlying factors include acute myocardial infarction, acute pancreatitis (the serum amylase concentration may be elevated in diabetic acidosis in the absence of pancreatitis), endocrine disorders (hyperthyroidism, acromegaly, pheochromocytoma, Cushing's syndrome), rarely severe emotional stress, and occasionally drugs (for example, thiazide diuretics, furosemide, ethacrynic acid).

SYMPTOMS AND SIGNS

These have already been described in Chapter 17. The temperature is usually normal or subnormal. Therefore, even a slightly elevated temperature suggests that an infection may be present.

LABORATORY FINDINGS

Blood

The electrolyte concentrations vary greatly, and depend on the duration and degree of the acidosis and the presence of associated decreased renal function. A constant and characteristic finding is a low serum bicarbonate concentration. Serum sodium is usually low. This is due either to sodium loss or to the increased osmolality of the extracellular water, caused by the high glucose concentration in the blood (Chap. 11). If an excessive amount of water has been lost, the serum sodium concentration will be high.

Serum chloride concentration is usually normal. It may be low as a result of urinary excretion, or vomiting.

Serum potassium concentration is usually normal, or high, due to the acidosis. Even if the total potassium supply of the body is depleted, the serum potassium concentration may be normal or high. Occasionally, a low serum potassium concentration occurs. This may be due to a loss of potassium ions from vomiting or inadequate food intake because of anorexia. Breakdown of muscle tissue and failure of glycogen deposition in the liver also tend to deplete the body stores of potassium ions. (When excessive potassium and chloride ions are lost, a metabolic alkalosis may replace the diabetic metabolic acidosis.) A normal or low serum potassium concentration in the presence of acidosis is a presumptive sign of potassium loss.

The blood sugar is characteristically high, and may reach or exceed 1500 mg/dl. Ketone acids are present in the blood and urine. A simple method of determining their presence is described below.

An elevated blood urea nitrogen concentration is found in the majority of patients. This is a result of increased protein catabolism and prerenal azotemia, secondary to the loss of extracellular fluids.

Urine

Ketonuria and glycosuria are present. Urinary ketone concentration may be high even when plasma ketone concentration is low. This is due to increased urinary excretion of the ketones, which results from the renal compensation for the metabolic acidosis.

The white blood count may be high, and values as high as 90,000/cu mm have been reported in uncomplicated diabetic patients with acidosis.

Serum amylase values may be abnormally high, even if acute pancreatitis is not present.

Example: Moderate diabetic acidosis
Blood sugar 450 mg/dl.
pH 7.34

P_{CO_2} 38 mm Hg
Standard bicarbonate 20.3 mEq/L
Actual bicarbonate 20 mEq/L
Base excess − 5 mEq/L
CO_2 content 21 mEq/L

The pH is slightly low. This indicates a mild acidosis. The negative base excess and the low standard bicarbonate indicate that a metabolic acidosis is present. The P_{CO_2} is normal, indicating respiratory balance. However, the actual bicarbonate is slightly lower than the standard bicarbonate. This indicates that a respiratory alkalosis is present. Therefore, a mild metabolic acidosis is present with a compensatory respiratory alkalosis (see Chap. 15).

This information can also be determined from the pH and P_{CO_2} by inspection of Figure 15–4, page 154.

Cation-anion balance:
Na 135 K 5 HCO_3 20 Cl 92 mEq/L
Anion gap = (Na + K) − (HCO_3 + Cl)
    = (135 + 5) − (20 + 92)
    = 140 − 112
    = 28 mEq/L. This is abnormally high. It is due to the accumulation of ketone acids.
Example: Patient with severe diabetic acidosis
Blood sugar 950 mg/dl
pH 7.2
P_{CO_2} 12.3 mm Hg
Standard bicarbonate 8.3 mEq/L
Actual bicarbonate 5 mEq/L
Base excess − 22.2 mEq/L

The pH is low, indicating a severe acidosis. The negative base excess and the low standard bicarbonate indicate that a metabolic acidosis is present. The low P_{CO_2} and the fact that the actual bicarbonate is lower than the standard bicarbonate indicate that a respiratory alkalosis is present. Therefore, a severe metabolic acidosis is present with a partially compensatory respiratory alkalosis (see Chap. 15).

This information can also be determined from the pH and P_{CO_2} by inspection of Figure 15–4, page 154.

Cation-anion balance:
Na 131 K 4.7 HCO_3 5 Cl 95 mEq/L
Anion gap = (Na + K) − (HCO_3 + Cl)
    = (131 + 4.7) − (5 + 95)
    = 135.7 − 100
    = 35.7 mEq/L. This is abnormally high. It is due to the accumulation of ketone acids.

DIAGNOSIS

It has already been pointed out that patients with renal tubular acidosis may also show glycosuria and ketonuria. However, in these patients, the blood sugar concentration is normal, and abnormal ketone acids are not found in the blood. Acetone and reducing substances which give a false positive test for glucose are also present in salicylate poisoning. In these patients, the blood sugar concentration is usually normal, or slightly elevated. In addition, a positive ferric chloride test for salicylates in the urine is present (also see Chap. 23).

Oxazepam (Serax) will also give a false-positive test reaction for glucose in the blood. Therefore, oxazepam intoxication may simulate diabetic coma.

Acetaminophen (paracetamol) overdosage can produce hypoglycemia and even hypoglycemic coma by injuring the liver. However, acetaminophen also can interfere with the measurement of the blood glucose concentration and indicate a spurious hyperglycemia. If insulin is given to such a patient, serious and even fatal complications can occur. The blood sugar should be checked with a Beckman glucose analyzer, if possible, if this is suspected.

Ethyl alcohol ketoacidosis may simulate diabetic acidosis because the patient may be comatose and the blood glucose concentration may be slightly elevated (even higher than 300 mg/dl). However, if blood or urine tests for ketones are done with Acetest (Ames), a negative result will be obtained because the Acetest is sensitive only to aceto-acetate ketones, whereas there is an excessive amount of beta-hydroxybutyrate ketones in alcoholic ketoacidosis. Beta-hydroxybutyrate ketone concentrations can be measured with enzymatic methods.

When these patients are treated with intravenous dextrose and water (the treatment of choice), the beta-hydroxybutyrates are converted into aceto-acetates, so that the ketosis will paradoxically seemingly become more severe as the patient's clinical condition is improving (if only aceto-acetate ketones are measured).

The differential diagnosis of diabetic patients who develop coma is shown in Table 22–1.

COURSE AND PROGNOSIS

In spite of recent advances in therapy, from 15 to 24% of patients with diabetic acidosis will die. However, many of these deaths are now due to associated pathological disturbances rather than to the diabetic acidosis.

PROPHYLAXIS

Every diabetic patient should be taught to test the urine for both sugar and acetone (ketone acids) and to report the presence of acetone to the physician immediately. The physician should also be aware that factors such as infection, trauma, surgical operation, irregular diet, inadequate

Table 22–1. Differential Diagnosis of Coma in Diabetic Patients

Laboratory tests	Diagnosis				
	Diabetic ketoacidosis	Hyperosmolal hyperglycemic nonketoacidosis	Hypoglycemia	Lactic acidosis	Ethyl alcohol ketoacidosis
Plasma					
Glucose	High	Very high	Low	Normal, or high	Slightly high
Ketones	4 plus*	Absent	Absent	Absent	Absent‡
pH	Low	Normal	Normal	Low	Low
CO$_2$ content (or bicarbonate)	Low	Normal	Normal	Low	Low
Osmolality	High	Very high	Normal	Normal	High
Lactate	Normal	Normal	Normal	Very high	Normal
BUN	Elevated	Elevated	Normal	Elevated	Normal or high
Urine					
Glucose	4 plus	4 plus	Absent†	Absent to 4 plus	Absent or present
Ketones	4 plus	Absent	Absent†	Absent	Absent‡

*4 plus or more in an undiluted sample.

†Urine that has been in the bladder for several hours may show glucose or ketones as a result of earlier hyperglycemia or ketonemia.

‡The Acetest reaction may be negative because the predominant ketone present is beta-hydroxybutyrate. A test for beta-hydroxybutyrate ketones will be positive.

Table 22–2.   *Schedule of Laboratory Tests Which Should be Done in the Treatment of Patients with Diabetic Acidosis*

Hours of Treatment	0	1	2	3	4	5	6	7	8	9	10	11	12
Blood sugar	*				*				*				*
Ketones	*		*		*		*		*		*		*
CO₂ content or bicarbonate	*				*				*				*
pH and Pco₂	*				*				*				*
Hematocrit	*		*		*		*		*		*		*
Urea nitrogen	*												*
Potassium, sodium, chloride (magnesium)	*				*				*				*
Urine													
Sugar	*		*		*		*		*		*		*
Ketone	*				*				*				*
Analysis	*				*				*				*
Electrocardiogram	*				*				*				*
Blood pressure	*	*	*	*	*	*	*	*	*	*	*	*	*

*Indicates intervals at which the respective studies are usually performed.

insulin dosage, vomiting or diarrhea from any cause, pregnancy, thyrotoxicosis, or the acute onset of diabetes can precipitate diabetic acidosis.

TREATMENT

The treatment of diabetic acidosis is complicated because several independent disturbances may be present simultaneously. For example, in addition to a lack of insulin, sodium loss, water loss, potassium loss, shock, accumulation of ketone acids producing a metabolic acidosis, a metabolic acidosis due to decreased renal function, even in the absence of previous renal disease, and a compensatory respiratory alkalosis which may persist even when the acidosis is corrected may be present.

The following plan of therapy can be used:

Emergency Treatment

A flow chart should be started (Table 22–2) to chart the results of laboratory tests. In addition notes should be made of the patient's vital signs and level of consciousness.

As soon as the patient is admitted to the hospital, the following tests should be done: blood sugar, plasma acetone, carbon dioxide content, pH, hematocrit and hemoblobin, blood urea nitrogen, potassium; urine sugar, acetone, and routine urine analysis; electrocardiogram; blood pressure and pulse. These tests can be repeated according to Table 22–2.

Treatment should include correction of the hyperglycemia and hyperosmolality, metabolic acidosis and ketosis, sodium loss, water loss, potassium loss.

Use of Low-Dose Regular, Rapidly Acting Insulin

It has been found that large doses of IV or subcutaneous insulin used previously are not necessary. Regular insulin can be given IV or IM. Then, when the acidosis is under control, the patient can receive insulin subcutaneously.

If the patient is hypotensive, insulin should be given IV rather than IM because the intramuscular absorption from poorly perfused muscles may be erratic. When the blood pressure is stable, insulin can be given IV or IM.

A continuous infusion of regular insulin at a rate of 6 to 10 units per hour is usually adequate.

When insulin is given IV, some of it may bind to the glass container and to the plastic tubing. This can be counteracted by adding 100 units regular insulin to 1 L full-strength (isotonic) saline solution and discarding the first 50 ml of the solution.

One ml per minute of this solution will deliver 6 units of insulin per hour. The solution should be given with an infusion pump if possible or with a pediatric microdrip bulb which delivers 1 ml with 60 drops.

> 100 units insulin in 1000 ml. (1 L).
> = 0.1 unit in 1 ml.
> If 1 ml is delivered per min, 60 ml will be delivered in 1 hour. Therefore 0.1 × 60 = 6 units of insulin will be delivered in 1 hour.

One must be careful not to lower the blood glucose concentration too fast. If this occurs, the plasma glucose concentration falls below the intracerebral glucose concentration because of the blood-brain barrier. This can lead to mental confusion and other neurologic abnormalities.

The IV insulin is given at the rate described above until the blood glucose concentration falls to approximately 250 mg/dl. (With adequate insulin therapy, the blood glucose concentration should fall from 75 to 100 mg/dl per hour).

When the blood glucose concentration reaches 250 mg/dl and when the ketosis disappears, the IV insulin can be stopped and regular insulin subcutaneously should be started every 2 hours.

The dose of regular subcutaneous insulin can be determined from blood glucose concentrations, or from double-voided urine specimens (to make certain that one is not checking the glucose concentration of residual urine in the bladder).

Regular insulin can be given subcutaneously every 2 hours on the basis of the following urinary findings:

Urinary Sugar		Regular Insulin Dosage
1/10%*	(trace)	0
1/4%	(trace)	0
1/2%	(1 plus)	0
3/4%	(2 plus)	5 units
1%	(3 plus)	10 units
2%	(4 plus)	10 units

*The American Diabetic Association recommends that this numerical system of reporting urinary blood sugar values should be used.

Determining the Degree of Ketosis

The degree of ketosis can be determined in a general way, using the effect of plasma (or serum) on a crushed Acetest tablet.

Acetone in the plasma is tested in the following way: Approximately 10 ml of blood is drawn, placed in a test tube with potassium oxalate, and shaken to prevent clotting. The tube is allowed to stand until a drop of clear plasma can be drawn off the surface, or the tube can be centrifuged immediately.

To get a drop of plasma more rapidly, absorbent cotton can be twisted around the tip of a pipette or dropper. The blood is sucked through the pipette. The cotton allows only plasma to be drawn into the pipette.

A drop of undiluted plasma is placed on a *crushed* Acetest tablet. (The undiluted plasma may not adequately wet an intact tablet, and this may cause a false-negative reading.) The result can be graded as 1 plus (faint), 2 plus (moderate), and 3 plus (marked). If a 3 plus reaction occurs, the plasma is diluted with an equal part of water or saline solution *(first dilution plasma)*, and tested again for acetone. If a 3 plus reaction still persists, it is diluted again with an equal part of water or saline solution *(second dilution plasma)*, and the acetone test is done again.

Captopril can give a false-positive ketone urine test.

When the blood glucose concentration has fallen to 250 mg/dl and the IV insulin is stopped, the patient can receive an infusion of 5 or 10% dextrose in water and is allowed to have oral fluids such as diluted orange juice, water, salted broth, or diabetic carbonated drinks.

Subcutaneous regular insulin can be continued for 24 to 36 hours, when an intermediate-acting insulin can be started.

Insulin Resistance

If, after the first 2 hours of IV insulin therapy, the plasma glucose concentration is not decreasing and the arterial pH is not increasing, then the insulin dosage should be doubled every 2 hours until a significant response is observed (Shade and Eaton).

An alternate therapy to combat such insulin resistance is to give the patient 100 units of regular insulin IV. The dose may be doubled every 1 to 2 hours (100, 200, 400 units, etc.) if no response is obtained (Kleeman and Narins).

Use of Regular Insulin IM

Six to 10 units of regular insulin can be injected IM preferably into the arms rather than the buttocks, hourly. The same conditions described for the use of IV insulin, see above, apply.

The blood sugar level should not be lowered too rapidly because, when severe hyperglycemia occurs, the glucose concentration of the interstitial spaces of the brain also rises, in spite of the blood-brain barrier. If the blood sugar concentration falls too rapidly with treatment, the osmotic pressure of the blood rapidly falls below that of the brain interstitial fluid. Therefore, water moves out of the blood and into the brain tissue and may cause cerebral edema and coma (Fulop, et al).

Sodium Loss

Most patients with diabetic acidosis show a loss of sodium ions as well as water. Therefore, intravenous fluids should be started with a sodium-containing solution such as isotonic saline (sodium chloride solution) (although some physicians prefer to start with half-strength sodium chloride solution). Two to 3 liters of isotonic sodium chloride solution can be given in the first 6 to 12 hours. The first 2 liters can be given at a rate of 500 to 1000 ml per hour. If more than 3000 ml of isotonic sodium chloride solution is given in the first 24 hours, a metabolic acidosis due to the high chloride content of the sodium chloride solution may be induced (page 173). Therefore, half-strength sodium chloride solution should be used after the first 3 to 4 liters of isotonic sodium chloride solution have been infused.

Patients may require as much as 6 or more liters of fluid to correct the water loss. If the patient is elderly or has organic heart disease, one should observe for signs of developing congestive heart failure such as increased respiratory rate, engorged liver, distented neck veins, edema.

Shock

Sodium chloride solution may cause the shock to disappear. If this does not relieve the shock, dextran, plasma, or whole blood (if anemia is present) can be used. The use of vasopressor drugs such as dopamine (Intropin), and so on, is now considered to be secondary to fluid replacement in the treatment of shock.

Alkalinizing Solutions

There is a difference of opinion as to whether an alkalinizing solution should be used routinely in the treatment of diabetic acidosis. I believe that it is usually not necessary for the following reasons:

1. The basic cause of the acidosis is the lack of insulin and the accumulation of ketone acids. Therefore, as insulin is given and the ketone acids are metabolized, the acidosis disappears.
2. Sodium bicarbonate may paradoxically increase spinal fluid acidosis and may precipitate coma (Ohman, et al).
3. When diabetic acidosis is treated the usual way, rises in CO_2 content, serum bicarbonate concentration, and pH are associated with the elimination of ketone acids from the blood. However, if sodium bicarbonate is given, it will cause only these values to rise and may obscure the persistence of a significant ketonemia.
4. When the CO_2 content or the serum bicarbonate concentration is raised too high with sodium bicarbonate therapy, a metabolic alkalosis may develop (Chap. 17).

However, when the CO_2 content is below 10 mEq/L, or the serum bicarbonate concentration is below 9 mEq/L, or the pH is 7.1 or less, insulin is less effective. Therefore, sodium bicarbonate can be used. The dosage of sodium bicarbonate is described in Chapter 17.

Sugar Solutions

As was pointed out above, dextrose in water infusion is not needed until the blood glucose concentration falls to approximately 250 mg/dl. This may not occur for four or more hours if the initial blood glucose concentration had been high.

When the blood glucose concentration has fallen to this level, there is danger that hypoglycemia may suddenly occur. If this occurs, neurologic complications, described above, may develop. Hypoglycemia can be avoided by starting an infusion of 5 or 10% dextrose in water at this time. One should try to maintain the blood glucose concentration between 200 and 300 mg/dl for the first day of therapy. From 1 to 3 liters may be needed in the next 24 hours.

Fructose (levulose) is the levorotatory isomer of dextrose. It does not require insulin for oxidation. For this reason, it has been used in the treatment of diabetic acidosis and in other patients in place of dextrose. However, fructose causes only a small increase in the utilization of carbohydrate and is therefore not essential. It can be used in a 10% concentration in water. Fructose may worsen the metabolic acidosis because it causes a rise in the serum pyruvic and lactic acid concentrations.

Neither dextrose in water nor fructose in water should be given subcutaneously, because such a solution can cause the serum electrolytes to pass into the solution in the subcutaneous tissue. When this happens, the circulating blood volume decreases and shock can be precipitated or aggravated.

Potassium Salts

A marked urinary (or gastrointestinal) loss of potassium ions often occurs in patients with diabetic acidosis, and it has been estimated that such patients have a total potassium deficit of usually 3 to 10 mEq per kg body weight. However, it is not necessary to restore this loss in the first 24 hours of treatment. In addition, it may be dangerous to give potassium chloride while the patient is in shock and is passing only a small volume of urine. However, when the blood sugar concentration begins to fall, as after the sixth hour of treatment, or when the urine output increases, or when the serum potassium concentration falls to 4 mEq/L or lower, or when the electrocardiogram begins to show signs of hypokalemia, potassium ions may be needed to prevent serious hypokalemia.

Approximately 40 mEq/L of potassium ions (3 g of potassium chloride) can be given intravenously in the saline or dextrose solution being infused. It is sometimes necessary to give as much as 200 to 300 mEq of potassium ions during the first 24 hours of treatment.

The electrocardiogram or preferably serum potassium concentrations can be used to determine the amount of potassium chloride needed and to prevent hypokalemia.

Phosphate and Magnesium Salts

It has been shown that patients with diabetic acidosis lose phosphate and magnesium ions during therapy. However, the addition of these ions does not seem to increase the rate of recovery.

If desired, potassium phosphate can be given at a rate of 2.5 mM per hour. Potassium phosphate is available in 1 mm vials (for dilution and intravenous use) that contain 3 mM phosphate and approximately 4.5 mEq potassium.

Magnesium sulfate can be given IV as 500 ml of a 2% solution, given over a period of 4 to 6 hours.

Other Therapy

Gastric aspiration with a Levin tube is indicated only if there is severe vomiting or gastric dilatation. Lavage of the stomach is not necessary, nor is the instillation of either a saline of sodium bicarbonate solution.

It is not necessary to catheterize the bladder routinely. This should be done only if the patient does not produce a urine sample after 3 or 4 hours of treatment, or is comatose.

REFERENCES

Abramson, E., and Arky, R.: Diabetic acidosis with initial hypokalemia. Therapeutic implications. JAMA, *196*:401, 1966.

Addis, G.J., Thomson, W.S.T., and Welch, J.D.: Bicarbonate therapy in diabetic acidosis. Lancet, *2*:223, 1964.

Alberti, K.G.M.M., Hockaday, T.D.R., and Turner, R.C.: Small doses of intramuscular insulin in the treatment of diabetic "coma." Lancet, *2*:515, 1973.

Androgué, H.J., et al.: Plasma acid-base patterns in diabetic ketoacidosis, N Engl J Med, *307*:1603, 1982.

Assal, J.P., et al.: Metabolic effects of sodium bicarbonate in management of diabetic ketoacidosis. Diabetes, *23*:405, 1974.

Bendezu, R., et al.: Experience with low-dose insulin infusion in diabetic ketoacidosis and diabetic hyperosmolarity. JAMA, *138*:60, 1978.

Bolli, G.B., and Gerich, J.E.: The "dawn" phenomenon. A common occurrence in both non insulin-dependent and insulin-dependent diabetes mellitus, N Engl J Med, *310*:746, 1984.

Carroll, P., and Matz, R.: Uncontrolled diabetes mellitus in adults, Diabetes Care, *6*:579, 1981.

Cobble, S.P.: Insulin: not recommended in infusions. JAMA, *230*:468, 1974.

Connors, J.M.: Insulin therapy in diabetic ketoacidosis, comments. Ann Intern Med, *86*:109, 1977.

Cooperman, M.T., et al.: Clinical studies of alcoholic ketoacidosis, Diabetes, *23*:433, 1974.

Farah, D., et al.: Paracetamol interference with blood glucose analysis. A potentially fatal phenomenon, Brit Med J, *285*:172, 1982.

Felig, P.: Diabetic acidosis. N Engl J Med, *290*:1360, 1974.

Felts, P.W.: Ketoacidosis, Med Clin N Am, *67*:831, July 1983.

Finn, R., and Cope, S.: The plasma amylase in diabetic coma. Diabetes, *12*:141, 1963.

Fisher, J.N., Shahshahani, M.N., and Kitabchi, A.E.: Diabetic ketoacidosis. Low-dose insuline therapy by various routes. N Engl J Med, *297*:238, 1977.

Foster, D.W., and McGarry, J.D.: The metabolic derangements and treatment of diabetic ketoacidosis, N Engl J Med *309*:159, 1983.

Fulop, M., et al.: Ketotic hyperosmolar coma. Lancet, *2*:635, 1973.

Gerich, J.E., et al.: Prevention of human diabetic ketoacidosis by somatostatin. Evidence for an essential role of glucagon. N Engl J Med, *292*:985, 1975.

Glasgow, A.M.: Hyperglycemic response to massive doses of commercial insulin. Diabetes, *19*:28, 1970.

Jenkins, D.W., Eckel, R.E., and Craig, J.W.: Alcoholic ketoacidosis. JAMA, *217*:177, 1971.

Jimenez, J.A., et al.: Metabolic alkalosis in diabetic ketosis. JAMA, *233*:1193, 1975.

Kleeman, C.R., and Narins, R.G.: Diabetic acidosis and coma, in Maxwell M.H. and Kleeman C.R., editors, *Clinical Disorders of Fluid and Electrolyte Metabolism,* 3rd ed, New York, McGraw-Hill Book Co., 1980.

Kreisberg, R.A.: Diabetic ketoacidosis. New concepts and trends in pathogenesis and treatment. Ann Intern Med, *88*:695, 1978.

Lucas, C.P., Grant, N., Daily, W.J., and Reaven, G.M.: Diabetic coma without ketoacidosis. Lancet, *1*:75, 1963.

Matz, R.: Diabetic coma. Guidelines in therapy. New York State J Med, *74*:642, 1974.

Matz, R.: Diabetic acidosis. Rationale for not using bicarbonate. New York State J Med, *76*:1299, 1976.

Metzter, A.L., and Rubenstein, A.H.: Reversible cerebral edema complicating diabetic ketoacidosis. Br Heart J, *3*:746, 1970.

Mishbin, R.I.: Insulin resistance in ketoacidosis, correspondence. N Engl J Med, *297*:893, 1977.

Molnar, G.D., and Service, F.J.: Low-dosage continuous insulin infusion for diabetic coma. Editorial notes. Ann Intern Med, *81*:853, 1974.

Munro, J.F., et al.: Euglycemic diabetic ketoacidosis. Br Med J, *2*:578, 1973.

National Diabetes Data Group: Classification and diagnosis of diabetes mellitus and other categories of glucose intolerance, Diabetes, *28*:1039, 1979.

Nuttall, F.Q.: Metabolic acidosis-diabetic. Arch Intern Med, *116*:709, 1965.

Ohman, J.L., Jr., et al.: The cerebrospinal fluid in diabetic ketoacidosis. N Engl J Med, *284*:283, 1971.

Page, M. McB., et al.: Treatment of diabetic coma with continuous low-dose infusion of insulin. Br Med J, *2*:687, 1974.

Pagliara, A.S.: Managing ketoacidosis in diabetic patients, Consultant P. 121, March 1981.

Peterson, L. et al.: Insulin absorbance to polyvinylchloride surfaces with implications for constant infusion therapy, Diabetes *25*:72, 1976.

Podolsky, S.: Nonketotic diabetic coma in the cardiac patient, Cardiovasc Rev & Reports. *4*:201, 1983.

Roggin, G.M., et al.: Ketosis and metabolic alkalosis in a patient with diabetes. JAMA, *221*:296, 1970.

Root, H.F.: Treatment of diabetic coma. J Chronic Dis, *2*:121, 1955.

Schade, D.S., and Eaton, R.P.: Diabetic ketoacidosis. Pathogenesis, prevention, and therapy, Clin Endocrino. & Metab. *12*:321, 1983.

Sherwin, R.S., and Felig, P.: Hyperglucagonemia in diabetes, letter. N Engl J Med, *299*:1366, 1978.

Siegel, A.J., Steinke, J., and Bell, W.R.: Insulin-resistant diabetic coma. Arch Intern Med, *134*:562, 1974.

Sussman, K.E., and Metz, R.J.S., editors: *Diabetes Mellitus,* 4th ed., American Diabetes Association, 1975.

Taylor, A.L.: Diabetic ketoacidosis, Postgrad Med *66*:161, 1980.

Trevor, R.W., and Cluff, L.E.: Problem of increasing azotemia during management of diabetic acidosis. Am J Med, *24*:368, 1958.

Warren, S.E.: False-positive urine ketone test with captopril, letter, N Engl J Med, *303*:1003, 1980.

Zileli, M.S., et al.: Oxazepam intoxication simulating non-ketoacidotic diabetic coma. JAMA, *215*:1986, 1971.

CHAPTER 23

METABOLIC ACIDOSIS SYNDROMES (Continued)

SALICYLATE POISONING

Salicylate poisoning is commonly observed in infants and children under the age of 1 year. However, it also occurs in adults. It can be produced by the oral ingestion of acetylsalicylic acid (aspirin), methyl salicylate (oil of wintergreen), salicylic acid, sodium salicylate, or even by the use of salicylic acid ointments.

PATHOPHYSIOLOGY

Salicylates cause two types of acid-base disturbances. First, a primary stimulation of the respiratory center of the brain occurs. This produces a marked hyperventilation and a primary respiratory alkalosis. Within 3 to 24 hours usually, sometimes within 1 hour, the salicylate disturbs carbohydrate metabolism and causes a depletion of liver glycogen. As a result, ketone and particularly lactic and pyruvic acids accumulate in the body. This causes a primary metabolic acidosis. Hyperglycemia may also develop. The salicylates also interfere with prothrombin and fibrinogen formation in the liver.

When the respiratory alkalosis develops, the renal compensatory mechanisms cause an excretion of bicarbonate and other basic salts. This tends to produce a compensatory metabolic acidosis superimposed on the lactic acidosis. The respiratory alkalosis can also produce hypokalemia, which may be severe and may persist even after the metabolic acidosis has developed.

(Eichenholz has shown that if the respiratory alkalosis is prevented, by having subjects who have received an excessive amount of salicylates inhale a high carbon dioxide mixture, the metabolic acidosis does not develop.)

The toxicity of salicylates is related more to their blood level than to the amount ingested. Ordinarily, the toxic blood salicylate level is 30 mg/dl. However, severe intoxication can occur at a lower blood concentration. Conversely, no toxicity may occur in other patients with a much higher blood salicylate concentration.

SYMPTOMS AND SIGNS

These vary with the age of the patients. In adults, the classic symptoms of salicylism occur—vertigo, tinnitus, impaired hearing, and visual blurring. Anorexia, nausea, vomiting, sweating, pallor, flushing, cyanosis and tetany may also occur.

Numbness and tingling of the face, lips and extremities may occur as a result of the hyperventilation. Fever is usually present. Bleeding may also develop. Later erythema, scarlatinal or desquamative rashes may appear.

Signs of central nervous toxicity are also common—hyperventilation, mental confusion, excitement or hyperactivity, disorientation, or delirium (salicylate "jag"). Muscle twitchings or convulsions can also occur, and may be followed by progressive central nervous system depression with lethargy, stupor, coma, and death (terminal respiratory acidosis). (This is probably due to an abnormally low glucose concentration in brain cells, produced by the salicylates.) Acute renal failure or injury to the liver may also develop.

LABORATORY FINDINGS

Blood

The blood findings depend on the presence of respiratory alkalosis, or metabolic acidosis, and on the occurrence of vomiting or other losses of water and electrolytes. Water loss and hypernatremia are common. Hyperglycemia or hypoglycemia may be present. The white blood count may be elevated.

Urine

Oliguria may be present, with albumin, red blood cells and casts. Positive tests for glucose or ketone acids and acetone may be present but may be false-positives. However, salicylate poisoning can cause a true diabetes-like condition to develop temporarily.

Salicylic acid can be detected in the urine by means of the ferric chloride test. A sample of urine is boiled to vaporize acetone and ketone substances. Then a 10% solution of ferric chloride is added. This causes a strong purple color in the presence of salicylic acid.

Example: An adult who has taken an excessive amount of acetylsalicylic acid (aspirin).
Blood salicylate concentration 60 mg/dl
pH 7.4

P_{CO_2} 18.4 mm Hg
CO_2 content 11.6 mEq/L
Standard bicarbonate 16.3 mEq/L
Actual bicarbonate 11 mEq/L
Base excess -10.5 mEq/L

The pH is normal. However, the P_{CO_2} is low. This indicates that a respiratory alkalosis is present. Similarly, the actual bicarbonate is lower than the standard bicarbonate, because of the respiratory alkalosis.

The low standard bicarbonate, and the negative base excess indicate that a metabolic acidosis is also present. Therefore, a respiratory alkalosis and a metabolic acidosis are present (Chap. 15).

This information can also be determined from the pH and P_{CO_2} by inspection of Figure 15–4, page 154.

Cation-anion balance:
Na 140 K 4.0 HCO_3 11 Cl 106 mEq/L
Anion gap $= (Na + K) - (HCO_3 + Cl)$
$= (140 + 4) - (11 + 106)$
$= 144 - 117$
$= 27$ mEq/L. This is abnormally high and is due to the accumulation of lactic and other metabolic acids.

DIAGNOSIS

Salicylate poisoning can be confused with diabetic acidosis and coma because both conditions may show hyperpnea, hyperglycemia, ketonemia, glycosuria and ketonuria. The urinary test for salicylic acid has been described above. One should also remember that a true diabetic-like state can be produced by salicylate poisoning.

The best way to make a diagnosis of salicylate poisoning is to obtain a history of salicylate ingestion, and to find a high blood salicylate concentration.

COURSE AND PROGNOSIS

Salicylate poisoning is a serious condition because death often occurs in spite of vigorous treatment. Death is probably due to a toxic encephalopathy.

PROPHYLAXIS

Salicylate toxicity does not usually occur in adults until a daily dose of aspirin, for example, exceeds 5 g (15 5-gr tablets). There is no direct correlation between salicylate dosage and the appearance of even mild toxic symptoms, such as tinnitus.

Salicylate dosage must be carefully regulated, especially in elderly patients. In addition, changes in the urine pH (due to changes in diet, medication, and so on) directly affect blood salicylate levels—the lower the urinary pH, the higher the blood salicylate level (Levy and Leonards).

TREATMENT

Serum salicylate concentration should be determined. If it is higher than 70 mg/dl, this is an indication for hemodialysis. (Peritoneal dialysis is relatively ineffective in removing salicylates.)

If the patient is seen early after the ingestion of salicylates, gastric lavage with isotonic saline solution, using a wide-bore Jacques, 30-gauge French tube, can be done (although the value of this has been questioned). Sodium bicarbonate should *not* be used for stomach lavage, because it increases the absorption of salicylates from the gastrointestinal tract.

Oral administration of an aqueous suspension of activated charcoal in an amount up to 10 times the amount of salicylates that have been ingested may also reduce the salicylate absorption. This should be done preferably within 30 minutes (or within several hours) after the salicylates have been ingested. Vomiting can be induced, using syrup of ipecac, if the patient is awake and alert. (Activated charcoal should not be given prior to the administration of ipecac, because it inactivates ipecac.)

During the stage of respiratory alkalosis, dextrose in water should be given intravenously to enhance the renal excretion of the salicylates. The dextrose also prevents excessive lowering of the glucose content of the brain cells. The water counteracts the water loss produced by hyperventilation and/or fever.

When metabolic acidosis develops, particularly when the pH is low, sodium bicarbonate should be given intravenously, because the metabolic acidosis is associated with increased ionization of the salicylate ions and their increased movement out of the blood and into cells. This increases the salicylate toxicity, even though the serum salicylate level falls when this happens.

The amount of sodium bicarbonate should be determined from changes in pH (page 182). However, because the respiratory alkalosis may persist longer than the metabolic acidosis, the pH should be raised to only 7.30—but not higher—to prevent the development of severe alkalosis (respiratory and metabolic).

Potassium chloride should be given intravenously in conjunction with the sodium bicarbonate. Large doses may be needed, particularly if hypokalemia develops.

Calcium gluconate or chloride can be given for tetany. Vitamin K_1 oxide can be given if bleeding occurs. Fever is treated symptomatically.

REFERENCES

American Hospital Formulary Service: Salicylates. Category 28: 08.

Anderson, R.J., et al.: Unrecognized adult salicylate intoxication. Ann Intern Med *85*:745, 1976.

Arena, F.P., et al.: Salicylate-induced hypoglycemia and ketoacidosis in a nondiabetic adult. Arch Intern Med, *138*:1153, 1978.

Beveridge, G.W., et al.: Acute salicylate poisoning in adults. Lancet, *1*:1406, 1964.

Cohen, A.S.: Differential diagnosis of salicylate intoxication and diabetic acidosis. N Engl J Med, *254*:457, 1956.

Dukes, D.C., Blainey, J.D., Cummung, G., and Widdowson, G.: Treatment of severe aspirin poisoning. Lancet, *2*:329, 1963.

Eichenholz, A.: Respiratory alkalosis. Arch Intern Med, *116*:699, 1965.

Eichenholz, A., Mulhausen, R.O., and Redleaf, P.S.: Nature of acid-base disturbance in salicylate intoxication. Metabolism, *12*:164, 1963.

Ferguson, R.K., and Boutros, A.R.: Death following self-poisoning with aspirin. JAMA, *213*:1186, 1970. Also JAMA, *15*:298, 1971.

Hill, J.B.: Salicylate intoxication. N Engl J Med, *288*:1110, 1973.

Koppes, G.M., and Arnett, F.C.: Salicylate hepatotoxicity. Postgrad Med, *56*:193, 1974.

Levy, R.I.: Overwhelming salicylate intoxication in an adult. Acid-base changes during recovery with hemodialysis. Arch Intern Med, *119*:399, 1967.

Levy, G., and Leonards, J.R.: Urine pH and salicylate therapy. JAMA, *217*:81, 1971.

Matthew, H.: Gastric aspiration and lavage. Clin Toxicol, *3*:179, 1970.

Mongan, E., et al.: Tinnitus as an indication of therapeutic serum salicylate levels. JAMA, *226*:142, 1973.

Robin, E.D., Davis, R.P., and Rees, S.B.: Salicylate intoxication with special reference to the development of hypokalemia. Am J Med, *26*:869, 1959.

Rupp, D.J., et al.: Acute polyuric renal failure after aspirin intoxication, Arch Intern Med, *143*:1237, 1983.

Singer, R.B.: Acid-base disturbance in salicylate intoxication. Medicine, *33*:1, 1954.

Temple, A.R.: Acute and chronic effects of aspirin toxicity and their treatment, Arch Intern Med, *141*:364, 1981.

Vivian, A.S., and Goldberg, I.B.: Recognizing chronic salicylate intoxication in the elderly, Geriatrics, *37*:91, 1982.

Zimmerman, H.J.: Effects of aspirin and acetaminophen on the liver, Arch Intern Med, *141*:333, 1981.

CHAPTER 24

METABOLIC ACIDOSIS SYNDROMES (Continued)

HYPERKALEMIA

Hyperkalemia is present when the serum potassium concentration is higher than 5.5 mEq/L.

Although it is possible to measure the total exchangeable body potassium experimentally, such measurements are not available for clinical purposes. Therefore, most physicians use the terms *hyperkalemia* (hyperpotassemia) and *hypokalemia* (hypopotassemia), which merely describe the serum potassium concentration, to indicate potassium excess and potassium loss. Unfortunately a change in serum potassium concentration does not always correspond to a similar change in total exchangeable body potassium. For example, a low, normal, or high serum potassium concentration may exist with a low or normal total exchangeable body potassium. However, it has been shown that an excess of total exchangeable body potassium does not occur in a patient with azotemic acidosis, for example, even though hyperkalemia may be present and even though the patient may die from the toxic effects of potassium.

One of the serious difficulties in studying potassium excess or potassium loss is that the potassium is essentially an intracellular ion. Measurement of serum potassium concentration merely indicates the extracellular concentration of the ion. For this reason, the electrocardiographic patterns of hyperkalemia and hypokalemia have been used instead of the serum potassium concentrations to determine whether hyperkalemia or hypokalemia is present. However, even this method is not completely accurate, as will be pointed out in this chapter and in Chapter 27.

Potassium balance is normally maintained by a daily dietary intake and excretion of about 50 to 100 mEq. This is equivalent to 3.73 to 7.46 g of potassium chloride. This is associated with a normal serum potassium concentration between 3.5 to 5.0 mEq/L.

248

PATHOPHYSIOLOGY

Both respiratory and metabolic acidosis (including diabetic and azotemic acidosis) are associated with hyperkalemia, which probably occurs as a compensatory mechanism. When the acidosis develops, the hydrogen ion concentration of the extracellular water increases. This causes potassium ions to move out of the cells into the extracellular water, and causes hydrogen and sodium ions to move into the cells. Conversely, the rapid infusion of a potassium salt, such as potassium chloride, will produce a metabolic acidosis.

The relations of potassium disturbances to muscle paralysis can be better understood by means of the following brief outline of the physiology of muscle contraction: The transmission of a nerve impulse from nerve endings to the motor end-plate of muscle is due to the release of acetylcholine. Further conduction of the stimulus along the muscle fiber is related to electrical currents produced by potassium. This occurs because there is a potential difference of 90 millivolts between the inner (negative) and outer (positive) surface of the muscle fiber membrane. In other words, the membrane of the muscle fiber is polarized. The polarization is due to the difference in the concentration of potassium inside and outside the cells. The potassium concentration in the cell is very high, approximately 150 mEq/L, whereas the extracellular potassium concentration is low, approximately 4 mEq/L. When the muscle is stimulated, potassium moves out of the cell, depolarizes the cell membrane, and causes a stimulus to spread along the length of the muscle fiber.

The importance of this polarized state of the muscle cell membrane is that a persistent increased or decreased polarization can block the spread of the stimulus along the muscle fiber. It can therefore cause either muscle weakness or paralysis.

Hypopolarization occurs when the concentration of potassium outside the cell is decreased, due to hypokalemia (or the concentration of potassium within the cell is increased). When the muscle is now stimulated, the degree of depolarization produced by acetylcholine is not sufficient to start the spread of the stimulus along the muscle fiber.

Hyperpolarization occurs with hyperkalemia (or when the potassium concentration within the muscle cell falls). When this occurs, the transmission of a stimulus along the muscle is also prevented.

Although potassium disturbances inside or outside the cell can cause muscle weakness or paralysis, measurements of potassium concentrations inside the cell cannot be done clinically. Therefore, muscle paralysis due to potassium disturbances is usually described in relation to hypokalemia or hyperkalemia.

The most serious effect of hyperkalemia is on the heart. Intraventricular conduction disturbance occurs with or without A-V dissociation.

Finally, ventricular fibrillation and cardiac arrest develop. Hyperkalemia also affects the peripheral nerves. Potassium is capable of stimulating pain receptors. This is the reason for the paresthesias which may develop.

ETIOLOGY

It has already been mentioned that an excess of total body potassium does not occur, in contrast to the retention and accumulation of sodium ions. However, hyperkalemia can occur in the following situations:

1. Spurious or artifactual causes. Artifactual hyperkalemia may occur if the blood sample hemolyzes, if there is venous stasis and muscular exercise of the extremity during a venipuncture, or if the venipuncture is done near the site of an intravenous infusion of potassium chloride. (A severe and dangerous hyperkalemia may occur if a bolus of potassium chloride solution is injected into the side arm of an intravenous infusion bottle and if the bottle is not inverted and agitated to disperse the potassium chloride throughout the bottle.)

   Hyperkalemia has been noted *in vitro* in patients with an abnormal elevation of the blood platelet count. These patients show no clinical or electrocardiographic signs of hyperkalemia.

2. Primary renal disease (acute or chronic renal failure). Hyperkalemia does not occur until the creatinine clearance decreases to approximately 10 ml per minute or less.

3. Acidosis (metabolic or respiratory). Acidosis is associated with a rise in serum potassium concentration, even to a hyperkalemic level. This is not associated with clinical signs in most patients. However, ventricular fibrillation and death due to hyperkalemia have been described in patients who develop acute respiratory acidosis, or in severely burned patients.

4. Adrenocortical insufficiency (Addison's disease). Most of these patients show neither clinical nor electrocardiographic signs of hyperkalemia. Rarely, severe and even fatal hyperkalemia may occur.

5. Hyperkalemia due to renin deficiency (hyporeninemic hypoaldosteronism). Hypokalemia can be caused by a deficiency of the salt-retaining hormone, aldosterone. This usually occurs in adrenal insufficiency as was just mentioned. However, hypoaldosteronism can occur as an isolated abnormality.

   When aldosterone deficiency occurs with total adrenal insufficiency, the progressive loss of sodium ions and water and the decreased plasma volume stimulate renin release. However, in isolated hypoaldosteronism, renin activity is low. The primary disturbance is a defect in renin secretion. The hypoaldosteronism is secondary to this. The defect in renin secretion is due to damage to the juxtoglomerular apparatus of the kidneys. Pathologically it is associated with pyelonephritis, nephrosclerosis, hyperparathyroidism, diabetes, gout. It can also be produced by nonsteroidal antiinflammatory drugs, such as indomethacin.

   Treatment includes adequate salt intake and the use of mineralocorticoids to lower the serum potassium concentration.

6. Drugs. Hyperkalemia can also occur as a result of potassium-sparing diuretics, such as triamterene (Dyrenium) or spironolactone (Aldactone),

and from other drugs (succinylcholine) when given to patients with neuromuscular disease, arginine, when given to patients with renal failure, aminocaproic acid, if renal function is decreased, antineoplastic drugs, probably as a result of destruction of neoplastic cells, arginine infusion if used in an azotemic patient, isoniazid (INH), if excessive doses are given, cephaloridine (Loridine), or penicillin G, potassium. (Each million units for intravenous use contains 1.7 mEq potassium ions.)

7. Exogenous sources.

   a. Diet. When foods containing an excessive amount of potassium salts are ingested, hyperkalemia may develop. Normally, potassium balance is regulated by the urinary excretion of potassium ions. About 80% of ingested potassium salts are excreted in the urine, and approximately 20% in the stool. A normal person can take a single oral dose of 10 g potassium chloride without toxic effects. The dose will be excreted in approximately 4 to 8 hours. Even when the urinary elimination of potassium ions is impaired, as in patients with renal failure, signs of hyperkalemia do not usually appear. However, when the urinary output falls below 400 or 500 ml a day, the ingestion of a diet which contains a normal amount of potassium ions can cause hyperkalemia.

   b. Excessive intravenous administration of potassium chloride (or any potassium salt). The concentrations of potassium chloride that can be safely given intravenously to patients are described in Chapter 27. However, if the potassium chloride is infused too rapidly, or if renal insufficiency, inadequate urinary output, or acidosis is present, hyperkalemia may develop from the infusion of a small concentration of potassium chloride.

      One should remember that salt substitutes contain potassium chloride as a major ingredient. A salt substitute will not cause hyperkalemia in a patient with normal renal function, but hyperkalemia can occur if the salt substitute is given to a patient with renal failure.

   c. A rapid transfusion of a large volume of bank blood (which may contain 20 mEq/L potassium ions or more, particularly if the blood is more than 10 days old).

8. Endogenous sources. Tissue trauma liberates intracellular potassium ions. For example, hyperkalemia has been noted in the *crush syndrome.* However, the hyperkalemia in these patients is probably due mostly to the acute renal tubular failure that is present.

Hyperkalemia can also be classified according to pathophysiology, according to the presence of decreased renal failure, decreased aldosterone secretion, potassium-sparing diuretics, and so on, or the presence of excessive exogenous potassium ions (diet, intravenous potassium salts, bank blood, and so on), or the presence of endogenous release of potassium ions (tissue trauma, succinylcholine, acidosis, and so on).

One should remember that hyperkalemia is frequently the result of numerous factors simultaneously present. For example, a patient with acute failure may also develop hyperkalemia due to acidosis, dietary excess of potassium salts, and tissue destruction.

SYMPTOMS AND SIGNS

Vague muscle weakness is usually the first symptom of hyperkalemia. Muscle paralysis develops over a period of several days. It is usually first noticed in the legs, then in the trunk and in the arms. The facial and respiratory muscles are affected last. The paralysis usually spares the muscles supplied by the cranial nerves.

The paralysis is flaccid, like that which occurs with hypokalemia. Paresthesias of the face, tongue, feet and hands may occur. Later, anesthesia may occur. In addition, the muscles are irritable and will respond to tapping or squeezing. Vibratory and position senses may be decreased or absent.

In spite of the muscle paralysis, the patient usually remains alert and apprehensive, and consciousness may persist until cardiac arrest and death occur. The heart rate may be slow and regular. In other patients, a slow or rapid irregular rate may be present.

There is no direct relation between the degree of muscle weakness or paralysis and the serum potassium concentration. However, when it reaches 10 to 12 mEq/L, ventricular fibrillation, cardiac arrest and death usually occur.

A rare hereditary type of periodic muscle paralysis is associated with hyperkalemia, *adynamia episodica hereditaria.* Attacks can be precipitated by the ingestion of potassium chloride, and can be relieved by intravenous calcium gluconate, or by glucagon (30 mcg per kg of body weight) intravenously, or epinephrine (0.25 to 0.4 ml of a 1:1000 dilution) subcutaneously. Dextroamphetamine sulfate in a daily dose of 10 to 15 mg (in the form of Dexedrine Spansules, S.K.F.) has been found helpful in preventing attacks. The way in which this drug causes a fall of serum potassium concentration is not known. Carbonic anhydrase inhibitors and other diuretics which promote the excretion of potassium have also been found helpful.

ELECTROCARDIOGRAM

The electrocardiographic changes which occur with hyperkalemia can be related in a general way to the serum potassium concentration:

At a concentration of approximately 6 to 7 mEq/L, tall peaked T waves with a narrow base and a normal or decreased Q–T occur (Fig. 24–1).

At approximately 8 mEq/L, the P waves disappear or wander in and out of the QRS *(B)*.

At approximately 10 mEq/L, wide, aberrant QRS complexes appear *(C)*.

At approximately 11 mEq/L, biphasic deflections, caused by a fusion of the QRS complex, ST segment and the T wave, appear *(D)*.

At 12 mEq/L (or even at a lower concentration of 10 mEq/L), ventricular fibrillation and cardiac standstill and death may occur *(E)*.

With the onset of the wide aberrant QRS complexes and the loss of

Fig. 24–1. Electrocardiographic patterns of hyperkalemia.

the P waves, an idioventricular rhythm develops which is similar to that which occurs in complete a-v block. The ventricular rate may be regular, irregular, slow or rapid, and the tracing may even resemble a ventricular tachycardia. In addition, the shape of the abnormal QRS complexes may vary from beat to beat.

Marked hyperkalemia is sometimes associated with transient electrocardiographic patterns that simulate myocardial infarction. Elevation of ST segments, coved or inverted T waves, and even transient Q waves may appear. These pseudo-infarct patterns should disappear when the serum potassium concentration is lowered.

These electrocardiographic findings do not occur in patients with Addison's disease and with adrenal cortical insufficiency in spite of the hyperkalemia which is present. The electrocardiogram may be normal, or the T waves may be flat or their direction reversed. In addition, when such patients are treated with desoxycorticosterone (DOCA) and the serum potassium concentration falls, the T waves may become large and normal again, in spite of the lowering of the serum potassium concentration. Alternatively, as in many patients with Addison's disease, the T-wave abnormalities may become more marked in spite of clinical improvement.

The presence of peaked T waves is not itself a pathognomonic sign of hyperkalemia, because such T waves may occur normally, or with myocardial infarction, intracranial hemorrhage, cardiac rupture, hemopericardium, and so on.

LABORATORY FINDINGS

The serum potassium concentration is elevated to 5.5 mEq/L, or higher. The serum sodium concentration is usually decreased. Serum calcium concentration may be normal or decreased. Other laboratory findings indicative of respiratory or metabolic acidosis are present.

If pseudohyperkalemia due to an increased platelet count is suspected, the potassium concentration of *plasma*, rather than serum, should be measured, because the potassium ions are released during clotting.

DIAGNOSIS

Hyperkalemia can be suspected in a patient with oliguria, anuria, or renal disease, or in a patient who is receiving potassium salts therapeutically who begins to complain of paresthesias. The serum potassium concentration will be 6 mEq/L, or higher. The electrocardiogram will show signs of hyperkalemia (except in patients with Addison's disease).

COURSE AND PROGNOSIS

The development of hyperkalemia is serious in patients with oliguria or anuria. Similarly, the cause of death in acute respiratory acidosis is probably the hyperkalemia which develops and causes ventricular fibrillation.

PROPHYLAXIS

Potassium should not be given to any patient with oliguria or anuria. In addition, even if a potassium deficit exists, as in a patient with diabetic acidosis, potassium should not be administered until the severity of the acidosis has decreased greatly, and the urinary output has increased.

One should also remember that the use of a low-sodium diet, such as the rice diet for a hypertensive patient who also has renal impairment, can cause a decrease in renal blood flow and a marked hyperkalemia. The hyperkalemia can be corrected in such patients by increasing the sodium content of the diet.

TREATMENT

Emergency Treatment

When the serum potassium concentration is 7.0 mEq/L or higher, or if the electrocardiogram shows serious changes such as disappearance of P waves or widening of the QRS complex, the following emergency treatment can be done:

1. Hypertonic 25% dextrose can be given intravenously into a large vein such as the superior vena cava with 1 unit of regular insulin per 4 or 5 g dextrose (1 unit insulin per 10 g dextrose if renal failure is present) (also see page 354). In a period of one-half hour 200 to 300 ml can be given. The serum potassium concentration will begin to fall in about one-half to 1 hour and will remain lowered for approximately 4 to 6 hours.

   An infusion of hypertonic dextrose causes the secretion of endogenous insulin. If the infusion is stopped suddenly, hypoglycemia may develop. This may be severe, if insulin had been added to the infusion bottle. For this reason, it is advisable to follow an infusion of hypertonic dextrose with an infusion of 250 to 500 ml of 5% dextrose in water.

2. Calcium gluconate or chloride can be given intravenously in a dose of 50 to 100 ml at a rate of 2 ml per minute. Chamberlain has given as much as 90 ml of a 10% calcium chloride solution intravenously in a period of 5 minutes, to treat hyperkalemia. When this is done, the patient should be monitored with an electrocardiograph, and the injection stopped as soon as electrocardiographic signs of hyperkalemia disappear. (The serum potassium concentration remains unchanged.) If necessary, the patient can then be given a daily dose of 100 mg of a 10% solution of calcium gluconate, as a prophylactic measure, if there is a possibility that the hyperkalemia will recur.

   The use of calcium salts to counteract hyperkalemia is contraindicated if the patient is receiving digitalis.

3. Hypertonic (7.5%) sodium bicarbonate solution given intravenously (Chap. 35) can lower the serum potassium concentration. The effect lasts 1 to 2 hours.

   Intravenous sodium bicarbonate can be combined with intravenous dextrose. After the patient has been given 1 ampul of hypertonic sodium bicarbonate intravenously, 1000 ml of 10% dextrose in water, with 2 to 3 ampuls of the hypertonic sodium bicarbonate, can be infused for 1 to 2 hours. Ten units of regular insulin may be given subcutaneously at the start of the infusion.

4. Hypertonic (5%) sodium chloride solution is also able to lower the serum potassium concentration in a few minutes. Its beneficial effects last only about 1 to 2 hours. Two hundred ml can be given rapidly (even in one-half hour). However, the solution must be used cautiously if the patient has hypertension or congestive heart failure.

5. Hemodialysis or peritoneal dialysis is also effective in lowering the serum potassium concentration.

6. Repeated electrocardiograms or serum potassium determinations should be used to check the therapy. However, the electrocardiogram cannot be used as a guide to the treatment of hyperkalemia in patients with Addison's disease.

Nonemergency Treatment

The following can also be done to lower the serum potassium concentration when a dangerous level of hyperkalemia is not present:

1. Low-potassium, high-carbohydrate diet can be prescribed. A low-potassium diet contains 40 mEq potassium ions or less daily. This is equivalent to approximately 3 g of potassium chloride daily. Table 24–1 lists foods

Table 24-1.   *Potassium Content of Foods.* *

Minimal Potassium Content: butter or margarine, carbonated water, cranberry juice or sauce, ginger ale, gumdrops or jelly beans, lollypops or Charms, root beer, salad oil, sugar or honey, water ices or popsicles. Also spices (allspice, anise, basil, bay leaf, caraway, celery flakes, celery salt, chili powder, cinnamon, cream of tartar, curry, garlic, garlic powder, ginger, horseradish, mace, marjoram, mint leaves, dry mustard, nutmeg, onion powder, paprika, pepper, poppy seeds, rosemary, sage, sesame seeds, tarragon, thyme, turmeric, vanilla extract).

High Potassium Content: chocolate, coffee, cocoa, tea, dried fruits, dried peas or beans, ice cream or sherbet, milk desserts, molasses, whole grain breads and cereals, wild rice (also see page 286).

The potassium content of other foods is as follows:

Dairy Products: 2 mEq potassium ions supplied by milk or cream, ½ cup, or sour cream, ¼ cup.
1.75 mEq potassium ions supplied by cottage cheese, ½ cup, or cream or processed cheese, 1 oz.

Breads and Cereals: 1.25 mEq potassium ions supplied by: bread, 1 slice; cooked cereal (cornmeal, farina, cream of wheat, hominy grits, oatmeal), ½ cup; dry cereal (corn flakes, puffed rice, puffed wheat, shredded wheat), ¾ cup; cooked macaroni, noodles, spaghetti, or rice, ½ cup; dry cereals (corn flakes, puffed rice, puffed wheat, shredded wheat), ¾ cup.

Fruits: 2.5 mEq potassium ions supplied by: apple, 1 small; apple juice, ½ cup; apple-sauce, ⅓ cup; blueberries, fresh, 1 cup; orange, ½ small; peaches, canned, ½ cup; pears, canned, ½ cup; pineapple, canned, ½ cup (or 1 slice).
3.5 mEq potassium ions supplied by: fruit cocktail, ½ cup; grapes, seedless, ½ cup; grape juice, ½ cup; grapefruit, ½ medium; grapefruit juice, ½ cup; peach, fresh, 1 small; pineapple juice, ½ cup; pear, fresh, ½ small; strawberries, fresh, 10 large; strawberries, frozen, slices, ½ cup; tangerine, 1; watermellon, ½ cup.

Eggs: 1.75 mEq potassium ions supplied by: 1 egg, medium, prepared any way.

Meat and Poultry: 3 mEq potassium ions supplied by: 1 ounce of beef, lamb, liver, veal, chicken, or turkey.

Seafood: 1.75 mEq potassium ions supplied by: lobster, fresh, 1 ounce; oysters, fresh, 4; shrimp, fresh, 1 ounce.
3 mEq potassium ions supplied by: 1 ounce cod, halibut, haddock, or salmon.

Vegetables: 3 mEq potassium ions supplied by: beans, green or waxed, canned, ½ cup; beets, canned, ¼ cup; carrots, canned, ⅓ cup; cucumber, 4 slices; corn, canned, ½ cup; lettuce, 2 large leaves; onions, cooked, ½ cup; peas, canned, ½ cup; summer squash, ½ cup; turnips, ½ cup.
6 mEq potassium supplied by: asparagus, frozen, 6 spears; broccoli, frozen, 1 stalk (or ½ cup); cabbage, raw, 1 cup; cabbage, cooked, ½ cup; cauliflower, cooked, 1 cup; corn, fresh, 1 4-inch ear; eggplant, cooked, ½ cup; okra, ½ cup; potato, boiled without skin, ¼ cup; potato, candied sweet, 2 halves; potato, baked sweet, ½ small; pumpkin, canned, ½ cup; rutabagas, cooked, ½ cup; winter squash, frozen, ½ cup; tomato, 1 small; tomato juice, ½ cup.

---

*A low-potassium diet contains 40 mEq potassium ions or less daily. This is equivalent to approximately 3 g of potassium chloride daily.

high in potassium which should be avoided, foods low in potassium which can be used as desired, and the potassium content of other foods.

2. A sodium polystyrene sulfonate (Kayexalate) resin can also be used to remove potassium ions from the colon. The sodium ions of the resin are partially released and replaced by potassium ions. The potassium-containing resin is then excreted in the stool. Each gram of resin binds approximately 1 mEq potassium ions. This can cause a significant decrease in serum potassium concentration. However, an effect may not be apparent for 24 hours; therefore, the resin cannot be used for the emergency treatment of hyperkalemia.

The average adult dose of the resin is 15 g (approximately 4 heaping teaspoonfuls) orally, 1 to 4 times daily. The resin can be suspended in 150 to 200 ml of water, flavored with syrup. It can also be given by nasogastric tube. Twenty ml of a 70% sorbitol syrup is often given with each dose of resin. The sorbitol can even be given every 2 hours. Its purpose is to produce a mild diarrhea and in this way to prevent fecal impaction.

The resin can also be given rectally, once or twice daily, in a dose of 30 g suspended in 200 ml of water, or in equal amounts of water and 2% methylcellulose suspension, or in 10% dextrose solution. The enema should be at body temperature and should be retained for 4 to 10 hours, if possible. If should be followed by a cleansing enema. Rectal administration is not as effective as oral administration.

When the resin is used in a patient with acute renal failure, the amount of water given with the resin should be measured. In this way, excessive administration of water will be prevented.

Serum potassium concentrations should be determined daily during resin therapy, and the resin should be stopped when the serum potassium concentration falls to 4 or 5 mEq/L. (The resin should be stopped when the serum potassium concentration falls to a level that is slightly higher than desired. The reason for this is that the resin which is already present in the gastrointestinal tract continues to remove potassium ions until it is eliminated in the stool.)

Adverse effects of the resin include anorexia, nausea, vomiting, hypokalemia, hypocalcemia, severe constipation, and even fecal impaction. Because hypokalemia may occur, the resin must be used cautiously in patients receiving digitalis preparations to avoid digitalis toxicity (which can be precipitated by hypokalemia). Similarly, when the resin is used for more than several days, it can cause a marked loss of calcium (and magnesium) ions. This can be prevented by determining the serum calcium concentration. If it begins to fall, calcium chloride or gluconate can be given intravenously.

Since sodium ions are released into the large intestine by the resin, they may be absorbed into the body. Therefore, the resin should be used cautiously if congestive heart failure is present.

REFERENCES

Bell, H., Hayes, W.L., and Vosburgh, J.: Hyperkalemic paralysis due to adrenal insufficiency. Arch Intern Med, *115*:418, 1965.

Bellet, S., and Wasserman, F.: The effects of molar sodium lactate in reversing the cardiotoxic effect of hyperpotassemia. Arch Intern Med, *100*:565, 1957.

Bostic, O., and Duvernoy, W.F.C.: Hyperkalemic cardiac arrest during transfusion of stored blood. J. Electrocardiol, *5*:407, 1972.

Burnell, J.M., Vallamil, M.F., Uyeno, B.T., and Scribner, B.H.: The effect in humans of extracellular pH change on the relationship between serum potassium concentration and intracellular potassium. J Clin Invest, *35*:935, 1956.

Bushinsky, D.A., and Gennari, F.J.: Life-threatening hyperkalemia induced by arginine. Ann Intern Med, *89*:632, 1978.

Chamberlain, M.J.: Emergency treatment of hyperkalemia. Lancet, *1*:464, 1964.

Cooperman, L.H.: Succinylcholine-induced hyperkalemia in neuromuscular disease. JAMA, *213*:1867, 1970.

Drescher, A.N., Talbot, N.B., Meara, P.A., Terry, M., and Crawford, J.D.: A study of the effects of excessive potassium intake upon body potassium stores. J Clin Invest, *37*:1316, 1958.

Egan, T.J., and Klein, R.: Hyperkalemic familial periodic paralysis. Pediatrics, *24*:761, 1959.

Fenech, F.F., and Solar, N.G.: Hyperkalemic periodic paralysis starting at age of 48. Br Med J, *2*:472, 1968.

Finch, C.A., Sawyer, C.G., and Flynn, J.M.: Clinical syndrome of potassium intoxication. Am J Med, *1*:337, 1946.

Goldfarb, S., et al.: Acute hyperkalemia induced by hyperglycemia. Ann Intern Med, *84*:426, 1976.

Haddad, A., and Strong, E.: Potassium in salt substitutes, letter. N Engl J Med, *292*:1082, 1975.

Herz, P., and Richardson, J.A.: Arginine-induced hyperkalemia in renal failure patients. Arch Intern Med, *130*:778, 1972.

Howard, J.A., and Kosowsky, B.D.: Electrocardiographic diagnosis of hyperkalemia in the presence of ventricular pacing and atrial fibrillation, Chest, *78*:491, 1980.

Hultgren, H.N., Swenson, R., and Wettach, G.: Cardiac arrest due to oral potassium administration. Am J Med, *58*:139, 1975.

Ingraham, R.H., and Seki, M.: Pseudohyperkalemia with thrombocytosis. N Engl J Med, *267*:895, 1962.

Levine, H.D., Wanger, S.H., and Merrill, J.P.: Dialyzable currents of injury in potassium intoxication resembling acute myocardial infarction or pericarditis. Circulation, *13*:29, 1956.

Levinsky, N.G.: Management of emergencies. Hyperkalemia. N Engl J Med, *274*:1076, 1966.

Marshall, M.: Potassium intoxication from blood and plasma transfusions. Anaesthesia, *17*:145, 1962.

McArdle, B.: Adynamia episodica hereditaria and its treatment. Brain, *85*:(I), 121, 1962.

Nicolis, G.L., et al.: Glucose-induced hyperkalemia in diabetic subjects, Arch Intern Med, *141*:49, 1981.

Nora, J.R., and Pilz, C.G.: Pseudo-infarction patterns associated with electrolyte imbalance. Arch Intern Med, *104*:300, 1959.

Perez, G., Siegel, L., and Schreiner, G.E.: Selective hypoaldosteronism with hyperkalemia. Ann Intern Med, *76*:757, 1972.

Pollen, R.H., and Williams, R.H.: Hyperkalemia neuromyopathy in Addison's disease. N Engl J Med, *263*:273, 1960.

Pongpaew, C., Na Songkhla, R., and Kozam, R.L.: Hyperkalemic cardiac arrhythmia secondary to spironolactone. Chest, *63*:1023, 1973.

Popovtzer, M.M., et al.: Hyperkalemia in salt-wasting nephropathy. Arch Intern Med, *132*:203, 1973.

Posner, J.B., and Jacobs, D.R.: Isolated analdosteronism. 1. Clinical entity with manifestations of persistent hyperkalemia, periodic paralysis, salt-losing tendency and acidosis. Metabolism, *13*:513, 1964.

Schambelan, M., et al.: Isolated hypoaldosteronism in adults. A renin-deficiency syndrome. N Engl J Med, *287*:576, 1972. Also ibid, p. 611.

Scherr, L., et al.: Management of hyperkalemia with a cation exchange resin. N Engl J Med, *264*:115, 1961.

Thomson, R.L.: Potassium penicillin G. N Engl J Med, *271*:1218, 1964.

Van Dellen, R.G., and Purnell, D.C.: Hyperkalemic paralysis in Addison's disease. Mayo Clin Proc, *44*:904, 1969.

Walker, B.R., et al.: Hyperkalemia after triamterene in diabetic patients. Clin Pharmacol Ther, *13*:643, 1972.

Williams, R.H.P.: Potassium overdosage. A potential hazard of nonrigid parenteral fluid containers. Br Med J, *1*:714, 1973.

Williams, F.A., Jr., et al.: Acquired primary hypoaldosteronism due to an isolated zona glomerulosa defect. N Engl J Med, *309*:1623, 1983.

CHAPTER 25

RESPIRATORY ALKALOSIS

Primary respiratory alkalosis occurs as a result of a decreased partial pressure of carbon dioxide in the alveolar air, due to hyperventilation. It is the least common type of acid-base disturbance.

A compensatory respiratory alkalosis can also occur as a result of a metabolic acidosis. In such patients, the respiratory alkalosis may continue even though the metabolic acidosis is corrected (page 170).

Synonyms: Carbonic acid deficit, hypocapnia.

PATHOPHYSIOLOGY

Respiratory alkalosis occurs as a result of hyperventilation. This should not be confused with an increased respiratory rate (tachypnea), which may or may not be associated with hyperventilation. Conversely, hyperventilation can occur with a normal respiratory rate. The characteristic findings of hyperventilation are an increased tidal volume and increased alveolar ventilation.

When hyperventilation occurs, a large amount of carbon dioxide is eliminated from the body. This causes the bicarbonate-carbonic acid ratio and the pH to rise.

Compensatory mechanisms occur to restore the pH. The normal excretion of an acid urine by the kidneys decreases. Instead the kidneys suppress hydrogen ion formation, suppress ammonia formation, suppress chloride ion excretion, and no longer conserve bicarbonate ions (page 128). In addition, potassium ions move from the extracellular water into the cells, and hydrogen and sodium ions move from the cells into the extracellular water. As a result of all these changes, a compensatory metabolic acidosis develops.

Respiratory alkalosis is also associated with an accumulation of lactate ions, which can lead to a metabolic acidosis independent of the usual compensatory metabolic acidosis.

ETIOLOGY

Respiratory alkalosis occurs as a result of stimulation of the respiratory center. The most common cause is the functional hyperventilation due to anxiety (hyperventilation syndrome). Other causes include: central nervous system lesions involving the respiratory center of the medulla, such as encephalitis, brain tumor, or intracranial surgery; hypermetabolic conditions due to fever, especially gram-negative sepsis, hyperthyroidism, alcoholic intoxication (delirium tremens), or exercise; salicylate or paraldehyde intoxication or disulfiram plus alcohol; conditions associated with increased cardiac output, such as anemia, beriberi, or cirrhosis of the liver; assisted respiration with either a pressure-cycled or volume-cycled respirator; hypoxia due to congestive heart failure, congenital heart disease with a right-to-left shunt, pulmonary atelectasis, high altitude residence, or pulmonary fibrosis (alveolar capillary block). In addition, the condition may occur in patients with serious abdominal disease such as peritonitis, ascites, or metastatic neoplasms. It also may occur after the administration of progestational drugs.

Acute respiratory alkalosis can also occur as a compensatory reaction in respiratory acidosis patients who have received a tracheotomy due to the sudden increase in alveolar ventilation.

SYMPTOMS AND SIGNS

The most characteristic clinical picture occurs in the *hyperventilation syndrome.* The patient may complain of dizziness, which is not true vertigo but lightheadedness, circumoral paresthesias, numbness and tingling of the fingers and toes, sweating, palpitation, tinnitus and tremulousness. In addition, dyspnea and air hunger, profuse sweating with a feeling of intense fear or panic or a feeling of unreality, muscle cramps, severe precordial chest pain including a sensation of tightness around the chest, or epigastric or lower abdominal pain with nausea, vomiting or diarrhea, blurred vision, loss of voice.

(Pitts and McClure have shown that the clinical picture of the hyperventilation syndrome can be experimentally produced in normal subjects by an intravenous infusion of sodium [DL] lactate.)

Signs include the hyperventilation and signs of tetany such as carpopedal spasm. Chvostek's and Trousseau's signs can also be elicited.

Atrial or ventricular tachyarrhythmias may also develop. These may be due to the alkalosis and/or the associated hypokalemia.

Convulsive tendencies are exaggerated by hyperventilation and grand mal or petit mal convulsions can be provoked. The electroencephalogram shows paroxysmal or continuous slow waves with high voltage. However, these changes cannot be correlated with the arterial pH.

Mental and neurological symptoms and signs are likely to occur when the pH rises to 7.54 or higher (Kilburn).

When acute respiratory alkalosis occurs as a result of tracheotomy, the patient may develop shock or arrhythmias, including ventricular fibrillation.

LABORATORY FINDINGS

The P_{CO_2} is characteristically low, the pH is high, and CO_2 content and the actual bicarbonate are low. However, the standard bicarbonate remains normal unless a compensatory metabolic acidosis occurs (Chap. 15).

The bicarbonate concentration is low and the chloride concentration is reciprocally elevated. The serum sodium concentration may be normal or low, due to a slightly increased sodium excretion by the kidneys. The serum potassium concentration is characteristically low. A variable elevation of the arterial lactate concentration occurs. The serum phosphate concentration falls, but the serum calcium concentration remains normal.

The electrocardiogram of respiratory and metabolic alkalosis is similar (Chap. 26).

Example: Respiratory alkalosis due to encephalitis.
P_{CO_2} 18 mm Hg
pH 7.5
CO_2 content 14.5 mEq/L
Standard bicarbonate 20.5 mEq/L
Actual bicarbonate 14 mEq/L
Base excess −4.5 mEq/L

The pH is high. This indicates an alkalosis. The P_{CO_2} is low. This indicates that a respiratory alkalosis is present. This is further indicated by the fact that the actual bicarbonate is lower than the standard bicarbonate. The negative base excess and the low standard bicarbonate indicate that a metabolic acidosis is present. Therefore, a primary respiratory alkalosis is present with a partially compensatory metabolic acidosis (page 155).

This information can also be determined from the pH and P_{CO_2} by inspection of Fig. 15–4, page 154.

Confidence bands are shown in Figure 13–1, page 135.

Cation-anion balance:
Na 136 K 4 HCO_3 14 Cl 109 mEq/L
Anion gap = (Na + K) − (HCO_3 + Cl)
         = (136 + 4) − (14 + 109)
         = 140 − 123
         = 17 mEq/L. This is normal.

DIAGNOSIS

The hyperventilation of primary respiratory alkalosis can be confused with the hyperventilation resulting from a compensatory metabolic acidosis. However, tetany does not occur with the compensatory hyperventilation of a metabolic acidosis.

The pH may also be helpful in differential diagnosis. For example, a high pH in association with the low P_{CO_2} suggests a primary respiratory alkalosis with (or without) a compensatory metabolic acidosis. A normal pH in association with the low P_{CO_2} suggests a simultaneous primary respiratory alkalosis and a primary metabolic acidosis. A low pH in association with the low P_{CO_2} suggests a primary metabolic acidosis and a compensatory respiratory alkalosis.

COURSE AND PROGNOSIS

The condition is usually self-limited. In severe cases, catatonia and coma may occur.

TREATMENT

Treatment of the hyperventilation syndrome is difficult. The physician can make the patient aware of the cause of the symptoms by having him or her hyperventilate and precipitate symptoms. Then the patient should breathe into a paper bag (not a plastic bag) held closed around the nose and mouth, to make the symptoms disappear.

A 5% carbon dioxide mixture with 95% oxygen has been used to treat patients with respiratory alkalosis. However, this can be dangerous because the respiratory center of patients with respiratory alkalosis is sensitive to carbon dioxide. Therefore, the inhalation of carbon dioxide may cause an increased hyperventilation. Patients with cerebral lesions can breathe a mixture of 5% carbon dioxide and 95% oxygen until clinical signs disappear.

If the P_{CO_2} is quickly restored to normal, the compensatory metabolic acidosis which is present may lower the pH to a dangerous level. It is therefore preferable to decrease the hyperventilation by using sedatives. In addition, it may be necessary to replace the bicarbonate ions which have been lost.

REFERENCES

Ackerman, S.H., and Sachar, E.J.: The lactate theory of anxiety. A review and reevaluation. Psychosom Med, *36*:69, 1974.

Andersen, M.N., and Svane, H.: Pattern of biochemical response to acute change in pCO$_2$. Ann Surg *156*:752, 1962.

Eichenholz, A., et al.: Primary hypocapnia. A cause of metabolic acidosis. J Appl Physiol, *17*:283, 1962.

Eichenholz, A.: Respiratory alkalosis. Arch Intern Med, *116*:689, 1965.

Eldridge, F., and Salzer, J.: Effect of respiratory alkalosis on blood lactate and pyruvate in humans. J Appl Physiol, *22*:261, 1967.

Gambino, S.R.: Acid-base balance in tetanus. JAMA, *187*:307, 1964.

Greene, N.M.: Fatal cardiovascular and respiratory failure associated with tracheotomy. N Engl J Med, *261*:846, 1959.

Halsam, M.T.: The relationship between the effect of lactate infusion on anxiety states and their amelioration by carbon dioxide inhalation. Br J Psychiat, *125*:88, 1974.

Harrop, G.A., and Loeb, R.F.: Uncompensated alkalosis in encephalitis. JAMA, *81*:452, 1923.

Karetzky, M.S.: Cause of hyperventilation and arterial hypoxia in patients with cirrhosis of the liver. Am J Med Sci, *254*:797, 1967.

Kiely, J.M.: Organic disease presenting as hyperventilation syndrome. Psychosomatics, *11*:326, 1970.

Kilburn, K.H.: Shock, seizures and coma with alkalosis during mechanical ventilation. Ann Intern Med, *65*:977, 1966.

Lane, D.J., Rout, M.W., and Williamson, D.H.: Mechanism of hyperventilation in acute cerebrovascular accidents. Br Med J, *3*:9, 1971.

Okel, B., and Hurst, J.: Prolonged hyperventilation in man. Associated electrolyte changes and subjective symptoms. Arch Intern Med, *108*:747, 1961.

Pitts, F.N., Jr., and McClure, J.N., Jr.: Lactate metabolism in anxiety neurosis. N Engl J Med, *277*:1329, 1967.

Saltzman, H., Heyman, A., and Sieker, H.: Correlation of clinical and physiological manifestations of sustained hyperventilation. N Engl J Med, *268*:1431, 1963.

Sattler, T.H., Marquardt, G.H., and Cummins, G.M., Jr.: Alkalosis due to hyperventilation. JAMA, *146*:1125, 1951.

Wilson, R.F., et al.: Severe alkalosis in critically ill surgical patients. Arch Surg, *105*:197, 1972.

CHAPTER 26

METABOLIC ALKALOSIS SYNDROMES

Metabolic alkalosis is an alkalosis that results from a loss of hydrogen (and chloride) ions, or an excess of base (bicarbonate ions).

PATHOPHYSIOLOGY

When hydrogen ions are lost, or bicarbonate ions are retained in the body, the bicarbonate-carbonic acid ratio increases and the pH rises. As a result of this, the kidneys compensate for the rise in pH, just as in respiratory alkalosis (page 128). In addition, breathing becomes more shallow and the PCO_2 rises, so that a respiratory acidosis develops to compensate for the metabolic alkalosis. In the past, it has been assumed that the compensatory respiratory acidosis was minimal, because respiratory acidosis might produce decreased oxygen saturation of the blood; in addition, the retention of carbon dioxide would serve as a stimulus for hyperventilation, which would reduce the PCO_2. However, studies have shown that the compensatory respiratory acidosis that develops in a patient with a primary metabolic alkalosis may be so severe that the PCO_2 may rise above a value of 55 mm Hg (Tuller and Mehdi, Lifschitz, et al, and others). (A PCO_2 value above 55 mm Hg has been considered a sign of primary respiratory acidosis, but this criterion is no longer valid.)

The electrolyte disturbances that occur in metabolic alkalosis are described below.

ETIOLOGY

Metabolic alkalosis can occur in the following situations:

1. When hydrochloric acid is lost from the body, due to vomiting, gastric suction, or villous adenoma of the sigmoid colon.

   Normally, the parietal cells of the stomach form carbonic acid from carbon dioxide and water by means of the enzyme carbonic anhydrase. The carbonic acid dissociates into hydrogen and bicarbonate ions. The hydrogen ions enter the lumen of the stomach along with chloride ions to form hydrochloric acid. The bicarbonate enters the bloodstream, producing the transient "alkaline tide" noted after meals.

In the alkaline medium of the intestines, the intestinal epithelial cells also form carbonic acid from carbon dioxide and water by means of carbonic anhydrase. However, the hydrogen ions pass back into the lumen of the gut. This restores the neutrality of the blood, because the hydrogen ions which enter the blood from the intestinal cells neutralize the bicarbonate which had passed into the blood from the stomach.

When hydrogen ions are lost from the gastrointestinal tract, as in vomiting, the bicarbonate which passes into the blood from the stomach is not neutralized. This causes the bicarbonate-carbonic acid ratio and the pH to rise, producing a metabolic alkalosis. In addition, the vomiting also causes a loss of chloride and potassium ions which aggravate the alkalosis.

Alkalosis due to vomiting can occur in an otherwise normal patient. In addition, vomiting can occasionally cause an alkalosis in a patient with chronic renal disease. It is comparatively uncommon, because there is a high incidence of achlorhydria in these patients. Therefore, even if vomiting occurs, little hydrochloric acid is lost.

The excessive use of milk and an antacid, such as sodium bicarbonate or particularly calcium carbonate, in the treatment of a patient with peptic ulcer, can produce not only a metabolic alkalosis, but also severe hypercalcemia with renal insufficiency and azotemia *(milk-alkali syndrome)*.

2. When excessive sodium bicarbonate, or other alkaline salts such as sodium or potassium acetate, lactate, or citrate, are given orally or parenterally.

    When sodium bicarbonate, for example, is ingested, the bicarbonate ions combine with the hydrochloric acid of the gastric juice, the hydrogen ions are neutralized, and carbon dioxide is formed and eliminated, *viz:*

    $$NaHCO_3 + HCl \rightarrow H_2CO_3 + NaCl + CO_2 \uparrow.$$

3. When excessive potassium ions are lost as a result of diarrhea, vomiting, cirrhosis of the liver, or any other condition (Chap. 28).

4. When hydrogen and chloride ions are lost from the body from excessive use of the thiazide diuretics, or from the use of the "loop" diuretics, furosemide (Lasix), or ethacrynic acid (Edecrin). (A metabolic alkalosis may also develop because of a loss of potassium ions in the urine [see Chapter 27].)

    The thiazides inhibit the reabsorption of sodium ions in the distal renal tubule, and in this way increase the excretion of sodium and chloride ions in the urine (see Chap. 10). However, more chloride than sodium ions are excreted. Potassium and ammonium ions are also excreted with the excess chloride ions.

    When the patient becomes refractory to the thiazide diuretics, due to a low sodium intake or decreased renal blood flow, or when excessive amounts of the diuretics are given, the excretion of chloride ions continues. However, a large amount of potassium or ammonium ions, instead of sodium ions, is excreted along with the chloride ions. The mechanism by which the loss of potassium ions produces a metabolic alkalosis is discussed in Chapter 27. The excretion of each ammonium ion is associated with a loss of a hydrogen ion.

    Furosemide and ethacrynic acid act by inhibiting active sodium reab-

Table 26–1. Causes of saline-responsive and saline-resistant metabolic alkalosis.

Saline-responsive	Saline-resistant
Loss of HCl by vomiting, etc.	Primary aldosteronism
Diuretics associated with loss of Cl ions through kidneys*	Bartter's syndrome
	Cushing's syndrome
Abrupt relief of chronic hypercapnia	Licorice ingestion
Villous adenoma of colon	Severe K^+ depletion

*These include thiazides and loop diuretics.

sorption in the ascending limb of the loop of Henle. They are associated with an excretion of sodium and particularly chloride ions, as well as with a lesser excretion of potassium ions. A large amount of water is also excreted from the kidneys.

When a large amount of water is excreted as a result of the action of either furosemide or ethacrynic acid, the bicarbonate-carbonic acid ratio may become higher because of the increased concentration of extracellular water. This is called a *contraction alkalosis* (page 268).

5. When prolonged hypercalcemia is associated with a metabolic alkalosis. This is probably due to loss of potassium ions in the urine resulting from disturbed renal tubular function produced by the hypercalcemia.

6. When metabolic alkalosis occurs during the diuretic phase of acute renal failure. This is also due to an excessive loss of potassium ions in the urine.

7. When metabolic alkalosis is due to the effects of aldosterone or a similar mineralocorticoid steroid, as in primary aldosteronism, Cushing's syndrome, malignant hypertension, renal artery stenosis, and so on (see Chap. 28).

Most metabolic alkalosis patients can be treated with chloride ions in the form of sodium chloride (*saline-responsive* metabolic alkalosis), rather than potassium chloride (which is preferable). This is due to the fact that these patients have a decreased (arterial) blood volume, from vomiting, for example. This stimulates the secretion of aldosterone, which causes an increased urinary loss of potassium ions. In addition, a decreased blood volume is associated with an increased reabsorption of bicarbonate ions from the tubular urine. When a large amount of sodium chloride is given to such a patient, either intravenously or even orally, chloride ions are supplied, the blood volume rises, the excessive secretion of aldosterone stops, the excessive urinary loss of potassium ions stops, and the excessive reabsorption of bicarbonate ions from the kidney tubules stops. As a result, metabolic balance reappears.

However, when the metabolic alkalosis is due to the effects of excessive aldosterone or another mineralocorticoid steroid, as in primary aldosteronism, and so on, the patient will not respond to sodium chloride and requires potassium chloride. This is known as a *saline-resistant* metabolic alkalosis. (A *saline-resistant* metabolic alkalosis can also occur when metabolic alkalosis is due to depletion of potassium ions and the serum potassium concentration is less than 2 mEq/L.)

Table 26–1 shows the different etiologies of saline-responsive and saline-resistant metabolic alkalosis.

The usual *saline-responsive* metabolic alkalosis can be differentiated from a *saline-resistant* metabolic alkalosis by means of the urinary chloride concentration, because in a *saline-responsive* metabolic alkalosis there are only minimal chloride ions in the urine (less than approximately 10 mEq/L unless the patient is receiving diuretics). However, when a *saline-resistant* metabolic alkalosis is present (and the patient is not receiving diuretics), the chloride concentration of the urine is more than approximately 10 mEq/L.

(The relative absence of chloride ions in patients with metabolic alkalosis due to the usual causes [loss of hydrogen and chloride ions resulting from a loss of gastric secretions, or from diuretic therapy] is as follows: When sodium ions are reabsorbed from the tubular filtrate into the blood, chloride ions are also usually reabsorbed, to preserve electroneutrality. However, when a metabolic alkalosis occurs due to a continued loss of chloride ions, most if not all of the chloride ions that reach the tubular filtrate are reabsorbed, so that little or none appears in the urine.)

8. Bartter's syndrome (see Chapter 28).
9. With *overcompensatory metabolic alkalosis (posthypercapnic metabolic alkalosis)*. Chronic respiratory acidosis is associated with a compensatory metabolic alkalosis, with a loss of hydrogen and chloride ions in the urine and a retention of bicarbonate ions, so that hypochloremia and an elevated serum bicarbonate concentration develop. If the cause of the respiratory alkalosis is suddenly removed and the Pco_2 suddenly decreases, a severe metabolic alkalosis may develop because of the elevated serum bicarbonate concentration. This will persist until the patient is given chloride ions (either in the form of sodium or potassium chloride or an acidifying salt such as ammonium chloride, 1-lysine monohydrochloride, or dilute hydrochloric acid).

Overcompensatory metabolic alkalosis usually occurs in patients with chronic pulmonary disease and congestive heart failure who are treated with a low-sodium diet and diuretics.

10. With *contraction alkalosis*. If the volume of extracellular water decreases rapidly, for example, as the result of the diuretic ethacrynic acid or furosemide, the concentration of extracellular bicarbonate will increase. Theoretically, the concentration of dissolved carbon dioxide should also similarly increase and the pH should remain unchanged. However, the increased concentration of dissolved carbon dioxide will raise the carbon dioxide pressure of the blood and increase the diffusion of carbon dioxide into the alveolar air, where it is removed during respiration. As a result, the bicarbonate-carbonic acid ratio and the pH rise. The metabolic alkalosis produced in this way has been called a *contraction alkalosis*. It is the reverse of a *dilution acidosis* (Chap. 17).

SYMPTOMS AND SIGNS

It is difficult to separate the clinical symptoms and signs of patients with metabolic alkalosis from those of their associated disease processes, and especially from the symptoms and signs of hypokalemia (Chap. 27). A characteristic clinical picture of metabolic alkalosis occurs after a large amount of absorbable antacid medication is taken over a long time. Anorexia, nausea, and painless vomiting may occur. The patient may become confused and mentally unreliable. These patients have been described as being "difficult." This stage may be followed by drowsiness and coma. Tetany is another common sign of either metabolic or respiratory alkalosis.

Tetany

Tetany can be caused by either an increased pH or a decreased serum calcium concentration. If the serum pH is normal, tetany may occur when the serum calcium concentration decreases to 7.5 to 7 mg/dl or lower (4.25 to 3.5 mEq/L or lower). However, a low pH decreases the tendency to tetany. This is the reason tetany does not appear in metabolic acidosis due to chronic renal disease, where the serum calcium concentration is low. When both the serum calcium and potassium concentrations are low, tetany is also inhibited. However, tetany will appear when the serum potassium concentration is elevated and the serum calcium concentration remains low. A high serum potassium concentration does not induce tetany when the serum calcium concentration is normal.

Tetany can therefore be corrected by either lowering the pH or raising the serum calcium concentration, if the pH is normal. If the low serum calcium is due to an increased serum phosphate concentration, the serum calcium concentration can be raised only by lowering the serum phosphate concentration.

In addition, when a patient is treated for hypokalemia, the serum calcium concentration should be checked. If hypocalcemia is also present, it should be treated along with the hypokalemia.

Electrocardiogram

Patients with metabolic and respiratory alkalosis may show a characteristic electrocardiographic pattern which results from sinus tachycardia and a relative prolongation of the Q-T interval. The pattern consists of a T (or U) wave which approaches or actually merges with the P wave which follows (T-P phenomenon).

Electroencephalogram

Gross slowing or rhythmic activity may be present.

LABORATORY FINDINGS

Blood

In a patient with uncomplicated metabolic alkalosis, the pH is high, indicating the alkalosis. The P_{CO_2} is normal.

The bicarbonate concentration is high and the chloride concentration is reciprocally low. Serum sodium concentration is normal or high. Serum potassium concentration may be normal or low.

Urine

The urine is usually alkaline, due to renal compensatory changes. However, if the alkalosis is due to potassium loss, the urine may be acid.

Example: Patient with metabolic alkalosis due to excessive vomiting.
pH 7.56
P_{CO_2} 46 mm Hg
CO_2 content 41.4 mEq/L
Standard bicarbonate 39 mEq/L
Actual bicarbonate 40 mEq/L
Base excess +16.2 mEq/L

The pH is high. This indicates an alkalosis. The positive base excess and the high standard bicarbonate indicate that a metabolic alkalosis is present. The P_{CO_2} shows a high normal value. Therefore, respiratory balance is present. However, the actual bicarbonate is higher than the standard bicarbonate. This indicates that some degree of respiratory acidosis is present. Therefore, a primary metabolic alkalosis is present with a partially compensatory respiratory acidosis (see Chap. 15).

This information can also be determined from the pH and P_{CO_2} by inspection of Figure 15–4, page 154.

Cation-anion balance:
Na 137 K 3.5 HCO_3 40 Cl 88 mEq/L
Anion gap = (Na + K) − (HCO_3 + Cl)
= (137 + 3.5) − (40 + 88)
= 140.5 − 128
= 12.5 mEq/L. This is normal.

DIAGNOSIS

A metabolic alkalosis should be suspected in any patient who has vomited, or who has received large amounts of absorbable alkaline salts, or who has lost potassium, or who shows electrocardiographic signs of hypokalemia, or who shows hypoventilation, or tetany. The diagnosis is confirmed by finding a high CO_2 content and a high pH.

COURSE AND PROGNOSIS

The course and prognosis depend on the etiology of the metabolic alkalosis.

PROPHYLAXIS

Absorbable alkali should be given cautiously to patients. This applies not only to those with peptic ulcer, for example, but also to those with metabolic acidosis who are being treated with alkalinizing solutions. In addition, electrolytes should be replaced in patients who vomit, or who are being treated with gastric suction.

Patients with congestive heart failure who receive daily doses of a diuretic, such as a thiazide, or furosemide or ethacrynic acid, should receive prophylactic potassium chloride to prevent a metabolic alkalosis. A carbonic anhydrase inhibitor (see page 274) can also be used to prevent the development of a metabolic alkalosis, because it increases the concentration of chloride ions in the body.

Potassium chloride can be given in a daily dose up to 5 to 10 g. Numerous stock potassium chloride solutions are now available (Chap. 27). Potassium chloride can also be used as a salt substitute for sprinkling on food. The only contraindications to its use are severe renal disease and acidosis, because if the potassium ions are not excreted, muscular and nerve paralysis and death may occur. When potassium salts are used for patients with congestive heart failure, the potassium concentration in the body should be periodically checked with serum potassium concentrations.

TREATMENT

The aim of treatment is to correct the disturbance which has produced the metabolic alkalosis. For example, if vomiting or gastric suction is the cause, solutions containing saline and potassium chloride (page 82) should be infused in a volume approximate to the volume of gastric juice which has been lost. If potassium deficiency is present, due to any other cause, the patient should also receive potassium in the form of potassium *chloride.*

Ammonium Chloride

Ammonium chloride has been used in the treatment of metabolic alkalosis due to vomiting or gastric suction. However, in these patients, potassium loss is also present. For this reason, solutions containing sodium chloride and potassium chloride (page 82) may be preferable.

Ammonium chloride can also be used to treat metabolic alkalosis due to diuretics such as the thiazides. (It is rarely used now for this purpose.) Uncoated tablets of ammonium chloride are prescribed orally in a daily dose of 6 to 12 g. (Enteric coated tablets should not be used. They may not dissolve in the intestines.) The ammonium chloride should be used for only 3 days each week, because the ammonium ions are metabolized to urea by the liver. The chloride ions are excreted along with sodium ions and water by the kidneys. The loss of sodium ions causes a diuresis and a loss of edema fluid. If the ammonium chloride is given for more than 3 days at a time, ammonia is produced by the kidneys and chloride ions are excreted along with the ammonia. As a result, sodium ions are not eliminated and no diuresis occurs. In addition, the ammonium chloride may be retained in the body, causing a metabolic acidosis.

If the patient cannot tolerate the ammonium chloride orally, it can be given intravenously in the form of a 2.14% solution. One should not attempt to raise the serum chloride concentration above 95 mEq/L with the intravenous solution. In addition, the serum chloride concentration should not be raised more than 15 mEq/L in one infusion in this way.

Either solution can be given at a rate up to 120 ml per hour.

Example: Man weighing 70 kg. Serum chloride concentration 75 mEq/L. It is desired to raise serum chloride concentration to 90 mEq/L. Extracellular water is 20% of body weight.
70 × .2 = 14 liters extracellular water.
Unit chloride deficit is 90 mEq/L − 75 mEq/L = 15 mEq/L.
Total chloride deficit is 14 × 15 = 210 mEq/L.
Each liter of the 2.14% ammonium chloride solution contains 399.5 mEq chloride.
Therefore, 210/399.5 liter or approximately 526 ml are needed.
The following rule, based on the above calculations, can also be used:
0.50 ml of the 2.14% ammonium chloride solutions per kg of body weight will raise the serum chloride concentration 1 mEq/L.
Thus, in the above example of a 70-kg man with a chloride deficit of 15 mEq/L, the amount of 2.14% ammonium chloride solution needed is 70 × 15 × 0.50 = 525 ml.

The positive base excess concentration has also been used to determine the amount of ammonium chloride which is needed (see page 151).

Dilute Hydrochloric Acid (U.S.P., 10%)

This is a satisfactory substitute for ammonium chloride. It can be conveniently given by mouth. The dose is 20 ml daily. The patient sips 5 ml of the acid in a full glass of water, 4 times a day, through a glass tube to protect the teeth. The 20 ml of hydrochloric acid has a chloride content equivalent to about 3 g of ammonium chloride.

The duration of therapy with chloride salts depends on the degree of chloride depletion. It may take several days to a week or more. The patient usually responds within 2 to 3 days.

Intravenous Hydrochloric Acid

Hydrochloric acid can also be given intravenously when extreme metabolic alkalosis is present, and the patient has not responded to the usual treatment.

Intravenous hydrochloric acid can be given as a 0.05 normal (N) to 0.2 N solution. A 0.15 N solution in water (150 mEq HCl/L of H_2O) is approximately isotonic. The 0.15 N solution can also be given in a 5% dextrose in water solution.

A 0.15 N solution is prepared by adding 150 ml of 1.0 N hydrochloric acid to 850 ml of sterile water, or by diluting 12.5 ml of reagent grade hydrochloric acid (35 to 38%) to a total volume of 1000 ml with sterile water (Duncan).

The 0.15 N solution can be given at a rate up to 125 ml per hour. A glass container should be used because hydrochloric acid may react with a plastic container.

The hydrochloric acid must be given through a central venous catheter. If it is given into a peripheral vein, it will cause sloughing of the surrounding tissues. Supplemental potassium chloride is given as needed to correct any associated hypokalemia.

Knutson has suggested that hydrochloric acid can be given into a peripheral vein if it is buffered in an amino acid solution and infused with a fat emulsion.

The dose of IV hydrochloric acid can be calculated in several ways:

1. from the plasma bicarbonate level:
   mEq HCl needed = (HCO_3 observed − 24) × 0.5 × body weight (kg)
2. from the plasma chloride concentration:
   mEq HCl needed = (100 − Cl observed × 0.2 × body weight (kg)

About ½ to ⅔ the calculated deficit should be given during the first 24 hours to prevent overcorrection.

When loss of hydrochloric acid is severe, as in postoperative patients or in the Zollinger-Ellison syndrome, a patient can lose a massive amount of gastric juice with a high hydrochloric content. Abouna et al. have given as much as 600 mEq IV hydrochloric acid per 24 hours.

Excessive ammonium chloride or hydrochloric acid can cause a severe acidosis, disorientation, confusion, and coma (page 172). It is also dangerous to give these agents to patients with a primary respiratory acidosis who develop a high CO_2 content as a result of a compensatory metabolic alkalosis. If the metabolic alkalosis is eliminated by the ammonium chloride, the patient may die from the respiratory acidosis. Ammonium chloride is also contraindicated in cirrhosis of the liver, or in patients with right-sided heart failure and liver damage, because it can precipitate hepatic coma.

Sodium Chloride

Sodium chloride, in the form of oral table salt or saline solution given intravenously, can be used to correct a metabolic alkalosis, unless sodium ions are contraindicated because of congestive heart failure, edema, ascites, or a *saline-resistant* metabolic alkalosis.

Carbonic Anhydrase Inhibitors

Patients with severe congestive heart failure may develop a metabolic alkalosis due to thiazide or other diuretic therapy, and may become refractory to the action of the diuretic. A carbonic anhydrase inhibitor such as acetazolamide (Diamox) may be effective in decreasing the alkalosis and in restoring the sensitivity of the patient to the diuretic. The following schedule may be beneficial:

Diamox, 250 mg 2 or 3 times a day for 3 days.
Ammonium chloride, 6 to 9 g a day for 3 days, simultaneously.

The diuretic can then be resumed on the fifth day.

The carbonic anhydrase inhibitors can produce drowsiness or paresthesias as side reactions. Disorientation has also been observed in edematous patients with impaired liver function. In addition, drug fever and rashes may occur, probably due to the sulfonamide structure of the carbonic anhydrase inhibitors.

Other Acidifying Agents

L-lysine monohydrochloride has also been used to produce a mild metabolic acidosis in order to increase the effect of diuretics in patients with heart failure. It increases the serum chloride concentration, which may be lowered as a result of the diuretics.

L-lysine monohydrochloride can be given in a dose of 10 to 40 g a day, for 3 to 5 days. Each gram yields 5 mEq chloride ions. Forty grams is equivalent to 11 g of ammonium chloride, or 12 g of calcium chloride. It can be given as a 40% solution in cold fruit juice or in regular or low-sodium milk. Therefore, 1 teaspoonful (5 ml) contains 2 g. It may cause side effects such as abdominal cramps or transient diarrhea.

Treatment of Metabolic Alkalosis Complicated by Severe Respiratory Acidosis

Mechanical ventilation, using a respirator, should be avoided. Instead, the primary metabolic alkalosis should be corrected.

REFERENCES

Abouna, G.M., et al.: Intravenous infusion of hydrochloric acid for treatment of severe metabolic alkalosis. Surgery, 75:194, 1974.

Alexander, C.S.: T-P phenomenon. An electrocardiographic clue to unsuspected alkalosis. Arch Intern Med, 116:220, 1965.

Ariel, I., et al.: Metabolic studies of patients with cancer of gastrointestinal tract. XVI. Treatment of hypochloremia refractory to administration of sodium chloride, especially in patients with gastrointestinal cancer. JAMA, 123:28, 1943.

Cannon, P.J., et al.: "Contraction" alkalosis after diuresis of edematous patients with ethacrynic acid. Ann Intern Med, 62:979, 1965.

Clark, R.G., and Norman, J.N.: Metabolic alkalosis in pyloric stenosis. Lancet, I:1244, 1964.

Coe, F.L.: Metabolic alkalosis. JAMA 238:2288, 1977.

Duncan, D.A.: Use of intravenous hydrochloric acid for the treatment of metabolic alkalosis in renal or hepatic failure, IM, 5:56, 1984.

Fulop, M.: Hypercapnia in metabolic alkalosis. New York State J Med, 76:19, 1976.

Garella, S., Chazan, J.A., and Cohen, J.J.: Saline-resistant metabolic alkalosis or "chloride-wasting nephropathy." Report of four patients with severe potassium depletion. Ann Intern Med, 73:31, 1970.

Goldring, R.M., et al.: Respiratory adjustment to chronic metabolic alkalosis in man. J Clin Invest, 47:188, 1968.

Heinemann, H.O.: The effect of hypercalcemia on acid-base metabolism in man. Ann Intern Med, 58:741, 1963.

Heinemann, H.O.: Metabolic alkalosis in patients with hypercalcemia. Metabolism, 14:1137, 1965.

Javaheri, S., et al.: Compensatory hypoventilation in metabolic alkalosis, Chest 81:296, 1982.

Kassirer, J.P., and Schwartz, W.B.: Correction of metabolic alkalosis in man without repair of potassium deficiency. Re-evaluation of the role of potassium. Am J Med, 40:19, 1966.

Kassirer, J., Berkman, P., Lawrenz, D., and Schwartz, W.: Critical role of chloride in correction of hypokalemic alkalosis in man. Am J Med, 38:172, 1965.

Knutsen, O.H.: New method for administration of hydrochloric acid in metabolic alkalosis, Lancet, 1:953, 1983.

Kraft, A.R., Tompkins, R.K., and Zollinger, R.M.: Recognition and management of the diarrheal syndrome caused by nonbeta islet cell tumors of the pancreas. Am J Surg, 119:163, 1970.

Kurtzman, N.A.: Metabolic alkalosis. The Kidney, 9: no. 6, November, 1976.

Kurtzman, N.A., White, M.G., and Rogers, P.W.: Pathophysiology of metabolic alkalosis. Arch Intern Med, 131:702, 1973.

Lifschitz, M.D., Brasch, R., Cuomo, A.J., and Menn, S.J.: Marked hypercapnia secondary to severe metabolic alkalosis. Ann Intern Med, 77:405, 1972.

MacLean, L.D., et al.: Alkalosis in septic shock. Surgery, 62:655, 1967.

Miller, P.D., and Berns, A.S.: Acute metabolic alkalosis perpetuating hypercarbia. A role for acetazolamide in chronic obstructive pulmonary disease. JAMA 238:2400, 1977.

Mulhausen, R.O., and Blumentals, A.S.: Metabolic alkalosis. Arch Intern Med, 116:729, 1965.

Mulhausen, R., Eichenholz, A., and Blumentals, A.S.: Acid-base disturbances in patients with cirrhosis of the liver. Medicine, 46:85, 1967.

Oliva, P.B.: Severe alveolar hypoventilation in a patient with metabolic alkalosis. Am J Med, 52:817, 1972.

Roberts, K., et al.: Evaluation of respiratory compensation in metabolic alkalosis. J Clin Invest, 35:261, 1956.

Roggin, G.M., et al.: Ketosis and metabolic alkalosis in a patient with diabetes. JAMA, 211:296, 1970.

Rubin, A.L., et al.: Use of l-lysine monohydrochloride in combination with mercurial diuretics in treatment of refractory fluid retention. Circulation, 21:332, 1960.

Seldin, D.W., and Rector, F.C., Jr.: The generation and maintenance of metabolic alkalosis. Kidney Int, 1:306, 1972.

Tuller, M.T., and Mehdi, F.: Compensatory hypoventilation and hypercapnia in primary metabolic alkalosis. Am J Med, *50*:290, 1971.

Van Goidsenhoven, G. M.-T., et al.: The effect of prolonged administration of large doses of sodium bicarbonate in man. Clin Sci, *13*:383, 1954.

CHAPTER 27

METABOLIC ALKALOSIS SYNDROMES (Continued)

HYPOKALEMIA

Hypokalemia (hypopotassemia) is present when the serum potassium concentration is lower than 3.5 mEq/L.

Serum potassium concentrations can be misleading because a loss of total body potassium can be present with a normal serum potassium concentration. This can occur in several different ways:

1. Hemoconcentration is present, due to either water loss or sodium loss.
2. When acidosis is present, there is a shift of potassium from the cells into the extracellular water. Therefore, serum potassium concentration may be normal or even high in the presence of potassium loss. This occurs, for example, during diabetic acidosis. Conversely, alkalosis causes potassium to move from the extracellular water into the cells. Therefore, the serum potassium concentration may appear to be low without loss of potassium from the body.

The average daily intake of the potassium ion ranges from 50 to 75 mEq. This is equivalent to 3.73 to 5.6 g of potassium chloride, and is adequate for the normal needs of the body.

PATHOPHYSIOLOGY

In Chapter 24 it was pointed out that a loss of total exchangeable body potassium is not necessarily associated with hypokalemia, and that the serum potassium concentration in such patients may be low, normal, or even high, depending on the associated presence of water loss or acidosis.

It can be stated as a general rule that potassium loss causes a metabolic alkalosis, and, conversely, that a metabolic or respiratory alkalosis causes hypokalemia.

Potassium loss causes a metabolic alkalosis in the following way: When potassium ions are lost from the cells, sodium and hydrogen ions move from the extracellular water into the cells to replace the potassium. However, for every 3 potassium ions lost from the cell, only 2 sodium ions enter the cell. The remaining potassium ion is replaced by a hydrogen ion. This causes a decreased hydrogen ion concentration of the extracellular water, and a metabolic alkalosis. A similar loss of potassium ions occurs through the kidneys. Normally, potassium ions are completely filtered by the glomeruli. Then they are completely reabsorbed in the proximal tubules. Finally, approximately 10% of the potassium ions that had been originally filtered are actively secreted by the distal tubular cells into the urine, and are excreted.

The secretion of potassium ions from the distal tubular cells into the urine occurs in association with a reabsorption of sodium ions from the tubular urine into the tubular cells (and into the blood), although these two processes do not occur at the same anatomical site. If the number of potassium ions available for exchange with sodium ions is decreased, hydrogen ions, instead of potassium ions, will be excreted into the tubular urine, while sodium ions are reabsorbed. The urinary loss of hydrogen ions also causes a metabolic alkalosis. In addition, the hydrogen ions in the urine cause the urine to show an acid pH even in the presence of a metabolic alkalosis. This is a characteristic finding of metabolic alkalosis due to potassium loss.

Alkalosis, conversely, causes a hypokalemia. Potassium ions move from the extracellular water into the cells, and hydrogen ions move from the cells into the extracellular water, in an attempt to raise the hydrogen ion concentration and lower the pH of the extracellular water toward normal.

The relation of hypokalemia to muscle paralysis is discussed in Chapter 24.

Hypokalemia causes an important abnormality of renal function, namely, an inability of the kidneys to concentrate urine normally. As a result, the osmolality of the urine falls to a value only slightly above that of the plasma *(hyposthenuria).* The urinary specific gravity also becomes low. (The hyposthenuria is characteristically resistant to the action of vasopressin.) As a result, nocturia, polyuria, thirst and polydipsia may occur.

Insulin is necessary for potassium ions to enter cells. Therefore, patients with diabetes mellitus may not be able to tolerate large doses of potassium salts. And, if renal insufficiency is present, a potassium-sparing diuretic such as triamterere may easily induce hyperkalemia.

The pathophysiologic mechanisms by which hypokalemia occurs in other clinical conditions are discussed below.

ETIOLOGY

The following conditions tend to decrease the serum potassium concentration and to cause hypokalemia. A loss of total exchangeable potassium may or may not be present.

1. Hypokalemia due to a loss of potassium ions from the body. This can occur in at least three ways:
   a. Loss of potassium ions from the gastrointestinal tract. This can cause two patterns of hypokalemia:
      i.   Hypokalemia associated with a loss of gastric juices *(upper GI syndrome)*. This occurs with persistent vomiting, particularly with pyloric obstruction. The hypokalemia is associated with a metabolic alkalosis, due to the loss of hydrogen ions from the gastric juice.
      ii. Hypokalemia associated with a loss of lower intestinal fluids. This can occur with diarrhea due to any cause, with intestinal fistulas, or with a *villous adenoma of the colon* (or from long-term surreptitious use of laxatives or excessive enemas). A large number of bicarbonate ions are lost, in addition to the potassium (and sodium) ions, so that the hypokalemia is associated with a metabolic alkalosis.

      Patients with *nonbeta islet cell tumor of the pancreas* often show a profuse watery diarrhea ("pancreatic cholera"), hypokalemia, and characteristic achlorhydria (WDHA syndrome). Excessive secretin secretion may be the cause of the syndrome. Secretin suppresses gastric acid secretion, but stimulates the secretion of bile and pancreatic juices, and may inhibit the intestinal absorption of fluids.

      Hypercalcemia is often present. This may be due to parathyroid hormone secretion, stimulated by the low serum magnesium concentration which occurs as a result of the diarrhea. In other patients, the pancreatic tumor may have parathyroid hormone-like activity. Hyperglycemia may also be present.

      Hypokalemia may also occur in patients with the Zollinger-Ellison syndrome (non-beta islet cell adenomas of the pancreas, excessive hydrochloric acid secretion by the stomach, peptic ulcers of esophagus, stomach, duodenum or jejunum, chronic diarrhea, and hypokalemia. Some of these patients also have hyperparathyroidism).

      Hypokalemia due to diarrhea has also been reported in *medullary carcinoma of the thyroid*. The carcinoma cells secrete prostaglandins, which stimulate intestinal secretions and produce the diarrhea. The syndrome may be a variant of the Zollinger-Ellison syndrome (see above). However peptic ulcers are not present.

      Another factor in producing hypokalemia with lower intestinal losses is that feces contain an appreciable amount of potassium ions. (From 8 to 15 mEq potassium ions are normally excreted in the feces daily. A much greater loss occurs with diarrhea.)

      In patients with hypokalemia due to gastrointestinal losses, the actual serum potassium concentration may be misleading because severe water loss, sodium loss, or acidosis may be present. Therefore, the serum potassium concentration may be normal (or high) in spite of a loss of total exchangeable body potassium and a low potassium concentration in the cells.

      The electrocardiogram will reflect the serum potassium concentration. In cholera, for example, where there may be a high serum potassium concentration due to the associated metabolic acidosis, the electrocardiogram may show signs of hyperkalemia. Conversely, patients with hypokalemia secondary to gastric losses may show the classic electrocardiographic patterns of hypokalemia.

b. Loss of potassium ions through the urine. This can occur in several ways:

    i.   Diuretics, such as the thiazides, ethacrynic acid, or furosemide. An important action of these diuretics is the excretion of chloride ions in the urine. The chloride is usually excreted with sodium, ammonium, or potassium ions. Potassium loss this way may be severe, especially in patients who are on a low-sodium diet and receive a large amount of the diuretics. Sodium ions are not available for urinary excretion, and the kidneys may not be able to form ammonium ions. Therefore, potassium is excreted with the chloride ions. (Surreptitious diuretic use is occasionally a cause of hypokalemia.)

    ii.   Excessive administration of bicarbonate or other alkaline salts. In these patients, the potassium loss is due to its urinary excretion in association with the urinary excretion of excess bicarbonate ions.

    iii.   Decreased intake of potassium ions (orally or parenterally). Malnourished or semistarved patients have a low intake of potassium salts, but a continued excretion of potassium ions occurs. Apparently, the kidneys do not have a homeostatic mechanism for the conservation of potassium ions, and as much as 20 mEq can be excreted in the urine daily for a long time, even if a person is on a potassium-free diet.

        When a patient is given a large volume of potassium-free fluids parenterally, the hypokalemia that occurs is partly due to dilution of the blood with the intravenous fluids. In addition, a large number of potassium ions is excreted in the urine, for reasons just mentioned.

    iv.   The effect of aldosterone or other mineralocorticoid hormones (see Chapter 28). Postoperative potassium loss and the potassium loss that occurs in Cushing's syndrome have the same mechanism. Large doses of corticosteroids can also cause a severe potassium loss.

    v.   Renal tubular dysfunction. Potassium loss can occur in patients with renal tubular acidosis (Chap. 18) and in patients with uretero-enterostomy. Renal tubular acidosis may be one of the mechanisms by which hypokalemia occurs in patients with cirrhosis of the liver.

    vi.   Diuretic phase of acute renal failure (Chap. 21).

    vii.   Massive doses of sodium penicillin G (100 million units a day) may be associated with potassium loss through the kidneys. Apparently, penicillin promotes the urinary excretion of potassium ions by interfering with distal tubular cation transport. Amphotericin B, gentamicin, and carbenicillin may also cause potassium loss through the kidneys. The hypokalemia that often occurs in patients with acute myeloid leukemia is also partly due to loss of potassium ions through the kidneys.

c. Loss of potassium ions through the skin. Excessive sweating, particularly in persons acclimatized to tropical climates (where the potassium loss in sweat may equal or exceed the sodium loss).

2. Intracellular shifts of potassium ions. This can occur in the following conditions:
   a. Hypokalemia due to the transfer of potassium ions from the blood into the liver and muscle cells. Potassium is needed by the liver to convert glucose to glycogen. The ingestion of food, particularly carbohydrates, causes the secretion of insulin, which stimulates the liver cells. As a result, the concentration of potassium in the blood falls. A similar lowering of serum potassium concentration occurs after the parenteral injection of insulin or epinephrine.
   b. Hypokalemic periodic paralysis. The fall in serum potassium concentration, by the mechanism described above, is probably the direct cause of attacks of familial periodic paralysis. This type of hypokalemia is not associated with a decreased total exchangeable body potassium. However, patients who experience attacks of periodic paralysis show a lowered muscle potassium concentration, even during periods between attacks. This suggests that chronic potassium loss is present in these patients. (This may be due to an intermittent aldosteronism [Chap. 28].)
   c. The action of an anabolic hormone, such as testosterone. Potassium ions enter the muscle cells, where they are utilized to build muscle protein. However, in these latter patients, the electrocardiogram does not show signs of hypokalemia. The reason for this is not known.
   d. Alkalosis, either respiratory (Chap. 25) or metabolic (Chap. 26). The low serum potassium concentration may or may not indicate a loss of potassium ions from the body.
   e. Treatment of megaloblastic anemia. When hematopoiesis starts, a large number of potassium ions enter the young red blood cells, and serious hypokalemia may result.
3. Combination factors. Numerous factors producing hypokalemia may be present simultaneously or in sequence. For example, hypokalemia may occur in uncomplicated cirrhosis of the liver, if diarrhea is present. Renal tubular acidosis may also be a factor in the potassium loss. When cirrhosis is associated with ascites, hypokalemia may be due to secondary aldosteronism, or to the effect of diuretics.
4. Pseudohypokalemia. This can occur with leucocytosis, thrombocytosis, hemolysis.

PATHOLOGY

When potassium loss occurs for a long time, it may cause hydropic and degenerative changes in the convoluted tubules of the kidneys, without significant glomerular or vascular changes. These renal changes are associated with a hyposthenuria which is resistant to vasopressin (ADH).

Potassium loss can also cause degeneration of the myocardium. Loss of striation of the cells occurs. This is followed by poor staining of the cytoplasm and finally by karyorrhexis and karyolysis. In addition, infiltration of the myocardium by neutrophilic polymorphonuclear leukocytes and large mononuclear cells occurs. Later, fibrosis occurs.

SYMPTOMS AND SIGNS

The clinical symptoms and signs of hypokalemia are mostly non-specific and may occur in seriously ill patients who do not show hypokalemia. They include: anorexia, nausea and vomiting, abdominal distention, decreased bowel sounds, paralytic ileus, muscle weakness, absent or diminished deep tendon reflexes, and a depressed mental state. Thirst and polyuria may also occur.

Neuromuscular symptoms and signs do not usually appear until the serum potassium concentration falls to approximately 2.5 mEq/L, and may not even be present when it reaches 2 mEq/L. Muscle weakness first develops, then paralysis. Paresthesias or severe pain in the muscles may also be present. The muscle weakness is most prominent in the legs, especially in the quadriceps muscles. Later, the respiratory muscles become weakened. The diaphragm becomes paralyzed before the intercostal muscles and the accessory muscles of respiration. As a result, a characteristic "fish-mouth" type of breathing, characterized by pursing of the lips, occurs. The muscles innervated by the cranial nerves are almost never affected. Instead of muscle weakness, a patient may complain of severely tender muscles or paresthesias. Chronic potassium loss may cause muscle weakness due to actual muscle atrophy. In spite of the muscle weakness, deep tendon reflexes and the abdominal and cremasteric reflexes remain normal. The electroencephalogram also is normal.

Central nervous symptoms may include lethargy, drowsiness, irritability, confusion. Rarely coma, delirium, and hallucinations occur.

Occasionally, tetany may occur when hypokalemia has been corrected. This is due to a concomitant hypocalcemia whose effects have been inhibited by the hypokalemia.

Postural hypotension is common.

Nocturia, polyuria, and polydipsia may occur because the kidneys lose their capacity to concentrate urine normally. The resultant loss of water through the urine also produces thirst.

The most characteristic signs of muscle paralysis associated with hypokalemia are seen in *familial periodic paralysis.* The attacks can occur spontaneously, or can be precipitated by substances such as epinephrine, desoxycorticosterone acetate, corticotropin (ACTH), insulin, dextrose, or a large carbohydrate meal, which reduce the serum potassium concentration. The attacks can occur when the serum potassium concentration is at a low normal level, such as 3.5 mEq/L, which would have no effect on the normal person. (Hyperthyroidism may also induce attacks.)

ELECTROCARDIOGRAM

Assuming that there are no local alterations of the potassium content of heart muscle (due to muscle injury or ventricular strain) the elec-

HYPOKALEMIA

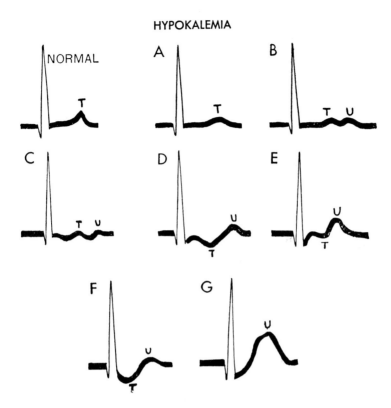

Fig. 27–1. Electrocardiographic patterns of hypokalemia.

trocardiographic changes which occur in hypokalemia can be correlated in a general way with the level of potassium in the serum.

Figure 27–1 shows some of the common changes seen, which include:

1. Lowering and broadening of the T wave *(A)*. The Q–T interval is also slightly prolonged. Such a pattern may occur when the serum potassium is merely at a low normal level, for example, 3.5 mEq/L.
2. Low, broad T waves with a double summit, due to superimposition of the U wave on the T *(B)*. The Q–T interval may appear markedly prolonged in such cases. However, the prolongation may be more apparent than real because it may be difficult to determine where the T ends and the U begins. As a consequence, The Q–U interval, rather than the Q–T interval, is often measured.
3. Downward T waves and prominent U waves *(D,E,F)*. Such a pattern is best seen in precordial leads such as V_1 through V_4, which overlie the right ventricle and thus have an rS or RS pattern.
4. Depression of the ST segment and slight lengthening of the Q–T interval *(D,E)*. The ST may be slightly depressed, or may show several small undulations *(C)*. D, E, F, G, show more marked ST deviations. These ST segments have a sagging appearance, characteristic of hypokalemia.
5. Increase in P wave amplitudes, and widening of the QRS interval.

6. Numerous arrhythmias, including sinus bradycardia, prolonged P–R interval, Wenckebach type of a-v block, paroxysmal atrial tachycardia with a-v block (PAT with block). Arrhythmias due to digitalis toxicity may be precipitated or worsened.

Although *A* through *G* show the progressive changes which can occur as hypokalemia becomes more marked, these progressive changes do not always occur, and it may be impossible to determine the exact degree of hypokalemia from the electrocardiogram.

LABORATORY FINDINGS

Blood

The normal serum potassium concentration varies from 3.5 to 5.0 mEq/L (13.7 to 19.5 mg/dl). Signs of hypokalemia are usually associated with serum concentrations of 3 mEq/L (12 mg/dl) or less. The serum calcium concentration may be normal, low, or high in association with the hypokalemia. (Serum potassium concentration should always be determined in hypocalcemic tetany. If the hypokalemia alone is corrected, tetany may be precipitated.)

With severe hypokalemia, laboratory findings of a metabolic alkalosis, including a high bicarbonate concentration and a high CO_2 content, are present (Chap. 26).

One should remember that if an acidosis is present the serum potassium concentration tends to be high, regardless of the total exchangeable body potassium. A normal or low serum potassium concentration in an acidotic patient therefore indicates a severe potassium loss. Conversely, in alkalosis, the serum potassium concentration tends to be low, even when the total exchangeable body potassium is normal. Significant potassium loss should be suspected in an alkalotic patient when the serum potassium concentration is below 2.5 mEq/L.

Potassium loss may cause decreased carbohydrate tolerance, so that an elevated fasting blood sugar level and a diabetic glucose tolerance test response may develop. (If this happens when a patient is receiving diuretics, it can be corrected by also giving potassium chloride in conjunction with the diuretic.)

Urine

Hypokalemia is associated with a decreased ability of the kidneys to concentrate urine normally. Therefore, when the hypokalemia is severe, the urine osmolality decreases to approximately that of the serum. The urine shows an acid pH, but it is rare for the urinary pH to decrease to 5.0 or lower.

The urinary potassium excretion is low (less than 30 mEq a day), in association with the hypokalemia. However, if the hypokalemia is due to diuretics, to renal tubular acidosis, or to the diuretic phase of acute renal failure, the urinary potassium excretion will be high (more than 40 mEq a day).

DIAGNOSIS

The sudden development of marked muscle weakness or paralysis, or loss of deep tendon reflexes, or paralytic ileus, is suspicious of potassium loss. The electrocardiogram will usually show signs of hypokalemia in these patients, even if the serum potassium concentration appears normal.

Hypokalemia due to aldosterone and other mineralocorticoid hormones is discussed in the next chapter.

COURSE AND PROGNOSIS

Severe potassium loss can cause death. This is probably one of the reasons that some diabetic patients with acidosis have died in the past, even though the acidosis was apparently corrected.

Hypokalemia may worsen the clinical status of a patient with cirrhosis of the liver, because the kidneys are unable to excrete ammonium ions normally. Therefore, hepatic insufficiency and coma may be precipitated if such a patient is treated vigorously with diuretics, such as the thiazides, furosemide, or ethacrynic acid, which cause an increased urinary excretion of potassium ions.

PROPHYLAXIS

Potassium loss should be anticipated. If the patient has severe losses of gastrointestinal fluids, or is receiving intravenous fluids, the serum potassium concentration should be determined and potassium chloride given as indicated (also see below).

One of the most common causes of potassium loss is the use of long-term diuretics without supplemental potassium chloride. If potassium chloride is contraindicated, potassium loss can be prevented in these patients by the concomitant use of a potassium-sparing diuretic, such as spironolactone (Aldactone) or triamterene (Dyrenium). Supplemental potassium chloride may also be necessary for patients who are receiving long-term corticosteroid treatment.

TREATMENT

Potassium loss must be treated with potassium salts. Potassium chloride is the salt of choice, although potassium phosphate or other potassium salts can be used if there is no serum chloride deficit. If an acidosis is present along with the hypokalemia, an alkalinizing potassium salt such as potassium acetate, bicarbonate, or citrate should be used. (Liquid Potassium Triplex, Lilly, contains these three salts.)

The average daily intake of potassium ions ranges from 50 to 75 mEq. This is equivalent to 3.73 to 5.6 g of potassium chloride. When hypokalemia is present, 100 to 300 mEq of potassium (7.46 to 21.38 g of potassium chloride) can be given daily.

The amount of potassium that is required to correct a potassium deficit cannot be determined by any fixed formula. Average deficits of 200 to 400 mEq are common. However, the deficit may amount to as much as 800 to 1000 mEq of potassium. The deficit should be corrected slowly over a period of days. It may take weeks or months to correct severe potassium loss. However, the patient responds even when a small part of the potassium loss is corrected. Often as little as 30 to 50 mEq potassium daily is adequate to ameliorate symptoms of hypokalemia.

Numerous stock preparations of potassium chloride are now available, including Kay Ciel (10%) Elixir, or Kaochlor (10%) Liquid (each 15 ml supplies 1.5 g potassium chloride, equivalent to 20 mEq potassium and 20 mEq chloride ions), K-Lyte-Cl powder (a unit dose supplies 25 mEq potassium and 25 mEq chloride ions), and many others.

If a patient needs potassium chloride and cannot tolerate it because of gastrointestinal symptoms (which commonly occurs), an extended-release tablet of potassium chloride in a wax matrix can be tried. The following tablets are available: Kaon-Cl (6.67 mEq potassium and chloride ions per tablet), Micro-K Extencaps (8 or 10 mEq potassium and chloride ions per capsule). Slow-K (8 mEq potassium and chloride ions per tablet) and many others. However, complications such as intestinal ulceration, stricture, or hemorrhage can occur with these tablets. The following recommendations may prevent complications from the use of these extended-release potassium chloride tablets: they should not be used if a patient has an enlarged left atrium (due to mitral valvular disease), or if esophageal displacement or compression is present, or if a patient has definite or suspected stasis or obstruction of any part of the gastrointestinal tract. In addition, they should be used with extreme caution, if at all, if a patient has a history of a peptic ulcer.

Foods high in potassium content should also be ingested (see Table 24–1, page 256 and Table 27–1).

So-called electrolyte replacement solutions, such a lactated Ringer's solution, contain only 4 mEq potassium ions per liter, and are not suitable to treat hypokalemia.

If the patient cannot take potassium chloride by mouth, it can be given intravenously in a solution containing 39 to 80 mEq potassium (3 to 6 g of potassium chloride) per liter. The rate of infusion should

Table 27–1. Potassium Content (in mEq) of Some Potassium-Rich Foods

Apricots, 3	11 mEq
Banana	15
Cantaloupe, ½	23
Dates, 1 cup	36
Fig, dried, 1 large (1″ × 2″)	20
Orange	9
Orange juice, 8 oz.	11
Raisins, 1 cup	29
Watermelon, ½ slice	10

not exceed 20 mEq (rarely 35 mEq) potassium per hour. If 2 liters of solution containing 60 mEq/L are given daily for 2 days, the patient will have received 240 mEq.

The potassium chloride can be added to an infusion of dextrose in water or dextrose in saline solution. When severe hypokalemia is present, it is preferable, if possible, to give the potassium without sodium, because sodium tends to aggravate the potassium deficiency.

Mulhausen and Blumentals have given up to 120 mEq/L in dextrose solutions, using an indwelling catheter in a vein, over a period of at least 6 hours.

Large doses of potassium chloride from 80 to 120 mEq of potassium chloride in 250 ml of 5% dextrose in water or normal saline solution can also be given through a central venous catheter and an infusion pump at a rate up to 20 mEq per hour. Usually 8 to 15 mEq per hour is infused (Cullen).

Clementsen has described 2 patients with hypokalemic metabolic alkalosis whom he treated with massive amounts of potassium chloride. One patient received 28 g of potassium chloride (375 mEq) in 2000 ml 5% dextrose in water, with 40 units of insulin, over a period of 5 hours, 45 minutes. (The insulin aids the cellular uptake of the potassium ions.) During the infusion of such a large amount of potassium chloride, the patient should be under close supervision with electrocardiographic monitoring, to avoid hyperkalemia.

The intravenous administration of potassium in dextrose solutions may be associated with a transient *lowering* of serum potassium concentration. Kunin and his associates have suggested that this is due to a cellular uptake of potassium with dextrose which is more rapid than the potassium being given. They therefore recommend that at least 30 mEq potassium chloride in 5% dextrose in water be given during each hour.

The rapid intravenous infusion of potassium chloride in a digitalis-toxic patient may precipitate ventricular arrhythmias, such as ventricular premature beats or ventricular tachycardia, or, if a-v block is present, it may become more marked. The reason for this is that digitalis toxicity may interfere with the uptake of potassium ions by skeletal muscles. Therefore, the potassium chloride which is infused remains in the bloodstream and may cause an abnormal elevation of serum potassium concentration.

Potassium can also be given rectally. Twenty milliliters of a 25% solution of potassium chloride (5 g) can be instilled into the rectum with a rubber bulb syringe, or a continuous rectal drip of a 10% potassium chloride solution can be given.

Familial periodic paralysis can be prevented by avoiding unusual stresses as much as possible and by avoiding high carbohydrate meals. An attack can be precipitated by rest, especially following vigorous exertion. Severe attacks often occur at night, or in the early hours of the morning. Some patients are able to "walk off" a mild attack. Acetazolamide (Diamox) is the most effective treatment available. Drugs such as epinephrine, thyroid extract, DOCA, and ACTH should be avoided.

REFERENCES

Aldinger, K.A., et al.: Hypokalemia with hypercalcemia. Prevalence and significance in treatment. Ann Intern Med, *87*:571, 1977.

Babior, B.M.: Villous adenoma of the colon. Study of a patient with severe fluid and electrolyte disturbances. Am J Med, *41*:615, 1966.

Bia, M.J., and DeFronzo, R.A.: Potassium chloride therapy, Questions and Answers. JAMA, *248*:2501, 1981.

Brunner, F.P., and Frick, P.G.: Hypokalemia, metabolic alkalosis and hypernatremia due to massive sodium penicillin therapy. Br Med J, *4*:550, 1968.

Brown, M.J., et al.: Hypokalemia from beta$_2$-receptor stimulation by circulating epinephrine, N Engl J Med, *309*:1414, 1983.

Cannon, P.R., Frazier, L.E., and Hughes, R.H.: Sodium as a toxic ion in potassium deficiency. Metabolism, *2*:297, 1953.

Clementsen, H.J.: Potassium therapy. Lancet, *2*:175, 1962.

Cullen, D.J.: Potassium chloride therapy, letter, JAMA, *247*:2780, 1982.

DeFronzo, R.A., and Bia, M.: Intravenous potassium chloride therapy, Questions and Answers. JAMA, *245*:2246, 1981.

DeGraeff, J., Struyvenberg, A., and Lameijer, L.D.F.: The role of chloride in hypokalemic alkalosis. Am J Med, *37*:778, 1964.

Dyckner, T., and Wester, P-O.: Potassium deficiency contributing to ventricular tachycardia. Acta Med Scandinav, *212*:89, 1982.

Feld, M., and Chang, E.B.: Pancreatic cholera. Is the diarrhea due to VIP? Editorial, N Engl J Med, *309*:1513, 1983.

Fisher, J.R.: Hypokalemia in leukemia, comments. Ann Intern Med, *86*:363, 1977.

Flear, C.T.G., Cook, W.G., and Quinton, A.: Serum potassium levels as an index of body content. Lancet, *1*:458, 1957.

Fleming, B.J., et al.: Laxative-induced hypokalemia, sodium depletion and hyperreninemia. Ann Intern Med, *83*:60, 1975.

Fletcher, G.F., Hurst, J.W., and Schlant, R.C.: Electrocardiographic changes in severe hypokalemia. A reappraisal. Am J Cardiol, *20*:628, 1967.

Garella, S., Chazan, J.A., and Cohen, J.J.: Saline-resistant metabolic alkalosis, or "chloride-wasting nephropathy." Report of four patients with severe potassium depletion. Ann Intern Med, *73*:31, 1970.

Gerstein, A.R., et al.: Potassium losing pyelonephritis. Response to spironolactone. Arch Intern Med, *123*:55, 1969.

Glazier, W.B., and Silen, W.: Acute potassium defect. Arch Surg, *112*:1165, 1977.

Gossain, V.V., and Werk, E.E.: Surreptitious laxation and hypokalemia. Ann Intern Med, 76:671, 1972.

Griggs, R.C., Engel, W.K., and Resnick, J.S.: Acetazolamide treatment of hypokalemic periodic paralysis. Ann Intern Med, 73:39, 1970.

Herrmann, R.A., Mead, A.W., Spritz, N., and Rubin, A.L.: Hypopotassemia with respiratory paralysis. Arch Intern Med, 108:169, 1961.

Hoffbrand, B.I., and Stewart, J.D.: Carbenicillin and hypokalemia. Br Med J, 4:476, 1970.

Jackson, H., and Glassburg, S.: Pancreatic cholera. NY State J Med, 84:31, 1984.

Jensen, R.T., et al.: Zollinger-Ellison syndrome, Ann Intern Med, 98:59, 1983.

Katz, F.H., Eckert, R.C., and Gebott, M.D.: Hypokalemia caused by surreptitious self-administration of diuretics. Ann Intern Med, 76:85, 1972.

Kraft, A.R., Tompkins, R.K., and Zollinger, R.M.: Recognition and management of the diarrheal syndrome caused by nonbeta islet cell tumors of the pancreas. Am J Surg, 119:163, 1970.

Kunin, A.S., Surawicz, B., and Sims, E.A.H.: Decrease in serum potassium concentrations and appearance of cardiac arrhythmias during infusion of potassium with glucose in potassium-depleted patients. N Engl J Med, 226:228, 1962.

Lai, F., et al.: Licorice, snuff, and hypokalemia, letter. N Engl J Med, 303:463, 1980.

Lawson, D.H., et al.: Hypokalaemia in megaloblastic anemias. Lancet, 2:588, 1970.

Lawson, D.H., et al.: Potassium supplements in patients receiving long-term diuretics for edema. Q J Med, 45:469, 1976.

Maronda, R.F., et al.: Response of thiazide-induced hypokalemia to amiloride, JAMA, 249:237, 1983.

Maronder, R.F., Milgrom, M., and Dickey, J.M.: Potassium loss with thiazide therapy. Am Heart J, 78:16, 1969.

McChesney, J.A., and Marquardt, J.F.: Hypokalemic paralysis induced by amphotericin B. JAMA, 189:1029, 1964.

McMahon, F., et al.: Upper gastrointestinal lesions after potassium chloride supplements, Lancet, 2:1059, 1982.

Mir, M.A., et al.: Hypokalaemia in acute myeloid leukaemia. Ann Intern Med, 82:54, 1975.

Muehrcke, R.C., and McMillan, J.C.: The relationship of "chronic pyelonephritis" to chronic potassium deficiency. Ann Intern Med, 59:427, 1963.

Nagy, M.: Dietary means of avoiding potassium deficiency. JAMA, 226:87, 1973.

Parker, M.S., et al.: Chronic hypokalemia and alkalosis. Arch Intern Med, 140:1336, 1980.

Re, R.: Hypokalemia in hypertension, Practical Cardiol, 9:103, 1983.

Resnick, J.S., et al.: Acetazolamide prophylaxis in hypokalemic periodic paralysis. N Engl J Med, 278:582, 1968.

Rovner, D.R.: Use of pharmacologic agents in the treatment of hypokalemia and hyperkalemia. Rational Drug Ther, 6:2, 1972.

Roy, A.D., and Ellis, H.: Potassium-secreting tumours of the large intestine. Lancet, 1:759, 1959.

Satoyoshi, E., et al.: Periodic paralysis in hyperthyroidism. Neurology, 13:746, 1963.

Schwartz, A.B., and Swartz, C.D.: Dosage of potassium chloride elixir to correct thiazide-induced hypokalemia. JAMA, 230:702, 1974.

Sirota, D.K., Gendelman, S., and Huschmand, F.: Thyrotoxic periodic paralysis. Mt Sinai J Med, 39:165, 1972.

Snively, W.D., Jr.: Potassium excretion and atavistic physiology. JAMA, 207:561, 1969.

Soffer, A.: Potassium therapy for digitalis toxicity. JAMA, 183:228, 1963. Also JAMA, 180:775, 1962.

Streeten, D.H.P.: Periodic paralysis. In *The Metabolic Basis of Inherited Disease* (Stanbury, J.B., Wyngaarden, J.B., and Fredrickson, D.S., Eds.). New York, McGraw-Hill Book Co., 1966.

Veldhuis, J.D.: The many faces of hypokalemia. Editorial, Arch Intern Med, 143:1521, 1983.

Verner, J.V., and Morrison, A.B.: Islet cell tumor and a syndrome of refractory watery diarrhea and hypokalemia. Am J Med, 25:374, 1958.

Walker, W.G., and Jost, L.J.: Relative roles of potassium and chloride in correction of hypokalemic alkalosis. Johns Hopkins Med J, 120:148, 1967.

CHAPTER 28

METABOLIC ALKALOSIS
SYNDROMES (Continued)
PRIMARY ALDOSTERONISM

In 1941, Ferrebee found that large doses of desoxycorticosterone (DOCA) produced sodium retention, potassium loss, polydipsia, polyuria, and intermittent muscular paralysis in dogs. Other investigators described similar but milder signs in humans who had been given excessive amounts of the DOCA. In 1955, Conn was able to show that a patient with similar signs had an excessive amount of a sodium-retaining hormone, which he identified as aldosterone. He described the patient as having "primary aldosteronism." The patient was cured by removing an adrenal cortical adenoma. Since then, numerous other reports of primary aldosteronism have been published.

PATHOPHYSIOLOGY

In Chapters 2 and 8 the mechanisms associated with the secretion of aldosterone are described. Aldosterone is the most potent mineralo-corticoid secreted by the zona glomerulosa of the adrenal cortex. Its major effect is to increase resorption of sodium ions and to promote the secretion of potassium ions in the distal tubules of the kidneys. (A similar effect occurs in thermal sweat, saliva, and in the stool, causing a decreased sodium-potassium ratio in these fluids.)

The usual stimulus for the secretion of aldosterone is a decrease in the circulating blood volume. However, in primary aldosteronism, aldosterone is secreted by adrenal cortical cells autonomously. This causes a chronic retention of sodium ions and water, and an increased circulating blood volume and extracellular volume. However, edema is typically absent in patients with primary hyperaldosteronism. The reason for this apparently paradoxical absence of edema despite an excessive secretion of a salt-retaining hormone is not clear. Somehow, there is a homeostatic "escape" from the increased sodium resorption.

The possibility that a natriuretic "third factor" is responsible for this escape phenomenon was mentioned in Chapter 2.

Renin activity is characteristically suppressed in primary aldosteronism, partly because of the increased circulating blood volume.

The diastolic hypertension which occurs in primary aldosteronism may be due partly to an increased concentration of sodium ions and water in the arteriolar walls. This causes the arterioles to swell and the lumina to become smaller. As a result, the peripheral resistance rises and hypertension develops.

The renal loss of potassium ions produced by aldosterone causes a loss of total exchangeable body potassium. This in turn causes a metabolic alkalosis and other disturbances which have been described in Chapter 27. Aldosterone also causes an increased urinary excretion of magnesium ions.

Primary aldosteronism produces a hypokalemic metabolic alkalosis. A similar metabolic alkalosis can occur with Cushing's syndrome, ACTH-secreting tumors (such as adrenal adenocarcinoma or oat-cell carcinoma of the lung), Bartter's syndrome (hyperplasia of the juxtaglomerular apparatus), with the administration of mineralocorticoid steroids such as DOCA, cortisone, hydrocortisone, prednisone, and particularly fludrocortisone (Florinef), or with the excessive ingestion of licorice (20 to 40 g daily). (Glycyrrhizic acid, the active principle of licorice extract, is structurally and chemically similar to aldosterone.) Estrogens can also cause a similar metabolic alkalosis.

The metabolic alkalosis that develops is characterized by the fact that it is *saline resistant;* it cannot be corrected by sodium chloride alone, and requires potassium chloride (see Chap. 26).

PATHOLOGY

Primary aldosteronism is usually produced by a unilateral, benign, adrenal cortical adenoma. Rarely, multiple or bilateral adenomas may be present. In about 15% of patients, the syndrome is associated with diffuse, bilateral, micronodular adrenal cortical hyperplasia. (This has been called idiopathic, nonadenomatous, pseudoprimary, or tertiary aldosteronism.)

The syndrome can also be caused by an adrenal carcinoma which may also produce significant amounts of corticosterone. If the urinary excretion of 17-hydroxycorticosterone is greatly increased, this suggests Cushing's syndrome associated with an anaplastic ACTH-secreting adrenal carcinoma.

Glucocorticoid-remediable hyperaldosteronism is a rare cause of primary aldosteronism. It may be familial and is associated with adrenal hyperplasia. It is characterized by the fact that the hypertension and metabolic abnormalities can often be reversed by a glucocorticoid drug, such as dexamethasone.

SYMPTOMS AND SIGNS

Primary aldosteronism is found most commonly in the fourth and fifth decades, more often in women than in men, although it can occur at any age and in either sex.

Common symptoms include severe "bursting" central headache, fatigue or muscle weakness, which may be episodic with flaccid paralysis, paresthesias, muscle cramps, or frank tetany, increased thirst, and polyuria or nocturia.

Hypertension is present. The blood pressure may be slightly elevated. Occasionally, the diastolic blood pressure may rise to 120 or 130 mm Hg, but, even when this occurs, other signs of malignant hypertension, such as advanced retinopathy, do not usually appear. Peripheral edema, as mentioned above, is not usually noted.

Signs of potassium loss *(potassium wasting)* such as muscle weakness, fatigue, hyposthenia, polydipsia, or polyuria are other common findings.

The electrocardiogram shows signs of hypokalemia.

LABORATORY FINDINGS

The characteristic laboratory findings in patients with primary aldosteronism are: increased plasma aldosterone level (however, urinary aldosterone excretion may be normal or increased), subnormal plasma renin activity, metabolic alkalosis with hypokalemia and hypochloremia, and a slightly elevated serum sodium concentration (usually 145 mEq/L or higher). (In the early stages, the serum electrolyte concentrations may be normal.) The 24-hour urinary excretion of 17-hydroxycorticosteroids is normal, unless the aldosteronism is due to Cushing's syndrome.

Other laboratory findings may include abnormal glucose tolerance (probably due to the hypokalemia) or a maturity-onset type of diabetes mellitus. The sodium-potassium ratio of saliva is characteristically less than 0.25. Serum calcium and magnesium concentrations are almost always normal although hypomagnesemia has been reported.

Urine

The specific gravity is typically below 1.010 because urine concentration ability is reduced. The urine pH is typically alkaline, because of the increased urinary excretion of bicarbonate ions. However, some patients can acidify the urine to a pH of 5.0. (The presence of an alkaline urine associated with hypokalemia does not necessarily indicate aldosteronism, because an alkaline urine can develop as a result of a urinary tract infection.)

The urinary potassium excretion has diagnostic importance. In the usual patient with hypokalemia (for example, secondary to diarrhea, decreased intake, cathartic abuse), urinary potassium excretion is low. However, if hypokalemia is due to primary aldosteronism, the daily urinary potassium excretion is 40 mEq or more.

When the patient has been taking diuretics, the daily urinary potassium excretion may also be abnormally high, and may continue this way for several days to weeks after the diuretic is stopped. Therefore, if primary aldosteronism is suspected, the patient must not receive diuretics for at least 3 or 4 weeks.

Example: Patient with primary aldosteronism
pH 7.54
P_{CO_2} 45 mm Hg
Standard bicarbonate 36.3 mEq/L
Actual bicarbonate 37 mEq/L
Base excess + 14 mEq/L
CO_2 content 38.4 mEq/L

The pH is elevated. This indicates an alkalosis. The positive base excess and standard bicarbonate indicate that a metabolic alkalosis is present. The P_{CO_2} is normal, indicating a respiratory balance. However, the actual bicarbonate is slightly higher than the standard bicarbonate. This indicates a slight respiratory acidosis. Therefore, a primary metabolic alkalosis is present with a partially compensatory respiratory acidosis (Chap. 15).

This information can also be determined from the pH and P_{CO_2} by inspection of Figure 15–4, page 154.

Cation-anion balance:
Na 146 K 2 HCO_3 37 Cl 103 mEq/L.
Anion gap = (Na + K) − (HCO_3 + Cl).
           = (146 + 2) − (37 + 96).
           = 148 − 133
           = 15 mEq/L. This is normal.

DIAGNOSIS

Primary aldosteronism must be suspected in any patient, particularly a relatively young person, who shows mild or moderate diastolic hypertension, metabolic alkalosis with a serum potassium concentration of less than 3.5 mEq/L, a urinary potassium loss of 40 mEq/L or more, and who has no obvious reasons (diuretic therapy, vomiting, etc.) for the metabolic findings. Other symptoms and signs include muscular weakness and fatigue, hyposthenuria, polyuria, or nocturia due to potassium loss. (Primary aldosteronism must also be differentiated from the metabolic alkalosis due to potassium loss from other causes (Chap. 27).)

The diagnosis of primary aldosteronism must be confirmed by showing that an increased aldosterone excretion in the urine or an elevated plasma aldosterone level cannot be suppressed by volume loading, together with a low and suppressed plasma renin activity, for example:

1. Testing the effect of volume loading on aldosterone excretion or secretion.

All diuretic drugs must be stopped for 3 to 4 weeks, because the volume-depleting effect of the diuretics may cause increased aldosterone secretion due to *secondary aldosteronism.*

An initial screening test for aldosterone production can be done as an out-patient procedure (Bravo et al). The patient adds 10 to 12 g of salt to the daily intake. After 5 to 7 days of increased salt intake the patient's serum potassium concentration is measured, along with a 24-hour urinary excretion of sodium, potassium, and aldosterone.

Patients who demonstrate nonsuppressible aldosterone production following the salt loading, namely, an excretion rate of 14.0 µg or more per 24 hours, when the urinary sodium excretion is more than 250 mEq per 24 hours, require further diagnostic tests to determine if primary aldosteronism is present.

A more specific test to determine whether aldosterone production cannot be suppressed with volume loading is to give the patient a high-sodium diet for 3 to 5 days. Then, 0.9% sodium chloride solution is infused over a 4-hour period in a dose of 25 mg/kg. Patients with primary aldosteronism show a high aldosterone excretion rate, greater than 14.0 µg per 24 hours.

A patient with primary aldosteronism will show an increased aldosterone excretion or an elevated plasma aldosterone level in spite of the volume loading. Other patients will show decreased aldosterone excretion or plasma levels.

2. Testing for low and suppressed plasma renin activity. It is important that the patient is not receiving any medications which can affect the plasma reinin activity for at least 2 weeks.

(Conditions and drugs that can cause decreased renin release include supine posture, sodium loading [volume expansion], drugs, such as potassium salts, propranolol, methyldopa, reserpine, ganglionic blockers (except guanethidine), clonidine, indocin, blockade of the autonomic nervous system. Conditions and drugs that can cause increased renin release include upright posture, sodium restriction [volume depletion], drugs such as diuretics, including spironolactone, diazoxide, nitroprusside, hydralazine, chlorpromazine, thyroxine, oral contraceptives, depletion of potassium [McGuffin and Gunnells]).

Abnormal suppressed supine plasma renin is less than 1.0 ng/ml per hour.

One should remember that finding a low or suppressed renin activity in a hypertensive patient is not necessarily a sign of primary aldosteronism, because it can occur in patients with low-renin essential hypertension. In order to establish a diagnosis of primary aldosteronism, it is also necessary to show that aldosterone excretion or secretion is nonsuppressible (see above).

It is also important to note that patients with primary aldosteronism may have normal or high plasma renin activity.

Differentiation of Primary Aldosteronism Due to Adrenal Tumor from That Due to Bilateral Adrenal Hyperplasia (idiopathic aldosteronism). When nonsuppression of aldosterone excretion, and suppressed plasma renin activity are present, this indicates primary aldosteronism. However, it does not differentiate patients who have an aldosterone-producing tumor from those who have bilateral adrenal hyperplasia (idiopathic aldosteronism). The differential diagnosis is important because patients with an adrenal tumor should have the tumor removed surgically, whereas patients with bilateral hyperplasia should be treated medically. However, the differential diagnosis can be difficult. It has been found (Bravo et al.) that when the spontaneous serum potassium concentration is less than 3.0 mEq/L in a patient with primary aldosteronism, this indicates that an adenoma is present. Another sign of an adenoma is a postural decrease in aldosterone production. However a postural increase in aldosterone production does not exclude an adenoma.

Measurement of plasma 18-hydroxycorticosterone concentration can also be used to differentiate an adenoma from adrenal hyperplasia. Biglieri et al. found that overnight recumbent values greater than 100 ng/dl were considered pathognomonic of an adenoma.

It is important to try to localize the adenoma. Three tests can be used: adrenal computerized tomographic scan, selective adrenal venography, and adrenal venous sampling for plasma aldosterone concentration.

Diagnosis of Normokalemic Primary Aldosteronism

Rarely, the serum potassium concentration is normal, in association with hypertension, in the early stages of primary aldosteronism. One can suspect that primary aldosteronism is present in such a patient if there are episodes of spontaneous hypokalemia, if hypokalemia develops shortly after thiazides are used, or if hypokalemia develops after a large amount of salt is ingested.

Low renin activity itself does not indicate primary aldosteronism, because low renin may be present in hypertensive patients who do not have aldosteronism. (These patients also have a normal or low urinary aldosterone excretion.)

Diagnosis of Secondary Aldosteronism

The term "secondary aldosteronism" describes patients in whom aldosterone levels are elevated due to extra-adrenal factors (primary increase in renin activity, decreased aldosterone clearance, etc.). Patients with hypertension associated with renal artery stenosis and patients with malignant hypertension may also have secondary aldosteronism and hypokalemia. Plasma renin activity in these patients with hypertension and secondary aldosteronism, however, will be *high*, in contrast to the low plasma renin activity in patients with primary aldosteronism.

(There have been several reports of aldosteronism secondary to a primary benign renin-secreting tumor of the kidney [juxtaglomerular cell tumor, renal hemangiopericytoma]. These patients show diastolic hypertension, increased plasma aldosterone level, increased plasma renin activity, and hypokalemia. Adrenal arteriography can be used to differentiate renal artery stenosis from a juxtaglomerular tumor. A unilateral high adrenal vein renin activity occurs in both conditions. However, a renal arteriogram will indicate if renal artery stenosis is present.)

Secondary aldosteronism (without hypertension) may also occur in the following situations: sodium depletion due to any cause, hypovolemia due to any cause, nephrotic syndrome, administration of large amounts of potassium salts, cirrhosis of the liver with ascites, congestive heart failure (particularly right-sided failure), idiopathic cyclic edema, Bartter's syndrome, and pregnancy. In all such patients, the plasma renin activity is high.

Differential Diagnosis of Patients with Hypertension, Hypokalemia, and Excessive Urinary Loss of Potassium Ions

These patients can be divided into two main types, depending on the plasma renin activity (Horton):

1. Patients with suppressed plasma renin activity include those with primary aldosteronism, aldosteronism due to Cushing's syndrome or tumors associated with excessive glucocorticoid production, excessive intake of licorice, tumors associated with the production of DOCA or corticosteroids, or excessive administration of mineralocorticoids or glucocorticoids, renal parenchymal disease, 11- or 17-hydroxylase deficiency.
2. Patients with elevated plasma renin activity include those with essential hypertension who have received diuretic therapy, malignant hypertension, renovascular hypertension, acute hydronephrosis, renin-producing juxtaglomerular tumors, or sodium-losing renal disease.

TREATMENT

Surgical removal of a single adrenal cortical tumor will cure the metabolic alkalosis and the hypokalemia. In addition, the hypertension will disappear in approximately one-half of the patients and will become significantly lower in the others. However, if bilateral adrenal hyperplasia is present, subtotal or total adrenalectomy will restore the metabolic balance, but will not relieve the hypertension. In addition, the surgery may produce adrenocortical insufficiency, which may require mineralocorticoid or glucocorticoid therapy indefinitely. It is preferable to treat such patients with spironolactone. A low-sodium, high-potassium diet may also be necessary.

Preoperatively, the serum potassium concentration should be raised to normal. This can be done with potassium chloride, or with the aldosterone antagonist, spironolactone (Aldactone). Large doses of 300 to 600 mg daily may be needed for even 1 week or more. As the serum potassium concentration rises, the blood pressure will fall and the weight will also fall because of a large urinary excretion of sodium ions (and water). (When the spironolactone is stopped, the serum potassium concentration will fall within 7 to 10 days. Also, when such large doses are used for chronic medical therapy, severe side effects—impotence, symptomatic gynecomastia, intermenstrual bleeding, mild azotemia, and so on—may occur.)

Immediately postoperatively, the patient usually shows signs of decreased aldosterone secretion, so that hyponatremia and hyperkalemia develop. In addition, the electrocardiogram may show ST and T changes which simulate myocardial ischemia. The patient should be treated with both mineralocorticoid and glucocorticoid steroids until aldosterone secretion returns to normal.

A renin-secreting kidney tumor is treated by surgical removal of the kidney.

BARTTER'S SYNDROME

Bartter's syndrome is a rare disorder in which patients show a hypokalemic metabolic alkalosis, occasionally with hyponatremia, due to aldosteronism with increased aldosterone levels but usually without hypertension. The plasma renin activity is characteristically elevated. The syndrome is associated with hyperplasia of the juxtaglomerular apparatus. The pathogenesis of Bartter's syndrome involves excessive production of prostaglandins. This in turn leads to the increased release of renin. Other characteristics include resistance to the pressor effects of intravenous angiotensin, a low serum magnesium concentration, megacolon, and dilated ureters.

The syndrome often begins in childhood. Patients may show retardation of growth, mental retardation, salt craving, tetany, and signs of hypokalemia.

The syndrome may be due to a form of salt wastage in the kidneys, due to defective reabsorption of sodium chloride in the loop of Henle. The loss of sodium chloride produces a sodium loss syndrome with a decreased blood volume. This stimulates the secretion of aldosterone. In addition, the reabsorption of potassium ions in the kidneys seems to be impaired, so that an excessive amount of potassium ions is lost in the urine. The combination of potassium loss and increased aldosterone secretion produces a metabolic alkalosis.

Bartter's syndrome can be simulated by pseudo-Bartter's syndrome. Patients with this disease are mostly women who have chronic potassium loss due to long-term use of diuretics, cathartics, and sometimes surreptitious vomiting. As a result there is a loss of potassium and sodium ions and extracellular water, and a resulting secondary aldosteronism.

Treatment of Bartter's syndrome includes the use of spironolactone (Aldactone), which blocks the action of aldosterone, or triamterene (Dyrenium), a potassium-sparing diuretic. Drugs that inhibit prostaglandin synthesis, such as indomethacin, may be helpful. Propranolol (Inderal), which inhibits renin activity, may also be helpful.

REFERENCES

Bartter, F.C.: Bartter's syndrome. Juxtaglomerular hyperplasia, normotension, hypokalemic alkalosis. JAMA, 216:152, 1971.

Bartter, F.C.: So-called Bartter's syndrome. N Engl J Med, 281:1483, 1969.

Bravo, D.L., et al.: The changing spectrum of primary aldosteronism, Am J Med, 74:641, 1983.

Biglieri, E.G., et al.: Plasma aldosterone concentration. Further characterization of aldosterone-producing adenomas. Circ Res, 34: suppl 11.1183, 1974.

Carey, R.M.: Screening for surgically correctable hypertension caused by primary aldosteronism, Editorial, Arch Intern Med, 141:1594, 1981.

Conn, J.W., et al.: Normokalemic primary aldosteronism. JAMA, 193:100, 1965.

Conn, J.W., et al.: The syndrome of hypertension, hyperreninemia and secondary aldosteronism associated with renal juxtaglomerular cell tumor (primary reninism). J Urol, 109:349, 1973.

Conn, J.W., Rovner, D.R., and Cohen, E.L.: Licorice-induced pseudoaldosteronism. Hypertension, hypokalemia, aldosteronopenia, and suppressed plasma renin activity. JAMA, 205:492, 1968.

Ganguly, A., and Donohue, J.P.: Primary aldosteronism, J Urol, 129:241, 1983.

Hoefnagels, W.H.L., and Kloppenborg, P.W.C.: Hazards of long-term dexamethazone treatment in primary aldosteronism, Letter, N Engl J Med, 306:427, 1982.

Goldsmith, R.S., et al.: Prominent peripheral edema associated with primary aldosteronism. J Clin Endocr, 20:1051, 1960.

Holifield, J.W., et al.: Renin-secreting clear cell carcinoma of the kidney. Arch Intern Med, 135:859, 1975.

Kaplan, N.M.: Primary aldosteronism with malignant hypertension. N Engl J Med, 269:1282, 1963.

Kassirer, J.P., et al.: On the pathogenesis of metabolic alkalosis in hyperaldosteronism. Am J Med, 49:306, 1970.

Mazzacca, G., et al.: Metoclopramide and secondary hyperaldosteronism, letter. Ann Intern Med, *98*:1024, 1983.

McGuffin, W.L., Jr., and Gunnells, J.C., Jr.: Primary aldosteronism. Urol Clin N Am *4*:227, 1977.

Modlinger, R.S., et al.: Some observations on the pathogenesis of Bartter's syndrome. N Engl J Med, *289*:1022, 1973.

Ram, C.V.S.: Primary aldosteronism. Comprehensive Therapy, *8*:60, 1982.

Vaisrub, S.: Simulacra of Bartter's syndrome. Editorial, JAMA, *243*:1075, 1980.

Weinberger, M.H.: Primary aldosteronism. Diagnosis and differentiation of subtypes, Editorial, Ann Intern Med, *100*:300, 1984.

White, M.G.: Bartter's syndrome. A manifestation of renal tubular defects. Arch Intern Med, *129*:41, 1972.

Wilson, D.M., Power, M.H., and Kepler, E.J.: Alkalosis and low plasma potassium in case of Cushing's syndrome. J Clin Invest, *19*:701, 1940.

CHAPTER 29

SIMULTANEOUS RESPIRATORY AND METABOLIC SYNDROMES OF ACID-BASE BALANCE

It has already been pointed out that a primary respiratory acidosis is usually associated with a compensatory metabolic alkalosis. The reverse is also true. Similarly, a primary respiratory alkalosis is usually associated with a compensatory metabolic acidosis. The reverse is also true. However, primary respiratory and metabolic disturbances of acid-base can occur simultaneously and independently.

SIMULTANEOUS RESPIRATORY AND METABOLIC DISTURBANCES CAUSING OPPOSITE CHANGES IN pH

Two types of such disturbances can occur: simultaneous respiratory acidosis and metabolic alkalosis: and simultaneous respiratory alkalosis and metabolic acidosis. When this happens, the two disturbances tend to neutralize the changes in pH. However, the P_{CO_2} and the CO_2 content, actual bicarbonate and standard bicarbonate concentrations indicate the two disturbances. This is shown below.

Simultaneous Respiratory Acidosis and Metabolic Alkalosis

This can occur, for example, in a patient with cor pulmonale who shows a respiratory acidosis and who also develops a metabolic alkalosis due to excessive diuretic therapy.

The simultaneous presence of the acidosis and the alkalosis tends to keep the pH within normal. However, the P_{CO_2} tends to be high due to the respiratory acidosis. The standard bicarbonate is high because of the metabolic alkalosis. The actual bicarbonate and the CO_2 content are necessarily high because of the standard bicarbonate. However, the actual bicarbonate is higher than the standard bicarbonate because of the respiratory acidosis.

Example: Simultaneous respiratory acidosis and metabolic alkalosis.
pH 7.4
P_{CO_2} 56 mm Hg
CO_2 content 35.1 mEq/L
Standard bicarbonate 30 mEq/L
Actual bicarbonate 33.4 mEq/L
Base excess +7 mEq/L

The pH is normal. However, the P_{CO_2} is high, indicating that a respiratory acidosis is present. Similarly, the actual bicarbonate is higher than the standard bicarbonate, because of the respiratory acidosis. The high standard bicarbonate and the positive base excess indicate that a metabolic alkalosis is also present. Therefore, a respiratory acidosis and a metabolic alkalosis are present (Chap. 15).

This information can also be determined from the pH and P_{CO_2} by inspection of Figure 15–4, page 154.

This type of acid-base pattern can occur as a result of a simultaneous respiratory acidosis and a compensatory metabolic alkalosis, or vice versa. However, in a patient such as this, the history and clinical course would enable one to diagnose that two independent acid-base abnormalities are present.

Confidence bands of pH-P_{CO_2} relationships have been constructed to differentiate acute from chronic respiratory acidosis or alkalosis patients (Fig. 13–1). These relationships describe 95% of patients. However, they are not diagnostic, particularly when simultaneous mixed respiratory and metabolic disturbances are present.

Simultaneous Respiratory Alkalosis and Metabolic Acidosis

This type of disturbance, for example, can occur in a patient with diabetes or (renal) acidosis who shows hyperventilation for any reason. It also occurs in salicylate poisoning.

Here again, the simultaneous respiratory alkalosis and the metabolic acidosis cause the pH to remain within normal. However, the P_{CO_2} will tend to be low because of the respiratory alkalosis. The CO_2 content and the actual bicarbonate will necessarily be low because of the low standard bicarbonate. However, because a respiratory alkalosis is present, the actual bicarbonate will be lower than the standard bicarbonate.

An example of a patient with simultaneous respiratory alkalosis and metabolic acidosis is given on page 245.

This type of acid-base pattern can occur in a patient with a primary respiratory alkalosis and a compensatory metabolic acidosis, or vice versa. However, in a patient such as this, the history and clinical course would enable one to diagnose that two independent acid-base disturbances are present.

SIMULTANEOUS RESPIRATORY AND METABOLIC DISTURBANCES CAUSING SIMILAR CHANGES IN pH

These patients may show a simultaneous respiratory acidosis and a metabolic acidosis, or a simultaneous respiratory alkalosis and a metabolic alkalosis.

In these patients, it is obvious that the respiratory and the metabolic disturbances are not related, because when a respiratory or a metabolic disturbance is compensated, the compensation tends to cause the pH to move in the opposite direction. This type of disturbance is serious because an extreme shift in pH occurs and the patient may die.

Two types of such similar respiratory and metabolic changes can occur: acidosis and simultaneous respiratory and metabolic alkalosis.

Simultaneous Respiratory Acidosis and Metabolic Acidosis

This is an unusual combination. It has been produced experimentally by administering carbon dioxide to a curarized mental patient. It can occur in a patient with a respiratory acidosis due to chronic pulmonary disease and a metabolic acidosis due to excessive treatment with ammonium chloride for congestive heart failure.

In such a patient, the pH may be lowered to an extreme value below 7. The standard bicarbonate will be low because of the metabolic acidosis. The CO_2 content and the actual bicarbonate will be necessarily low because the standard bicarbonate is low. However, the actual bicarbonate will be higher than the standard bicarbonate because of the respiratory acidosis.

Example: Simultaneous respiratory acidosis and metabolic acidosis
pH 7.04
P_{CO_2} mm Hg
CO_2 content 21.9 mEq/L
Standard bicarbonate 14.8 mEq/L
Actual bicarbonate 20.5 mEq/L
Base excess −12.8 mEq/L

The pH is low. This indicates an acidosis. The low standard bicarbonate and the negative base excess indicate that a metabolic acidosis is present. However, the high P_{CO_2}, and the fact that the actual bicarbonate is higher than the standard bicarbonate indicate that a respiratory acidosis is also present. Therefore, a metabolic acidosis and a respiratory acidosis are simultaneously present.

This information can also be determined from the pH and P_{CO_2} by inspection of Figure 15–4, page 154.

Figure 15–3, page 148, shows another example of a simultaneous respiratory acidosis and metabolic acidosis. The slightly elevated P_{CO_2} of 49.7 mm Hg indicates the respiratory acidosis. The low standard bicarbonate of 19.2 mEq/L and the negative base excess of -6.1 mEq/L indicate the metabolic acidosis. The information about the respiratory and metabolic acidosis can also be determined from the pH and P_{CO_2} by inspection of Figure 15–4, page 154.

Simultaneous Respiratory Alkalosis and Metabolic Alkalosis

This type of disturbance also occurs rarely. Singer and Hastings produced it experimentally by having a subject ingest sodium bicarbonate (causing a metabolic alkalosis) and simultaneously having the subject hyperventilate (causing a respiratory alkalosis).

It can also be produced therapeutically if metabolic acidosis is treated with an excessive amount of an alkalinizing solution. The patient shows a compensatory respiratory alkalosis, which often persists even when the pH returns to normal. The excessive alkalinizing solution causes the metabolic alkalosis. Such a patient is described on page 170.

In such a patient, the pH rises to a high level. The standard bicarbonate is high because of the metabolic alkalosis. The CO_2 content and the actual bicarbonate are necessarily high because of the high standard bicarbonate. However, the actual bicarbonate is lower than the standard bicarbonate, because a respiratory alkalosis is also present.

Example: Simultaneous respiratory alkalosis and metabolic alkalosis.
pH 7.64
P_{CO_2} 28 mm Hg
CO_2 content 30 mEq/L
Standard bicarbonate 32.5 mEq/L
Actual bicarbonate 29 mEq/L
Base $+9.3$ mEq/L

The pH is high. This indicates an alkalosis. The high standard bicarbonate and the positive base excess indicate that a metabolic alkalosis is present. However, the low P_{CO_2} and the fact that the actual bicarbonate is lower than the standard bicarbonate indicate that a respiratory alkalosis is also present. Therefore, a metabolic alkalosis and a respiratory alkalosis are simultaneously present.

This information can also be determined from the pH and P_{CO_2} by inspection of Figure 15–4, page 154.

SIMULTANEOUS MIXED METABOLIC DISTURBANCES

A primary metabolic acidosis can be complicated by a primary metabolic alkalosis, or vice versa. This can occur, for example, in a patient with diabetes (or renal) acidosis who develops severe vomiting or receives gastric lavage which causes a metabolic alkalosis.

Example: Simultaneous metabolic alkalosis and metabolic acidosis.
pH 7.54
P_{CO_2} 49.4 mm Hg
CO_2 content 42 mEq/L
Standard bicarbonate 38.8 mEq/L
Actual bicarbonate 40.5 mEq/L
Base excess +16 mEq/L

The pH is high. This indicates an alkalosis. The standard bicarbonate is high, and the base excess is positive. This indicates that a metabolic alkalosis is present. The high P_{CO_2} and the fact that the actual bicarbonate is higher than the standard bicarbonate indicate that a respiratory acidosis is present. Therefore, a primary metabolic alkalosis is present with a partially compensatory respiratory acidosis.

This information can also be determined from the pH and P_{CO_2} by inspection of Figure 15–4.

It is not possible from this data to indicate that a metabolic acidosis is present. However, the high anion gap (see below) does indicate the metabolic acidosis:

Cation-anion balance:
Na 139 K 4 HCO_3 40.5 Cl 50 mEq/L.
$$\text{Anion gap} = (Na + K) - (HCO_3 + Cl)$$
$$= (139 + 4) - (40.5 + 50)$$
$$= 143 - 90.5$$
$$= 52.5 \text{ mEq/L. This is abnormally high, and is due to the accumulation of metabolic acids.}$$

REFERENCES

Elkinton, J.R.: Clinical disorders of acid-base regulation. Med Clin N Am, *50*:1325, 1966.

Fulop, M.: Metabolic acidosis with alkalemia, New York State J Med, *80*:1365, 1980.

Fordham, C.C., and Relman, A.S.: Mixed respiratory and metabolic acidosis: Report of a case showing deceptively little change in carbon dioxide content of the blood. N Engl J Med, *256*:698, 1957.

Gamble, J.L.: *Chemical Anatomy, Physiology and Pathology of Extracellular Fluid,* 6th ed. Cambridge, Harvard University Press, 1954.

McCurdy, D.K.: Mixed metabolic and respiratory acid-base disturbances. Diagnosis and treatment. Chest, *62*:355, 1972.

Singer, R.B., and Hastings, A.B.: Improved clinical method for estimation of disturbances of acid-base balance of human blood. Medicine, *27*:233, 1948.

CHAPTER 30

SYNDROMES ASSOCIATED WITH CALCIUM AND PHOSPHATE DISTURBANCES

A detailed discussion of syndromes associated with calcium and phosphorus metabolism is outside the scope of this book. However, a few important aspects of the problem can be considered.

CALCIUM

Bone consists of an organic matrix in which a complex calcium phosphate salt, hydroxyapatite ($Ca_{10}[PO_4]_6[OH]_2$), is deposited. Bone has bone-resorbing and bone-forming surfaces. The kidneys normally regulate the composition of the extracellular fluid in contact with bone in such a way that bone is constantly being resorbed. The rate at which this occurs depends on minor fluctuations in the composition of the extracellular fluid. Bone deposition, on the other hand, occurs in response to stresses and strains whenever bone is needed; this is usually in areas where the bone has been resorbed. As a result of these two processes, about 0.5 g of calcium is renewed each day. This mechanism keeps the structure of the skeleton strong but not bulky. The average adult requires about 0.65 g of elemental calcium a day. A child needs 1 g, and a pregnant or lactating woman needs more.

The major factors which regulate bone resorption and formation are the presence or absence of vitamin D, the availability of parathyroid hormone, the serum concentrations of calcium and phosphate ions, and the ability of the kidneys to excrete or hold calcium or phosphate ions.

Level of Organic Phosphate Ions in the Serum

Normally, calcium and phosphate ions exist in a supersaturated state in the serum. The solubility constant of these ions is relatively fixed, so that an increase or decrease in serum phosphate concentration will tend to be associated with a reciprocal decrease or increase in serum calcium concentration, and vice versa.

Vitamin D

Necessary for the intestinal absorption of calcium, vitamin D also has the capacity to increase phosphate excretion by the kidneys to a lesser degree. Its presence may also be necessary for parathyroid hormone function.

Inactive vitamin D precursor in the skin is transformed into vitamin D_3 (cholecalciferol) as a result of ultraviolet radiation. It is also derived from foods such as milk, eggs, and fish. The vitamin D_3 is transported to the liver where it is hydroxylated to 25-OH-D_3 (25-hydroxycholecalciferol), which is more potent than vitamin D_3. (Anticonvulsive therapy with phenobarbital or phenytoin [Dilantin] interferes with the hydroxylation of vitamin D_3 and can lower the circulating level of 25-OH-D_3 and in this way can produce osteomalacia.) The 25-OH-D_3 is then carried through the blood to the kidneys where it is transformed into 1,25-$(OH)_2D_3$ (1,25 dihydroxy-vitamin D_3), which promotes the absorption of calcium ions in the intestines and mobilizes calcium ions from the bones. 1,25-$(OH)_2D_3$ is the most potent vitamin D metabolite.

When chronic renal disease is present, 1,25-$(OH)_2D_3$ is not formed in adequate amounts. Impaired vitamin D_3 metabolism is probably a significant factor in the pathogenesis of the hypocalcemia, osteomalacia, and secondary hyperparathyroidism which occur in chronic renal disease.

Other causes of a deficiency of vitamin D or its metabolites include dietary deficiency, hyperphosphatemia, intestinal malabsorption, nephrotic syndrome, chronic renal failure, etc.

It is now possible to measure the blood level of 25-OH-D_3. In patients with overt rickets or osteomalacia, the serum 25-OH-D_3 levels are essentially not detectable. Subnormal blood levels of 25-OH-D_3 can occur when there is a dietary deficiency of vitamin D, or decreased intestinal absorption due, for example, to gastrectomy or intestinal malabsorption, or long-term anticonvulsant therapy.

Parathyroid Hormone

Parathyroid hormone responds to the serum calcium concentration. A low serum calcium concentration stimulates parathyroid secretion, and a high concentration stops its secretion. Parathyroid hormone also is indirectly under the influence of the serum phosphate concentration. A high serum phosphate concentration will cause a secondary lowering of serum calcium concentration, which in turn stimulates the parathyroid hormone. This occurs in patients with severe renal disease and phosphate retention who develop secondary hyperparathyroidism (renal rickets).

The primary action of the parathyroid hormone is to increase the renal excretion of phosphate ions. Normally, most of the phosphate which is lost from the body appears in the urine. The amount excreted depends on the degree of glomerular filtration and the degree of tubular reabsorption. Parathyroid hormone reduces the amount of phosphate ions which are reabsorbed by the kidney tubules. As a result, an increased amount of phosphate is excreted in the urine, and the serum phosphate concentration falls. When parathyroid hormone is absent, the kidney tubules reabsorb an increased amount of phosphate, and the serum phosphate concentration rises. These changes in serum phosphate concentration cause reciprocal changes in serum calcium concentration and thus stimulate or depress the parathyroid gland. Parathyroid hormone also stimulates bone resorption directly, and can raise the serum calcium concentration in this way.

Rasmussen and his associates have suggested that at a cellular level one of the primary actions of parathyroid hormone may be to stimulate phosphate uptake in mitochondria, independently of the presence of vitamin D. However, when vitamin D is present, it influences calcium transport into the cells. Conversely, vitamin D influences calcium transport in the absence of parathyroid hormone, but does not have a direct effect upon primary phosphate transport.

Calcitonin

In 1961, Copp described a new calcium-lowering hormone which he called *calcitonin.* More recently, investigators have shown that calcitonin is secreted by specialized parafollicular cells which are embryonically related to the ultimobranchial bodies of birds.

The main action of calcitonin is to control calcium balance by counteracting some of the hypercalcemic effects of parathyroid hormone. For example, parathyroid hormone affects calcium metabolism by increasing resorption of bone, by increasing absorption of calcium ions from the gastrointestinal tract, and by increasing the reabsorption of calcium ions by the renal tubules. Calcitonin prevents the action of parathyroid hormone on bone by inhibiting the *osteoclastic* resorption of bone. Therefore, the serum calcium concentration decreases. Calcitonin secretion is directly stimulated by a high serum calcium concentration.

Calcitonin is a polypeptide and is inactivated by gastric juices. It is now available for clinical use and can be given parenterally. It may be useful in the treatment of hypercalcemic patients with hyperparathyroidism, hypervitaminosis D, osteoporosis, and a tendency to calcium stone formation, although it is recommended only for the treatment of patients with symptomatic Paget's disease. Conversely, the excessive production of calcitonin may be associated with hypocalcemia and increased density of bone.

Renal Excretion of Calcium

Most of the ingested calcium is excreted in the intestines. Less than 1% is excreted in the urine. In an adult, this amounts to about 100 to 150 mg a day. The amount of calcium excreted in the urine depends approximately on the serum calcium concentration. Parathyroid hormone is also able to increase directly calcium reabsorption by the renal tubules.

SIGNIFICANCE AND DETERMINATION OF SERUM CALCIUM CONCENTRATION

Disturbances in calcium metabolism are usually described in terms of hypocalcemia or hypercalcemia. However, determinations of serum calcium concentration may be misleading. The reason for this is that calcium is present in the blood primarily in two forms: (1) ionized calcium, which is physiologically active, and (2) calcium bound to protein. The concentration of bound calcium depends on the concentration of the plasma proteins. Normally, about 50 to 75% of the serum calcium is ionized; the remainder is bound to protein, mostly to the serum albumin. As the total protein in the blood rises, more of the calcium becomes bound.

Clinically it is important to correlate serum calcium concentration with the serum albumin level, because a larger percentage of the serum calcium becomes ionized as the total protein in the blood decreases. Therefore, a low serum calcium concentration in the presence of a low serum albumin level (this can occur with starvation, cirrhosis of the liver, or in the nephrotic syndrome) is associated with an increased concentration of ionized calcium ions, and symptoms of hypocalcemia do not appear. However, a low serum calcium concentration in the presence of a normal serum albumin level is associated with a decreased ionized calcium concentration, so that symptoms and signs of hypocalcemia may develop.

The following simple rule can be used to determine if the measured serum calcium concentration is significant:

Each fall (or rise) of serum albumin level by 1.0 g/dl (beyond the normal range of 4 to 5 g/dl) is associated with a fall (or rise) of serum calcium concentration of approximately 0.8 mg/dl.

In 1935, McLean and Hastings devised a nomogram to determine the ionized calcium concentration from the total protein and the total calcium values of serum. It is now possible to measure the ionized calcium ion concentration directly, using a special calcium ion electrode.

HYPOCALCEMIA

Hypocalcemia exists when the serum calcium concentration falls below the lower normal value of 9 mg/dl (4.5 mEq/L). It may be associated with a loss of calcium in both the extracellular fluid and bone (for example in osteomalacia). In other patients, the hypocalcemia may be associated with a retention of phosphate (as in chronic renal disease), or with other factors localized in the extracellular fluid, such as an abnormal increase of citrate, or acute pancreatitis which results in the binding of calcium in the inflammatory exudate in the peritoneal cavity.

Serum calcium determinations should always be made simultaneously with a serum albumin determination, for reasons discussed above.

Etiology

Hypocalcemia can occur in the following situations:

1. Deficiency of vitamin D. This is the cause of childhood rickets, or osteomalacia (adult rickets). It also appears in malabsorption states, such as steatorrhea due to pancreatic insufficiency, sprue, celiac disease, biliary obstruction, or small bowel disease. These patients have decreased fat absorption and an increased amount of fat in the stool. This causes a loss of calcium due to the excretion of calcium salts of fatty acids. Vitamin D is also lost in this way. An excess of phytic acids, a constituent of cereals, can cause a loss of calcium in a similar way.

   In vitamin D deficiency, as in patients with steatorrhea, the poor absorption of calcium from the intestinal tract causes hypocalcemia, and a resultant secondary hyperparathyroidism. This in turn counteracts the decrease in serum calcium concentration. However, it produces a low serum phosphorus concentration.

2. Deficiency of parathyroid hormone *(hypoparathyroidism)*. This may be idiopathic (where it may also be associated with adrenocortical insufficiency, or with pernicious anemia), or it may develop after thyroid or parathyroid surgery.

3. Inadequate response of the renal tubules to parathyroid hormone *(pseudohypoparathyroidism* and *pseudopseudohypoparathyroidism,* see below).

4. Acute pancreatitis. Hypocalcemia is a common finding in acute pancreatitis. In the past, it was attributed entirely to the precipitation of calcium esters in areas of fat necrosis. It has also been suggested that the hypocalcemia might be due to the excessive secretion of glucagon from the inflamed pancreas, which in turn stimulates the secretion of calcitonin. Recent studies by Weir and associates indicate that the hypocalcemia of acute pancreatitis is secondary to sequestration of calcium ions outside the skeleton and/or is due to a yet undefined defect of bone metabolism.

   Clinically, a fall in serum calcium concentration below 7 mg/dl is a sign of poor prognosis in acute pancreatitis. A normal or high serum calcium concentration suggests that hyperparathyroidism may be present.

5. Hyperphosphatemia. This occurs in renal insufficiency where phosphate ions are retained in the body. (The hyperphosphatemia is one of the causes of hypocalcemia in these patients.)

   Recently, hyperphosphatemia and hypocalcemia have been reported in patients with acute lymphoblastic leukemia 24 to 48 hours after chemotherapy has been started.

6. Magnesium deficiency. The magnesium deficiency may prevent the action of parathyroid hormone on bone, so that hypocalcemia develops.

7. Excessive secretion of adrenocortical hormones, as in Cushing's syndrome, or when corticosteroids are given therapeutically.

8. Neoplasms of the breast, lung, prostate, associated with *osteoblastic* (bone-forming) metastases. Also, medullary thyroid carcinoma, if calcitonin is secreted by the carcinoma.

9. Renal tubular acidosis.

10. Acute intermittent porphyria with inappropriate secretion of ADH. The usual electrolyte disturbance is hyponatremia, due to water excess. However, hypocalcemia and hypomagnesemia may also occur.

11. Drugs, such as the chelating agent disodium ethylenediaminetetraacetate (disodium EDTA), corticosteroids, mithramycin, glucagon, heparin, loop diuretics, sodium fluoride, sodium nitroprusside, theophylline. Angiographic contrast material may also contain a calcium chelating salt, which can precipitously lower the blood calcium level after arteriography.

   Hypocalcemia may also develop after an infusion of phosphate or sulfate salts (used to treat hypercalcemia).

12. Nephrotic syndrome or cirrhosis of the liver. The low serum calcium concentration is due to the low protein concentration. The ionized calcium concentration is normal, and there are no symptoms or clinical signs of hypocalcemia.

13. Infusion of ACD (acid-citrate-dextrose) blood. This can occur as a result of the transfusion of a large volume of blood-bank blood which is citrated.

   When sodium citrate is infused, it is usually oxidized to sodium bicarbonate. (This can produce a transfusion alkalosis.) However, if a large amount of sodium citrate is infused rapidly, or in the presence of shock or liver damage, the excess citrate ions may bind calcium ions, producing hypocalcemia. This may cause tetany and even shock. In addition, blood-bank blood contains an increased amount of potassium ions, which can cause serious hyperkalemia, especially in the presence of hypocalcemia.

14. Causes of parathyroid hormone deficiency include;

   genetic disturbances, such as congenital absence of parathyroid glands, multiple endocrine deficiency, autoimmune-candidiasis (MEDAC syndrome) where patients show chronic mucocutaneous candidiasis, Addison's disease, and other disturbances in association with hypoparathyroidism; acquired disturbances, such as surgical removal of the parathyroid glands, irradiation to the glands, iron overload, neoplastic infiltration, suppression by hypercalcemia, hypomagnesemia, transient maternal hyperparathyroidism.

Pathophysiology

Calcium is needed by all tissues. It is needed for normal cardiac function, for the normal functioning of the nervous system, for the normal development of bone, and for normal blood clotting. The characteristic sign of hypocalcemia is an increased neuromuscular irritability which may cause tetany or even epileptiform seizures (see discussion of tetany below). In addition, the intracranial pressure may become elevated, with choked discs. When hypocalcemia persists for any length of time, calcium deposits may occur in abnormal locations, such as the eye lens or the basal ganglia. In addition, the bones may be more dense if the hypocalcemia is due to a lack of parathyroid hormone.

Symptoms and Signs

Tetany is the most characteristic sign of hypocalcemia. This can be caused either by a decreased serum calcium concentration, as in the above patients, or by an increased pH, as in patients with metabolic or respiratory alkalosis. A low pH decreases the tendency to tetany. This is the reason that tetany does not appear in metabolic acidosis due to chronic renal disease, even when the serum calcium concentration is very low. When the pH is increased, as in alkalosis, tetany occurs even if the serum calcium concentration is normal. When both the serum calcium and potassium concentrations are low, tetany is also inhibited. However tetany will appear if the serum potassium concentration is raised in such a patient, but the serum calcium concentration is allowed to remain low. Tetany can also be associated with hypokalemia, hypomagnesemia, or primary aldosteronism.

The patient may show carpopedal spasm, Trousseau's sign, Chvostek's sign, facial muscle spasm, paresthesias, or even convulsions which are often misdiagnosed as idiopathic epilepsy. (However, there is no aura and the patient does not get relief with anticonvulsive drugs.) Spasm of the bronchial muscles can produce an asthmatic attack. Spasm of the muscles of the abdominal viscera can simulate the symptoms and signs of an acute surgical abdominal condition.

Trousseau's sign to detect latent tetany is elicited by applying a blood pressure cuff to an upper extremity and inflating the cuff above the systolic level for 3 minutes. A positive reaction is the development of carpal spasm. However, Trousseau's sign is often absent in patients with latent tetany, and may be present in normal persons.

Chvostek's sign to detect latent tetany is elicited by percussing the facial nerve anterior to the ear. A positive reaction is unilateral contraction of the facial muscles and the muscles of the eyelids. (Contraction of the facial muscles alone may occur normally.)

Mental changes include changes in mood, emotional depression, impairment of memory, confusion, delirium, or even hallucinations.

Hypoparathyroid patients may show *defects in ectodermal structures,* including the skin, nails, hair and teeth. Coarse dry skin with patchy or absent axillary or pubic hair may be noted. Various degrees of hypoplasia of the teeth may be present, depending on when the hypoparathyroidism started. Fingernails may be deformed and brittle. Monilial infections of the nails, pharynx, or vagina are common. *Cataracts* may develop within one year. *Papilledema,* with or without an increased cerebrospinal fluid pressure, may also develop and may be associated with symptoms and signs, including convulsions, suggestive of a brain tumor. *Congestive heart failure* which responds to treatment with calcium salts may occur. *Diarrhea,* due to intestinal malabsorption of vitamin B_{12} or fats, may also manifest itself.

Laboratory Tests

When parathyroid hormone is totally absent, the serum calcium concentration may fall to 4.5 mg/dl, and the serum phosphate concentration may rise even to 12 mg/dl especially in children.

Parathyroid Hormone (iPTH) Immunoassay in Blood. It is now possible to measure the parathyroid hormone level in serum, using a radioimmunoassay technic. Serum levels obtained in this way should be correlated with the serum calcium level to differentiate different conditions that may be associated with either hypocalcemia or hypercalcemia (Table 31–1).

One should be aware that the sensitivity of iPTH analyses from different laboratories can vary widely.

A metabolic alkalosis may develop. (Barzel and others have pointed out that the parathyroid hormone increases the urinary excretion of bicarbonate ions, in association with changes in serum calcium and phosphate concentrations. When hypoparathyroidism is present, the lack of the parathyroid hormone causes a retention of bicarbonate ions and a rise in pH.)

Hypokalemia, hyperphosphatemia, and hypomagnesemia may also occur.

In the urine, there is a threshold for calcium excretion. As a result, calcium will be absent from the urine when the serum calcium concentration falls below 7 to 8 mg/dl. In some diseases, such as sarcoidosis, a high urinary calcium excretion can occur in spite of a normal serum calcium concentration.)

The electrocardiogram shows a characteristic prolongation of the Q–T interval, with normal ST segments and normal T waves.

X-ray examination of the bones may not show abnormal findings. Occasionally, thickening of the lamina dura or calcification in various regions of the brain may occur. (Subcutaneous calcification rarely occurs in idiopathic hypoparathyroidism, but is common in pseudohypoparathyroidism.)

The electroencephalogram may show nonspecific changes.

Table 30–1. Serum Parathyroid Hormone Assays (iPTH) Correlated with Serum Calcium Levels

Serum calcium concentration (mg %)	Serum parathyroid hormone Level (pg/ml)**	Parathyroid function	Common clinical conditions
8.8 to 10.8	100 to 600	Normal parathyroid function	
11.0 to 16.2	more than 300	Primary hyperparathyroidism	Benign adenoma (81%), parathyroid hyperplasia (15%), parathyroid carcinoma (4%)
11.2 to 21.0	less than 280	Nonparathyroid hypercalcemia	Thiazide diuretics, milk-alkali syndrome, sarcoidosis, osteolytic metastases, multiple myeloma, vitamin D intoxication, hyperthyroidism, adrenal insufficiency, Paget's disease with immobilization
less than 9.4	more than 800	Secondary hyperparathyroidism	Chronic renal disease
less than 7.5	less than 300	Hypoparathyroidism	Removal of parathyroid glands during thyroid surgery
less than 7.0	350 to 700	Pseudohypoparathyroidism	Genetic—inadequate response of renal tubules to parathyroid hormone

* Adapted from Medpath Laboratories: Test of the month, May 1978.
** pg/ml, picograms per ml.

Diagnosis

Common causes of symptomatic hypocalcemia include azotemia, hypoparathyroidism, osteomalacia (or rickets), and malabsorption syndromes. (Hypocalcemia associated with hypoalbuminemia is asymptomatic, as has been pointed out above.)

The serum phosphate concentration may be helpful in the differential diagnosis of hypocalcemia. For example, it is normal or low in most patients with vitamin D deficiency or with intestinal malabsorption, and is elevated in most patients with hypoparathyroidism or azotemic patients (who are hypocalcemic).

Hypoparathyroidism can be simulated by *pseudohypoparathyroidism.* Such patients show a low serum calcium and a high serum phosphate concentration, due to a genetic lack of response of the renal tubules to parathyroid hormone rather than to a lack of the hormone. In addition, patients may show short metacarpals, characteristic thickset figure and round face, demonstrable presence of parathyroid gland on biopsy, subcutaneous calcification (this is rare in idiopathic hypoparathyroidism), calcification of the basal ganglia, cataracts, tetany, dental defects, and often mental retardation. Treatment is the same as for hypoparathyroidism.

These patients can be differentiated from those with hypoparathyroidism by means of the Ellsworth-Howard test. The test is based on the fact that parathyroid hormone normally causes a markedly increased urinary excretion of phosphate ions in hypoparathyroid patients and in normal persons, but only a small increased excretion in pseudohypoparathyroid patients.

The term *pseudopseudohypoparathyroidism* has been used to describe patients who show physical signs similar to the pseudohypoparathyroid patients. However, there is no tetany, and the serum calcium and phosphate concentrations are normal. The Ellsworth-Howard test shows a normal phosphate diuresis. This condition is now considered to be merely a variant of pseudohypoparathyroidism.

Treatment

Tetany can be treated by either lowering the pH, if alkalosis is present, or raising the serum calcium concentration, if it is low. Calcium gluconate in a dose of 10 to 20 ml of a 10% solution can be given intravenously. It should be given slowly at a rate not exceeding 2 ml per minute.

If symptoms are severe, calcium gluconate can be given by continuous intravenous solution. An average adult will require approximately 100 ml of 10% calcium gluconate dissolved in 1 liter of 5% dextrose in water, given slowly over a period of 4 hours.

Calcium salts should also be given orally. Calcium lactate (which contains 13% calcium ions) can be given in a daily oral dose of 12 g. Calcium gluconate (which contains 9% calcium ions) can be given in a daily oral dose of 16 g. (A level teaspoonful of calcium lactate or calcium gluconate contains approximately 3 g.)

If tetany does not respond to the injection of a calcium salt, this may be a sign that the tetany is due to hypomagnesemia, particularly if the patient shows chronic alcoholism or malabsorption, or is poorly nourished. In such a case, 2 ml of a 50% solution of magnesium sulfate can be given intramuscularly.

Hypoparathyroidism is treated with large doses of calcium salts orally (16 to 32 g calcium lactate daily) plus vitamin D. Usually, large doses of vitamin D (25,000 to 100,000 IU daily) are needed. Various vitamin D preparations can be used. Ergocalciferol (Vitamin D_2: Drisdol, Winthrop) is satisfactory.

One can start with a dose of 50,000 IU daily. However, ergocalciferol may not cause the serum calcium concentration to rise for 2 or more weeks.

If the hypocalcemia appears to be resistant to the action of ergocalciferol, dihydrotachysterol (Hytakerol, Winthrop) can be substituted. Conversely, patients who are resistant to dihydrotachysterol may respond to ergocalciferol. One should also remember that apparent resistance to the action of vitamin D may be due to hypomagnesemia. In such a case, the serum calcium concentration will rise only when the magnesium deficit is correct. Vitamin D requirements will also be higher if the patient is taking estrogens.

If hypercalcemia develops as a result of the vitamin D therapy, it may last 2 or more months after the vitamin D is stopped.

Calcitriol (1,25-$(OH)_2D_3$. Rocaltrol, Roche) has also been used to treat hypoparathyroidism.

The hypocalcemia of hypoparathyroidism can also be treated with a thiazide or similar diuretic, such as chlorthalidone (Hygroton), in conjunction with a salt-restricted diet, because the thiazides cause the serum calcium concentration to rise (Porter and associates). (Conversely, a diuretic such as furosemide, which can lower the serum calcium concentration, may worsen hypoparathyroidism.)

(Rarely, a patient will respond to calcium salts, without vitamin D. However, it may take 1 or 2 weeks for the oral calcium salts to cause a rise in serum calcium concentration.).

Patients may respond clinically even when they remain slightly hypocalcemic (serum calcium concentration 8.5 to 9.0 mg/dl). The effectiveness of calcium supplements and vitamin D should be checked with periodic serum calcium determinations every 3 to 4 months indefinitely. (In this way, the development of drug-induced *hypercalcemia* can be prevented.) The use of the Sulkowitch test to measure urinary calcium excretion is therefore not necessary.

When a patient is given large doses of oral calcium salts, it is not necessary to use a high-calcium diet. It is also not necessary to place the patient on a low-phosphorus diet, or to use aluminum hydroxide gels to prevent absorption of phosphate ions from the gastrointestinal tract.

Hypocalcemia due to hypomagnesemia must be treated by raising the serum magnesium concentration.

Calcium salts should be given cautiously to digitalized patients because there is evidence that the calcium can precipitate digitalis toxicity.

Hypocalcemia due to citrate toxicity can be prevented when no more than 1000 to 1500 ml of blood bank blood is given per hour to an adult, and when 10 ml calcium gluconate is given intravenously with each 1500 ml blood. (Howland and his associates found that the administration of calcium salts with blood-bank transfusions of 2500 ml or more can be associated with ventricular fibrillation. They therefore suggest that calcium salts should not be used even with blood bank blood. More recent studies by Olinger and associates and others indicate the value of calcium salts during transfusion of blood bank blood.)

OSTEOPOROSIS

Osteoporosis is due to excessive bone resorption. It is often seen in postmenopausal women, in hypogonadic males, or in elderly persons. However, it may occur at any age (idiopathic osteoporosis). Other causes include long-term corticosteroid therapy, Cushing's syndrome, hyperthyroidism, long-term heparin therapy, steatorrhea and other intestinal malabsorption syndromes, rheumatoid arthritis, vitamin C deficiency, and gastrectomy. It can also be precipitated by long-term immobilization. The mechanism by which it occurs is not clearly understood. A deficiency of calcium absorption from the gastrointestinal tract may be a factor, because there is an abnormally high fecal excretion of calcium ions in osteoporosis, regardless of the cause.

In spite of this, serum calcium, phosphate and alkaline phosphatase levels are normal in most patients with postmenopausal, senile, or idiopathic osteoporosis. In hyperthyroidism, the serum calcium concentration may become elevated; the serum phosphate concentration may be normal or low. In Cushing's syndrome, the patient may show slight hypocalcemia and hypophosphatemia, with a slight increase in alkaline phosphatase level.

Clinical signs are related to compression of one or more vertebral bodies (however, compression of the spinal cord does not occur) or fracture, particularly of the lower end of a radius, rib, or neck of a femur.

Treatment includes a high calcium intake, approximately 1 to 1.5 g of calcium ions daily. (One quart of milk provides 1 g of calcium ions, plus phosphate ions, which are also helpful in alleviating osteoporosis.) Other foods which have a high calcium content include broccoli, turnip greens (raw or cooked), watercress (raw or cooked), almonds, mackerel, molasses, and dried brewer's yeast.

Estrogens in postmenopausal women are also beneficial. However, there is an increased risk of uterine cancer even with small doses of estrogens.

Vitamin D is also helpful, particularly when the osteoporosis is due to corticosteroid therapy. As much as 5,000 to 10,000 IU daily may be needed. (One must check the serum calcium concentration every several months, to prevent hypercalcemia, when such high doses of vitamin D are given.

Fluoride salts have also been used but can induce changes in bone structure and can cause secondary hyperparathyroidism.

OSTEOMALACIA

Osteomalacia in adults (or rickets in children) is due to a defective mineralization of osteoid bone. The usual explanation for its development is a decrease of the serum Ca × P product below the critical level of approximately 30 to 40, which is necessary for the growth of hydroxyapatite crystals in bone matrix and epiphyseal cartilage. Therefore, osteomalacia can occur when the serum calcium concentration is low, as in vitamin D deficiency (this may occur as a result of a dietary deficiency of vitamin D, or from steatorrhea or other intestinal malabsorption syndromes, or after gastrectomy), or when the serum phosphate concentration is low (as after excessive intake of aluminium hydroxide gels, or in the Fanconi syndrome, or in familial hypophosphatemia [*vitamin D-resistant rickets*]). In addition, osteomalacia can occur when the Ca × P product is normal, as in renal osteodystrophy, renal tubular acidosis, or uretero-enterostomy with acidosis, for reasons which are not clear. Osteomalacia and osteoporosis can co-exist.

In the beginning of this chapter it was pointed out that phenobarbital or phenytoin (Dilantin) interferes with the metabolism of vitamin D and can cause osteomalacia. When acetazolamide is given to a patient who is taking phenytoin, the tendency to osteomalacia is increased.

Symptoms include muscular weakness, severe bone pains, worsened by weight lifting, and a waddling gait. Tetany may also occur. Characteristic findings on x-ray examination are linear translucencies (pseudofractures, Looser's zones, Milkman's syndrome). These can be seen in the wings of the scapulae, ribs, pubic and ischial rami, neck of the femurs, proximal third of the ulnae, and other bones. Actual fractures may also develop through these pseudofractures. (X-ray findings of secondary hyperparathyroidism [Chap. 31] may also develop.)

Characteristic laboratory findings include an elevated alkaline phosphatase level and a marked decrease or absence of calcium in the urine. (Hypophosphatemia may be more marked than the hypocalcemia. This is probably due to the development of secondary hyperparathyroidism, which raises the low serum calcium concentration.)

When the osteomalacia is due to vitamin D deficiency or to renal osteodystrophy, vitamin D is effective. Patients with the Fanconi syndrome, renal tubular acidosis, or ureteroenterostomy acidosis can be treated with alkaline salts to correct the acidosis, and with oral phosphate supplements (page 330), to correct the hypophosphatemia. Vitamin D is probably not necessary in these patients. If osteomalacia due to inadequate calcium absorption from the intestines is also present, the patient should be given a high calcium intake.

Postmenopausal osteoporotic hypertensive women with adequate kidney function can be treated with thiazides, which conserve the urinary excretion of calcium ions, rather than with furosemide which increases calcium excretion through the kidneys (Norenberg).

Hyperphosphatemia

An excess of phosphate ions and hyperphosphatemia are usually due to renal insufficiency. However, hyperphosphatemia may occur as a result of hypoparathyroidism. Clinically, it is associated with tetany. The hyperphosphatemia is usually associated with some degree of hypocalcemia and signs of renal impairment, such as acidosis, azotemia, or high serum creatinine level. Hyperphosphatemia also occurs with excessive bone growth activity, as in acromegalic patients.

The treatment of hyperphosphatemia is described on page 209.

REFERENCES

Ajlouni, K., et al.: Hyperphosphatemia and hypocalcemia in myeloproliferative disorders. Ann Intern Med, *81*:119, 1974.
Albright, F., and Reifenstein, E.C., Jr.: *Parathyroid Glands and Metabolic Bone Disease.* Baltimore, Williams & Wilkins, 1948.
Austin, L.A., and Heath, H. III: Calcitonin. Physiology and pathophysiology, N Engl J Med, *304*:269, 1981.
Avioli, L.V., guest editor: Vitamin D metabolites. Their clinical importance. Arch Intern Med, *138*:835, 1978.
Barragry, J.M., et al.: Vitamin D metabolism in nephrotic syndrome. Lancet *2*:629, 1977.
Bartter, F.C.: Pseudohypoparathyroidism and pseudo-pseudohypoparathyroidism. In *The Metabolic Basis of Inherited Disease,* 2nd ed. (Stanbury, J.B., Wyngaarden, J.B., and Fredrickson, D.S., Eds.). New York, McGraw-Hill Book Co., 1966.
Barzel, U.: Systemic alkalosis in hypoparathyroidism. J Clin Endocr, *29*:917, 1969.
Barzel, U.S.: Treatment of hypoparathyroidism. New York State J Med, *76*:579, 1976.
Bashour, T.T., et al.: Hypocalcemic cardiomyopathy, Chest, *78*:663, 1980.

Bashour, T.T., et al.: Hypocalcemic acute myocardial failure secondary to rapid transfusion of citrated blood, Am Heart J, *108*:1040, 1984.

Baylink, D.J.: Glucocorticoid-induced osteoporosis, Editorial, N Engl J Med, *309*:306, 1983.

Bikle, D.D.: Fluoride treatment of osteoporosis, Editorial, Ann Intern Med, *98*:1013, 1983.

Carpenter, T.O., et al.: Hypoparathyroidism in Wilson's disease. N Engl J Med, *309*:874, 1983.

DeLuca, H.F.: Vitamin D endocrinology. Ann Intern Med, *85*:377, 1976.

Dent, C.E.: Osteomalacia due to phosphate depletion from excessive aluminum hydroxide ingestion. Br Med J, *1*:551, 1974.

Editorial: Calcium or phosphate? Lancet, *2*:895, 1964.

Foster, C.V.: Calcitonin (thyrocalcitonin) N Engl J Med, *279*:349, 1968.

Frame, B., and Marel, G.M.: Clinical disorders of bone and mineral metabolism, Symposium, Ann Intern Med, *99*:725, 1983.

Frame, B., and Parfitt, A.M.: Osteomalacia. Current concepts. Ann Intern Med, *89*:966, 1978.

Frame, B., and Sudhaker, R.D.: Calcium-regulating hormones. Symposium, Ann Intern Med, *93*:928, 1980.

Fraser, D.R.: The physiological economy of vitamin D, Lancet, *1*:969, 1983.

Freitag, J., et al.: Impaired parathyroid hormone metabolism in patients with chronic renal failure. N Engl J Med, *298*:29, 1978.

Fulop, M.: Hypoparathyroidism after ^{131}I therapy. Ann Intern Med, *75*:808, 1971.

Gabow, P.A., et al.: Furosemide-induced reduction in ionized calcium in hypoparathyroid patients. Ann Intern Med, *86*:579, 1977.

Hall, T.C., et al.: Hypocalcemia—an unusual metabolic complication of breast cancer. N Engl J Med, *275*:1474, 1966.

Horsman, A., et al.: The effect of estrogen dose on postmenopausal bone loss, N Engl J Med, *309*:1405, 1983.

Howland, W.S., Boyan, C.P., and Schweizer, O.: Massive blood replacement without calcium administration. Surg Gynecol Obstet. *118*:814, 1964.

Juan, D.: Vitamin D metabolism, Postgrad Med, *68*:210, 1980.

Kalu, D.N., and Foster, C.V.: Calcitonin. Its physiologic roles. New York State J Med, *76*:230, 1976.

Lane, J.M., et al.: Osteoporosis, Current diagnosis and treatment. Geriatrics, *39*:40, 1984.

Laymon, C.W., and Zelickson, A.: Pseudohypoparathyroidism: The Seabright Bantam syndrome. Arch Derm, *79*:194, 1959.

Ludbrook, J., and Wynn, V.: Citrate intoxication. Br Med J, *2*:523, 1958.

Lutwak, L., Singer, F.R., and Urist, M.R.: Current concepts of bone metabolism. Ann Intern Med, *80*:630, 1974.

McLean, F., and Hastings, A.B.: Clinical estimation and significance of the calcium ion concentration in the blood. Am J Med Sci, *189*:601, 1935. Also J Biol Chem, *108*:285, 1935.

Moore, F.D.: The citrate lesion. In *Metabolic Care of the Surgical Patient.* Philadelphia, W.B. Saunders Co., 1959.

Morgan, D.B., et al.: Osteomalacia after gastrectomy. Lancet, *2*:1085, 1089, 1965.

Nealon, T.F., Ching, N.P.H., and Gibbon, J.H., Jr.: Prevention of citrate intoxication during exchange transfusions. JAMA, *183*:459, 1963.

Newmark, S.R., and Himathongkam, T.: Hypercalcemic and hypocalcemic crises. JAMA, *230*:1438, 1974.

Norenberg, D.D.: Furosemide, hypertension, and osteoporosis, letter, JAMA, *241*:237, 1979.

Olinger, G.N., et al.: Acute clinical hypocalcemic myocardial depression during rapid blood transfusion and postoperative hemodialysis. J Thoracic Cardiovascular Surg, *72*:503, 1976.

Parfitt, A.M.: Adult hypoparathyroidism. Treatment with calcifediol. Arch Intern Med, *138*:874, 1978.

Parfitt, A.M., and Kleerekoper, M.: Clinical disorders of calcium, phosphorus, and magnesium metabolism. In *Clinical Disorders of Fluid and Electrolyte Metabolism.* 3rd ed. (Maxwell, M.H., and Kleeman, C.R., Eds.), McGraw-Hill Book Co. New York, 1980.

Payne, R.B., et al.: Interpretation of serum calcium in patients with abnormal serum proteins. Br Med J, 4:643, 1973.

Pepper, G.M., et al.: Hypocalcemia in metastatic bone disease, NY State J Med, 84:41, 1984.

Porter, R.H., et al.: Treatment of hypoparathyroid patients with chlorthalidone. N Engl J Med, 298:577, 1978.

Raisz, L.G.: The pharmacology of bone. Rational Drug Ther, 5:6, 1971.

Raisz, L.G., and Kream, B.E.: Regulation of bone formation, N Engl J Med, 309: 29:83, 1983.

Raskin, P., McClain, C.J., and Medsger, T.A., Jr.: Hypocalcemia associated with metastatic bone disease. Arch Intern Med, 132:539, 1973.

Robertson, G.M., et al.: Inadequate parathyroid response in acute pancreatitis. N Engl J Med, 294:512, 1976.

Rushton, A.R.: Pseudohypoparathyroidism, cimetidine, and neurologic toxicity, letter, Ann Intern Med, 98:677, 1983.

Rude, R.K., et al.: Functional hypoparathyroidism and parathyroid hormone end-organ resistance in human magnesium deficiency. Clin Endocrinol, 5:209, 1976.

Silva, O.L., et al.: Ectopic secretion of calcitonin by oat-cell carcinoma. N Engl J Med, 290:1122, 1974.

Spencer, H., and Kramer, L.: Antacid-induced calcium loss. Editorial, Arch Intern Med, 143:657, 1983.

Spiegel, A.M., et al.: Pseudohypoparathyroidism. Editorial, N Engl J Med, 307:679, 1982.

Tapia, J., Stearns, G., and Ponseti, I.V.: Vitamin D-resistant rickets. J Bone Joint Surg, 46A:935, 1964.

Uhr, N., and Bezahler, H.B.: Pseudo-pseudohypoparathyroidism. Ann Intern Med, 54:443, 1961.

Weir, G.C., et al.: The hypocalcemia of acute pancreatitis, Ann Intern Med, 83:185, 1975.

Zimmerman, J., et al.: Normocalcemia in a hypoparathyroid patient with sarcoidosis. Evidence for parathyroid-hormone-independent synthesis of 1,25 dihydroxyvitamin D, Ann Intern Med, 98:338, 1983.

Zsigmond, E.K.: Hypocalcemic hypotension. JAMA, 226:355, 1973.

Zusman, J., Brown, D.M., and Nesbit, M.E.: Hyperphosphatemia, hyperphosphaturia and hypocalcemia in acute lymphoblastic leukemia. N Engl J Med, 289:1335, 1973.

CHAPTER 31

SYNDROMES ASSOCIATED WITH CALCIUM AND PHOSPHATE DISTURBANCES (Continued)

HYPERCALCEMIA

Hypercalcemia exists when the serum calcium concentration rises above the upper normal value of 10.5 mg/dl (5.25 mEq/L). It may be associated with an excess of calcium in both extracellular fluid and in bone (for example, due to excessive intake of vitamin D or calcium). In other patients, the hypercalcemia is associated with a localized or generalized deficit of calcium in bone (as in hyperparathyroidism).

Etiology

The most common causes of hypercalcemia are neoplasms (with or without bone metastases), hyperparathyroidism, multiple myeloma, sarcoidosis, excessive vitamin D therapy, the milk-alkali syndrome, and prolonged immobilization.

Hypercalcemia can also be classified in the following ways:

1. More calcium is absorbed from the gastrointestinal tract than can be stored in the bones, or excreted by the kidneys. This occurs in:
   a. Excessive administration of vitamin D (usually 50,000 IU or more daily) for several months or more. The hypercalcemia may occur as early as 2 weeks or as late as years after the vitamin D therapy has started.
   b. Sarcoidosis. Hypercalcemia can occur in the absence of bone involvement. It is probably due to excessive absorption of calcium from the bowel, related to increased sensitivity to exogenous or endogenous vitamin D. (Hypercalciuria is also common and may occur in sarcoid patients who do not have hypercalcemia.).
   c. Milk-alkali syndrome. This can occur in patients with peptic ulcer treated with an excessive amount of milk and alkaline antacids, particularly calcium carbonate, for a long time. (Excessive calcium car-

bonate intake, without milk, can also cause the syndrome.) These patients show a metabolic alkalosis in association with the hypercalcemia. If the syndrome persists, the hypercalcemia may cause severe renal failure. Vomiting is common and aggravates the metabolic alkalosis.

(The hypercalcemia, due to the increased intake of calcium salts, suppresses the secretion of parathyroid hormone. As a result, the urinary excretion of phosphate salts decreases, so that hyperphosphatemia may develop. The combination of hypercalcemia and hyperphosphatemia can produce nephrocalcinosis, metastatic calcification, and progressive renal failure.)

2. Bone destruction may exceed bone production so much that the kidneys are unable to excrete the excessive calcium ions. This occurs in:

   a. Primary hyperparathyroidism. This is usually due to a single parathyroid adenoma. In about 10% of patients, it is due to hyperplasia of the four parathyroid glands. Carcinoma of the parathyroid is a rare cause of hyperparathyroidism.

   Occasionally, hyperparathyroidism occurs in association with other endocrine disorders (multiple endocrine adenomatosis). For example, Sipple's syndrome refers to the triad of hyperparathyroidism, pheochromocytoma, and medullary carcinoma of the thyroid. Hyperparathyroidism also may occur in association with a pituitary adenoma. Severe peptic ulcer may be present, because parathyroid hormone induces hyperplasia of pepsin-secreting cells in the stomach. Other hyperparathyroid patients may show signs of a Zollinger-Ellison syndrome and WDHA syndrome (page 279).

   b. Osteolytic metastases, especially in carcinoma of the breast or lung (also see below).

   c. Disseminated tuberculosis of the bones.

3. Decreased bone formation may be present. This can occur if a patient is immobilized for a long time, particularly if Paget's disease is present. It can occur, however, in any patient who is immobilized.

4. A persistent, excessive secretion of parathyroid hormone may be present. This occurs in:

   a. Primary hyperparathyroidism.

   b. Secondary hyperparathyroidism. This can occur when the serum calcium concentration is lowered by such conditions as renal glomerular insufficiency with phosphate retention, renal tubular insufficiency with urinary loss of calcium, rickets or osteomalacia, or pregnancy. However, even when secondary hyperparathyroidism develops and the serum calcium concentration rises, it does not become abnormally high.

   c. Irreversible secondary hyperparathyroidism. This has previously been called "tertiary" hyperparathyroidism. This may develop in patients with secondary hyperparathyroidism, when the parathyroid glands become autonomous. These patients show both hypercalcemia and hyperphosphatemia. Davies has suggested a clue that irreversible secondary hyperparathyroidism is developing, namely, when vitamin D is given to control osteomalacia in a patient with secondary hyperparathyroidism, it also produces hypercalcemia.

   d. Malignant neoplasms. Hypercalcemia may occur in many types of neoplastic patients, especially carcinoma of the breast and lung, hypernephroma, multiple myeloma, and lymphomas and leukemias. The hypercalcemia of these patients may be due to diverse causes. In some patients, the hypercalcemia occurs with osteolytic metastases. Immobilization of a cancer patient may also contribute to the hypercalcemia. Some neoplasms may produce a parathormone-like hormone. Other neoplastic patients can produce a hormonal substance (or substances), such as prostaglandins, not related to parathormone, which causes calcium resorption from bone. In many neoplastic patients, hypercalcemia is present without obvious signs of bony metastases.

5. Hypercalcemia due to inadequate renal excretion of calcium salts.
6. Familial hypocalciuric hypercalcemia. This is a genetic disturbance showing an autosomal dominant syndrome of hypercalcemia, hypophosphatemia, and signs of parathyroid overactivity. In contrast to hyperparathyroidism, there is a markedly reduced urinary excretion of calcium. Chondrocalcinosis and pancreatitis are common. Ordinarily, no treatment is needed. However, if acute pancreatitis develops, total parathyroidectomy is recommended (Marx et al.).
7. Hypercalcemia may also occur as a result of the following miscellaneous causes:
   a. Endocrine disturbances such as hyperthyroidism, hypothyroidism, adrenocortical insufficiency, acromegaly, pheochromocytoma. Patients treated with radioiodine for hyperthyroidism seem to be at increased risk to develop hyperparathyroidism.
   b. Diuretics. Thiazides and chlorthalidone potentiate the action of parathyroid hormone on the kidneys, resulting in a retention of calcium ions. They are therefore helpful in treating idiopathic hypercalciuria. They rarely cause hypercalcemia. (When this occurs, hyperparathyroidism should be suspected.)
   c. Hypervitaminosis A. Hypercalcemia may occur as a result of increased bone resorption.
   d. After the use of calcium exchange resins in hemodialysis, the diuretic phase of acute renal failure, after renal transplantation, and in hypophosphatasia.
   e. Lithium salt intake.
   f. After the use of oral isotretinoin for acne.
   g. Tuberculosis, beryllosis.
   h. Artifactual hypercalcemia. This can occur, for example, in multiple myeloma, where one of the abnormal globulin molecules binds calcium ions. In such cases, the value of ionized calcium is normal.

Pathophysiology

Hypercalcemia causes decreased neuromuscular excitability, in contrast to hypocalcemia. In addition, marked hypotonicity of the muscles occurs.

Hypercalcemia may be associated with an increased calcium excretion in the urine (hypercalciuria). As a result, calcium stones can form in the kidney pelves, and calcium deposits can develop in the collecting tubules of the kidneys. These tubular injuries are probably the cause of the decreased ability of the kidneys to form a concentrated urine.

Hypercalcemia can cause severe anatomical injury to the kidneys, especially in the ascending limb of Henle, the distal convoluted tubules, and the collecting tubule. Epithelial degeneration, necrosis, and calcification have also been found.

In addition, metastatic calcification in various organs of the body (the lung, gastric mucosa, and kidneys) may develop, particularly where the local pH of the body is elevated. Calcification can also occur in arterial walls, around joints, in the cornea (producing a 'band' keratitis), and in the conjunctiva.

If the hypercalcemia is due to hyperparathyroidism and if the patient is in negative calcium balance due to a low-calcium diet, osteolytic bone lesions may develop.

Hypercalcemia (or parenteral calcium salts) can precipitate digitalis toxicity.

Symptoms and Signs

Some of the symptoms, such as muscular weakness or incoordination, loss of appetite, and constipation, may be due to decreased tone in smooth and striated muscle. Generalized muscle weakness is common, with or without muscle incoordination. The patient may drop things with the hands or trip with the feet. Ataxia may be present, and the patient may develop a loss of pain or vibration sense. Hypotonia may be present, and the patient may show hyperextensible limbs. Muscle aches and pains may be severe. Deep tendon reflexes may be increased or abnormal, and a positive Babinski reflex may be present. The electroencephalogram may show diffuse slow activity.

The cerebrospinal fluid protein level may be elevated. Therefore, when a patient with cancer develops disturbed consciousness, headache, and increased cerebrospinal fluid protein, this may be due to hypercalcemia alone rather than to cerebral metastases.

Gastrointestinal symptoms are also common—anorexia, nausea, vomiting, and constipation. Occasionally, increased salivation and dysphagia may be noted. Severe abdominal pain, abdominal distention, and ileus may simulate an abdominal emergency. (However, acute pancreatitis may develop as a complication of hyperparathyroidism.) Thirst may be severe. The increased incidence of peptic ulcers in hyperparathyroid patients has already been mentioned.

Itching may develop with chronic hypercalcemia. This may be due to calcium deposits in the skin.

Characteristic ocular signs of hypercalcemia may be found, including gray or white opaque granular bands in the cornea (band keratopathy). These have a crescent shape and follow the arc of the limbus. They resemble arcus senilis, but are more marked in the lateral and medial margins of the cornea. (Arcus senilis is more prominent at the superior and inferior borders of the cornea.) Small clear glass-like deposits may also develop in the conjuntivae, near the palpebral fissures.

Incomplete or complete a-v block may occur. Cardiac standstill occurs when the serum calcium concentration is approximately 18 mg/dl.

Psychoneurotic and neurological signs are often prominent. The patient may show mental confusion, impairment of memory, slurred speech, acute psychotic behavior, lethargy, or coma. Convulsions are rare. The more severe signs occur when the serum calcium concentration is approximately 16 mg/dl or higher. If hypercalcemia persists for a long time, mental retardation may occur.

Polyuria and polydipsia, with clinical signs of water loss, may occur, due to disturbed renal tubular function produced by the hypercalcemia. When kidney damage is marked, azotemia may develop. This may then cause a secondary hyperparathyroidism.

Renal colic, due to kidney stones, is very common. (X-ray signs of calcification in the kidneys may also be present.) The stones are usually composed of calcium oxalate or calcium phosphate, or both. However, if a chronic urinary tract infection has been present, the stones may be covered with a layer of triple phosphates.

If hyperparathyroidism is present, a palpable mass, often tender, may be found in the region of the thyroid gland in possibly one-third of patients.

Hyperparathyroid patients may also show other endocrine abnormalities (see Etiology, above).

Hypercalcemic Crisis. Hyperparathyroid and other hypercalcemic patients may develop a hypercalcemic crisis associated with an acute rise in serum calcium concentration. The critical level of serum calcium is approximately 17 mg/dl. At this concentration, calcium salts precipitate in the kidneys and in other organs.

Symptoms include muscular weakness, intractable nausea, abdominal cramps, obstipation or diarrhea, peptic ulcer symptoms, or bone pain. Severe thirst and polyuria are characteristic. These findings may quickly lead to signs of severe water loss, including fever, lethargy, mental confusion, delirium, or coma. Azotemia is present. The serum phosphate concentration may be normal or high. Hypokalemia or hypomagnesemia may be present, due to increased urinary excretion of these ions. Hypernatremia may be present, due to a loss of water from vomiting, or from the excessive volume of urine.

Emergency hydration with saline infusions are very helpful. Phosphate or sulfate salts and other drugs can be used (see Treatment, below).

Laboratory Tests

Blood. The serum calcium concentration is usually elevated above 11 mg/dl. However, Yendt has pointed out that the serum calcium concentration is *below* 11 mg/dl in approximately one-third of hyperparathyroid patients. He believes that the normal upper range of serum calcium concentration is 10.3 to 10.5 mg/dl for males, and slightly lower for females.

(Occasionally, primary hyperparathyroidism may occur with periods of normal calcium concentration. However, these patients will show an increased urinary excretion of calcium ions—see idiopathic hypercalciuria, below.)

(The blood should be drawn without a tourniquet around the extremity, if possible, because a tight tourniquet, applied for several minutes, can increase the serum concentration. In addition, the test tube should *not* be stoppered with a cork, because it contains calcium salts which can produce a factitious hypercalcemia [Stone].)

The serum phosphate concentration is often low when hyperparathyroidism is present. However, hyperphosphatemia may be present if the hypercalcemia is due to vitamin D intoxication, the milk-alkali syndrome, sarcoidosis, multiple myeloma, or hyperthyroidism. The serum alkaline phosphatase level varies. It is high when bony changes are present. However, it may be high when bone disease is not evident. It is normal or low when vitamin D intoxication is present. It is normal in multiple myeloma. It often is elevated if the hypercalcemia is due to sarcoidosis or osteolytic metastases.

For serum parathyroid hormone assay, see page 313.

A hyperchloremic metabolic acidosis with a low serum bicarbonate concentration is often present in patients with hypercalcemia due to hyperparathyroidism. This is due to increased urinary excretion of bicarbonate ions produced by parathyroid hormone. Patients with hypercalcemia due to other causes tend to show instead a metabolic alkalosis with a low serum chloride concentration and a high serum bicarbonate concentration. Therefore, the presence of a metabolic alkalosis in a patient with hypercalcemia who has no other cause for the alkalosis suggests that hyperparathyroidism is not the cause of the hypercalcemia.

Similarly, the serum chloride-phosphate ratio can also be used to differentiate hypercalcemia due to hyperparathyroidism from hypercalcemia due to other causes. In hyperparathyroidism, the chloride-phosphate ratio ranged from 31.8 to 80 and was almost always more than 33, whereas in hypercalcemia due to other causes it ranged from 17.1 to 32.3 and was almost always less than 30 (Palmer and associates). (These investigators also found a high chloride-phosphate ratio in some neoplastic patients, due to the ectopic secretion of parathormone by the neoplasm.)

Urine. The urine may show an increased calcium content. (Normally, the daily urinary calcium excretion is less than 300 mg in males, and 250 mg in females, when the diet is unrestricted.) However, an increased calcium excretion in the urine can occur in idiopathic hypercalciuria (page 333), after excessive calcium intake, excessive vitamin D ingestion, as a result of furosemide or ethacrynic acid. It may also occur in the Fanconi syndrome, renal tubular acidosis, and in some cases of osteoporosis. (Urinary calcium excretion is usually less than 400 mg a day in primary hyperparathyroidism, but is usually more than 500 mg a day in cancer, sarcoidosis, or with excessive vitamin D intake.)

The urine osmolality and specific gravity are low, secondary to the decreased ability of the kidneys to concentrate water produced by the hypercalcemia.

The urinary excretion of cyclic AMP (cAMP) is usually high in primary hyperparathyroidism. However, it may also be abnormally high in other causes of hypercalcemia.

The electrocardiogram shows a characteristic shortened Q-T interval, with rounding of the T waves and normal ST segments.

X-Ray Findings. Hyperparathyroid patients usually show characteristic x-ray findings, including areas of subperiosteal demineralization, especially on the lateral aspects of the middle phalanges. Similar periosteal demineralization may also occur in other bones, including the lateral ends of the clavicles, symphysis pubis, and sacroiliac joints. Generalized osteitis fibrosa cystica may also develop. The lamina dura of the teeth may disappear. (However, this is not pathognomonic of hyperparathyroidism and may occur in osteomalacia or even in pyorrhea.)

Diagnosis

Hyperparathyroidism should be suspected when the serum calcium concentration is elevated in a patient with peptic ulcer, pancreatitis, kidney stones (consisting of calcium salts), renal insufficiency where the cause is not obvious, or when generalized weakness or vague psychoneurotic symptoms are present.

X-ray findings of generalized osteitis fibrosa, such as subperiosteal resorption of bone in the phalanges, are further diagnostic signs.

The serum chloride concentration and the serum chloride-phosphate ratio (just discussed) are also helpful in differential diagnosis.

Sarcoidosis can simulate hyperparathyroidism because hypercalcemia and bony changes may be present. (However the pulmonary hilar adenopathy of sarcoidosis does not appear in hyperparathyroidism.)

The preoperative use of new diagnostic technics (parathormone radioimmunoassay, thyroid arteriography, computed tomography, and selective venous catheterization of the thyroid veins) has been very helpful. Discussion of these technics, however, is outside the scope of this book.

The *milk-alkali syndrome* can be differentiated from primary or secondary hyperparathyroidism because the urinary calcium excretion remains normal in spite of hypercalcemia. In addition, there is the history of prolonged milk and alkali ingestion.

Course and Prognosis

The course and prognosis depend on the etiology of the hypercalcemia. However, an acute hypercalcemic crisis may occur, especially in hyperparathyroid patients, with intractable nausea, vomiting, decreasing urine volume, progressive azotemia with rising serum calcium and phosphate concentrations, progressive drowsiness, and coma. Such patients may die in a few days.

Treatment

The serum calcium concentration can be used as a general guide to determine the urgency of treatment. A serum calcium concentration less than 12 mg/dl indicates that treatment of the hypercalcemia can be postponed while one searches for the cause of the hypercalcemia, unless azotemia or hypercalcemic symptoms or signs are present. A serum calcium concentration more than 12 mg/dl should be treated. A serum calcium concentration of 15 mg/dl or higher requires emergency treatment.

Hyperparathyroidism, acute adrenocortical insufficiency, or hyperthyroidism, if present, should be promptly treated. If a neoplastic patient has been receiving estrogens or androgens, these should be promptly stopped. If the patient has been immobilized, he or she should be made ambulatory as quickly as possible.

Symptomatic primary hyperparathyroidism requires surgical removal of the parathyroid tumor. One must remember that removal of a parathyroid tumor does not always cure the patient—a hyperfunctioning gland may still be present, or an aberrant parathyroid gland (or glands) may be present in the mediastinum, within or near the thymus. Such a patient may require reoperation.

After a successful parathyroidectomy, the serum calcium concentration usually falls to normal within 24 hours. Transient hypocalcemia may also develop approximately 4 to 10 days after surgery. This hypocalcemia usually does not require treatment. However, if hypocalcemic symptoms develop, calcium salts and vitamin D should be started. (Postoperative hypoparathyroidism and hypocalcemia may last as long as 4 years.)

Hypomagnesemia may also develop postoperatively, particularly if bone disease is present. Acute pancreatitis, acute hyperchloremic acidosis, or pseudogout may also occur postoperatively.

If surgical exploration of the neck has been done and no parathyroid tumor has been found but symptoms continue, long-term medical treatment with phosphate salts may be helpful.

The treatment of secondary and tertiary hyperparathyroidism is discussed in Chapter 20.

If the patient is taking digitalis, the dosage should be temporarily reduced until the serum calcium concentration falls.

If the patient has been taking too much vitamin D, calcium salts, or milk, these should be stopped immediately. In addition, the daily dietary calcium intake should be reduced to approximately 150 to 200 mg. The following is an example of a low-calcium diet which can be used:

A LOW-CALCIUM DIET

(Approximately 150 mg)

Breakfast

Orange juice—1 small glass
Cooked farina or rice—1/3 cup after cooking
Uneeda biscuits—4 (or 1 to 2 slices of Italian or French bread which is made without milk)
Oleomargarine
Coffee or tea
Sugar
Coarse salt (ordinary table salt often contains calcium to prevent lumping)

Lunch

Lean meat or chicken—medium sized serving
Potato—1 medium sized
Uneeda biscuits—2 (or 1 to 2 slices of Italian or French bread)
Oleomargarine
Apple—1
Coffee or tea
Sugar
Coarse salt

Supper

Lean meat or chicken—medium sized serving
Macaroni—1/3 cup (cooked)
Uneeda biscuits—4 (or 1 to 2 slices of Italian or French bread)
Banana—1 medium sized
Coffee or tea
Sugar
Coarse salt

Use oleomargarine and sugar generously to maintain weight. No butter, milk, cheese, cream, or egg yolk allowed. Avoid cereals, oleomargarine or other foods to which calcium has been added.

Emergency Treatment of Hypercalcemia. Drugs can also be used to treat hypercalcemia. Dosage and route will depend on the urgency of the clinical situation. A serum calcium concentration of 15 mg/dl or higher is an indication for emergency treatment.

Isotonic sodium chloride infusion is particularly helpful in a hypercalcemic crisis, particularly if the BUN concentration is less than 50 mg/dl. The sodium chloride increases urinary calcium excretion and lowers the serum calcium concentration, and the water alleviates the marked water loss that is present. (Dextrose in water infusions may also be necessary.) Two to 3 liters daily can be used, for 1 to 2 days. However, the sodium chloride solution may precipitate acute congestive heart failure. Therefore, it may be advisable to use CVP (central venous pressure) monitoring. If the CVP rises above 15 cm water, half-strength sodium chloride solution can be used instead. In addition, the patient can be given a diuretic such as furosemide or ethacrynic acid concomitantly.

Suki and associates have also used large doses of intravenous furosemide alone (80 to 100 mg at intervals of 1 to 2 hours) to increase urinary calcium excretion and to lower the serum calcium concentration. However, such large doses produce severe losses of water, sodium, potassium, magnesium, and chloride ions, and require continued measurement of urinary and serum electrolytes so that the excreted electrolytes (with the exception of calcium) can be replenished intravenously.

Inorganic phosphate salts can be given orally or intravenously. They are contraindicated when hypocalcemia is due to vitamin D intoxication, because of the dangers of metastatic calcification. They are also contraindicated if renal failure and hyperphosphatemia (serum phosphorus concentration more than 5 mg/dl before treatment) are present. The phosphate salts lower the serum calcium concentration by inhibiting bone resorption and by forming a calcium-phosphate complex which is deposited in soft tissue and/or bone.

Fleet Phospho-Soda is a palatable phosphate preparation. Each teaspoonful (5 ml.) contains approximately 645 mg elemental phosphorus. One-half teaspoonful (2.5 ml), 2 times a day, can be prescribed as a starting dose. Not more than 5 ml 3 times a day (approximately 2 g of elemental phosphorus) should be prescribed. (Vomiting or diarrhea will occur when a large dose is used, and may even occur with very small doses.) The serum calcium concentration begins to decrease in approximately 1 to 3 days. However, a normal calcium concentration may not appear for approximately 10 days. Long-term oral phosphate therapy has been given to hyperparathyroid patients who cannot be treated surgically. However, extraskeletal calcification and pancreatitis may develop.

Other phosphate preparations are listed in Table 31–1.

Inorganic phosphate salts can also be given intravenously if an acute hypercalcemic crisis is present, or if the patient is comatose or is vomiting. A 0.1 molar solution of sodium phosphate and potassium biphosphate can be prepared in the hospital pharmacy. This contains 0.081 mole of dibasic sodium phosphate and 0.019 mole of monobasic potassium phosphate, dissolved in 1 liter of distilled water. The solution has a pH adjusted to 7.4, an osmolality of 240 mOsm/kg, and each liter contains 100 millimoles (3.1 g) of elemental phosphorus, 162 mEq sodium, and 19 mEq potassium ions.

The solution is given slowly intravenously over a period of approximately 12 hours. Not more than one infusion of phosphate salts should be given in a 24-hour period, and treatment should not be continued for more than 2 days. If renal disease is present, 15 to 30 millimoles of phosphorus, rather than 100 millimoles, should be infused, and the serum calcium and phosphorus concentrations should be checked frequently during the infusion.

The serum calcium concentration may begin to decrease in a few minutes. A normal calcium concentration usually appears within 24 hours. However, in some patients, the serum calcium concentration may not decrease to normal for almost a week. The serum phosphorus concentration rises because of the infusion of the phosphate salts. The effects of the phosphate infusions may last as long as 2 weeks.

Intravenous phosphate therapy can cause calcification in the vein used for the infusion, and metastatic calcification in various tissues. In addition, hypocalcemia with tetany or hypotension or shock may occur. Acute renal failure may also occur if the serum calcium concentration decreases acutely.

Sodium sulfate intravenously also lowers the serum calcium concentration rapidly by increasing the urinary excretion of calcium ions, similar to the action of sodium chloride infusion. It is less effective than the phosphate salts, and is probably no more effective than isotonic saline. It is given intravenously in an isotonic solution (38.9 g of sodium sulfate decahydrate per liter of water), in a dose of 1 to 4 L over a period of 9 to 5 hours. The infusion can be repeated the following day. The serum calcium concentration falls rapidly, but rises again within 72 hours.

Hypokalemia and hypomagnesemia may result from the sodium sulfate infusion. The hypokalemia can be prevented by adding 20 mEq potassium chloride to each liter of solution. The high sodium content of the solution (each liter contains 242 mEq sodium) can cause a marked rise in serum osmolality, associated with a high serum sodium concentration. This can produce mental confusion, stupor, convulsions, or coma. Congestive heart failure may also develop, because of the large amount of sodium ions infused.

Sodium sulfate solution must be prepared in the hospital pharmacy.

Corticosteroids have been found helpful in treating the hypercalcemia of patients with sarcoidosis, myelomas, lymphomas and leukemias. Patients with solid carcinomas are less responsive, and hyperparathyroid patients usually do not respond. The corticosteroids probably act by decreasing resorption of bone and reducing the intestinal absorption of vitamin D. The serum calcium concentration may not decrease for 1 to 2 weeks after the corticosteroids are given. In addition, prolonged use of corticosteroids will produce osteoporosis. Therefore, they should be used only for a limited time.

Prednisone can be given orally in a daily dose of 40 to 80 mg until a satisfactory decrease in serum calcium concentration occurs. Then the dosage is gradually reduced. Parenteral corticosteroid therapy is used mostly in patients with renal insufficiency and hypercalcemia who have not responded to other medical therapy. Hydrocortisone sodium succinate, 100 to 500 mg daily, or prednisolone sodium phosphate, 20 to 100 mg daily, can be given intramuscularly, intravenously, or preferably by intravenous infusion.

Mithramycin (Mithracin), a cytotoxic drug, is also able to lower the serum calcium concentration, probably by acting directly on the bones. One-fifth to one-tenth of the antineoplastic dose is used to minimize toxic reactions. The serum calcium concentration may not decrease for 24 to 48 hours after an intravenous injection, but it may remain normal for one to three weeks. Mithramycin is useful to treat hypercalcemia associated with neoplastic diseases.

Mithramycin can cause severe thrombocytopenia and bleeding, and liver and renal toxicity. It should not be used if the patient has pancytopenia, decreased liver function, or severe renal insufficiency.

Disodium EDTA (disodium edetate, endrate, sodium versenate), a chelating agent, can lower the serum calcium concentration rapidly. However, its effects are transient and it is nephrotoxic. This seriously limits its usefulness. A dose of 40 to 50 mg per kg body weight is infused in a liter of 5% dextrose in water or isotonic saline solution over a period of 4 to 6 hours. The total dose must not exceed 3 g.

Calcitonin can transiently lower the serum calcium concentration within several hours. However, its use for this purpose is still investigational. It also has been used, in conjunction with prednisone, to treat the hypercalcemia of parathyroid carcinoma.

Propranolol has recently been used to treat hypercalcemia due to hyperthyroidism (Rude and associates).

Treatment of Hyperparathyroidism. If a patient with primary hyperparathyroidism has significant hypercalcemia (greater than 1 mg/dl above the upper limits of normal and shows symptoms or signs of hypercalcemia, surgical removal of the parathyroid adenoma should be done.

Surgery for hyperparathyroidism is not always successful because an aberrant parathyroid adenoma may be missed at operation. In addition, a patient may refuse surgery. Also, a patient may have a coexisting medical problem that makes a neck operation a serious risk.

If medical therapy for hyperparathyroidism is necessary, the patient must be adequately hydrated and encouraged to walk. Diuretic therapy may be dangerous if dehydration develops. Thiazide diuretics particularly should be avoided because they reduce urinary calcium excretion and may cause the serum calcium concentration to rise. Also the patients should be on a low-calcium diet (p. 329).

Oral phosphates may be helpful (Table 31–1). Estrogens may be helpful in postmenopausal women with primary hyperparathyroidism. Diphosphonates have been used experimentally.

IDIOPATHIC HYPERCALCIURIA

Idiopathic hypercalciuria is a metabolic abnormality characterized by excessive 24-hour urinary calcium excretion (greater than 300 mg in males, 250 mg in females, on a normal diet). Hypercalcemia is *not* present, alkaline phosphatase level is normal, and the serum phosphate concentration is usually normal. Occasionally it is low.

Idiopathic hypercalciuria is the most common cause of calcium-containing kidney stones. An effective treatment is the long-term use of the thiazide diuretics, for example, hydrochlorothiazide (Hydro-DIURIL, Esidrix) 50 mg orally, twice a day. (Some patients may develop hypercalcemia on this regimen. If this occurs, it suggests that the hypercalciuria is not idiopathic but is due to latent hyperparathyroidism.)

PHOSPHORUS

Just as potassium ions are the major intracellular cations, phosphorus ions are the major intracellular anions. Phosphorus is found in the body in the form of inorganic and organic phosphate salts. However, only inorganic phosphate salts are present in the extracellular water and blood.

Phosphorus is needed in many stages of intermediary metabolism, in bone formation. It is a constituent of nucleic acids. It has an important role in the delivery of oxygen to the tissues by regulating the levels of 2,3, DPG (2,3 diphosphoglycerate), and ATP (adenosine triphosphate) in red blood cells. Therefore, when hypophosphatemia is present, these levels fall. This interferes with the oxygen exchange in the red blood cells. Greater binding of oxygen to hemoglobin occurs and there is a decreased release of oxygen from the red blood cells. This leads to cellular anoxia. The lowering of the ATP content of the bed blood cells may also cause hemolysis and a hemolytic anemia.

Phosphate ions are also an important buffer mechanism in the kidneys for the elimination of fixed acids. Hypophosphatemia also depresses the bactericidal, phagocytic, and chemostatic activity of the white blood cells and is one of the factors that decrease resistance to infections.

Phosphate homeostasis is affected by several hormonal mechanisms: Growth hormone and probably vitamin D increase phosphate reabsorption from the gastrointestinal tract and kidneys. Parathyroid hormone increases the excretion of phosphate ions by the kidneys. Parathyroid hormone and vitamin D shift phosphate ions from bone to the extracellular water.

Phosphate balance is maintained by an intake of approximately 1 gram of elemental phosphorus a day. Pregnant and lactating women have a greater need for phosphorus than other adults.

HYPOPHOSPHATEMIA

Hypophosphatemia or depletion of phosphate stores (phosphorus depletion syndrome) can occur from a loss of phosphate ions in the urine or intestines, from decreased absorption from the intestines, or from intracellular shifts of phosphate ions, and can be found in the following conditions:

1. Low intake of phosphorus-containing foods, such as milk, meat, vegetables, due to anorexia, starvation, vomiting, prolonged diarrhea.
2. Poor absorption from the gastrointestinal tract, due to a lack of vitamin D, or to steatorrhea.
3. Increased renal excretion of phosphate ions, as in primary or secondary hyperparathyroidism, hypokalemia, hypomagnesemia.
4. Excessive ingestion of phosphate-binding antacids, suh as magnesium-aluminum hydroxides (Amphogel, Gelusil, Maalox, and many other preparations).
5. Diabetic acidosis. The osmotic diuresis that occurs with the diabetic acidosis is associated with an increased excretion of phosphate ions in the urine.
6. Hyperventilation and acute respiratory alkalosis. When respiratory alkalosis occurs, carbon dioxide moves out of the cells to compensate for the loss of carbon dioxide in the extracellular water. As a result, the pH of the cells becomes higher. This is associated with an increased formation of phosphorylated carbohydrate compounds in the cells. As a result, the serum phosphate concentration falls.

    Hyperventilation is one of the causes of hypophosphatemia seen in patients with bacteremia due to gram-negative sepsis.
7. Renal tubular acidosis (Chap. 18).
8. Administration of insulin, glucose, glucagon, lactate salts, fructose, intravenous sodium chloride, sodium bicarbonate, or sodium lactate solutions, diuretics, anabolic steroids, corticosteroids, androgens, epinephrine.
9. Intravenous hyperalimentation. As the patient receives the intravenous nourishment, extensive tissue repair occurs, and phosphate ions are withdrawn from the blood and extracellular water into the cells.
10. Nutritional recovery syndrome. This occurs when persons who have been starved or severely malnourished, such as military prisoners or concentration camp victims, are suddenly given food with a high carbohydrate content. Edema, ascites, pleural effusions, and even death may occur, unless foods with a high phosphate content are included in the diet.

11. Alcoholic withdrawal. Chronic alcoholics who eat well do not show hypophosphatemia. However, severe hypophosphatemia can occur when alcohol is withdrawn suddenly. The mechanism by which this occurs is not clearly understood. Chronic alcoholics often have hypomagnesemia, which may be a factor in the loss of an excessive amount of phosphate ions in the urine.
12. Salicylate poisoning.
13. Acute gout.
14. The diuretic-recovery phase after a severe burn (see Chap. 9).
15. Primary hypophosphatemia.

Symptoms and Signs

Since phosphate ions are found in all cells, the symptoms and signs of phosphate loss and hypophosphatemia can involve numerous organ systems:

Central nervous system symptoms include mental irritability, apprehension, malaise, numbness, paresthesias around the mouth, dysarthria, confusion, obtundation, convulsive seizures, or coma. The clinical findings may resemble delirium tremens, but characteristic hallucinations of delirium tremens do not appear. (Both conditions may coexist.) Cranial nerve palsies may also develop.

Muscle weakness, myopathy, or rhabdomyolysis may occur. EMG abnormalities may be present. Gastrointestinal symptoms include anorexia and dysphagia. Skeletal symptoms include joint stiffness and aching bone pains. Osteomalacia and pseudofractures may also occur. Severe congestive heart failure may develop.

Laboratory Tests

The normal serum phosphate concentration ranges from 2.7 to 4.5 mg per dl. (The blood should be drawn before breakfast, to prevent a high phosphate concentration due to food.) When moderate hypophosphatemia is present, the serum phosphate concentration ranges from 1.0 to 2.5 mg per dl. When severe hypophosphatemia is present, the serum phosphate concentration is less than 1.0 mg per dl and may fall to even less than 0.2 mg per dl.

A hemolytic anemia may develop.

Treatment

An attempt should be made to eliminate the factors that can contribute to the hypophosphatemia (see Etiology, above). Phosphate salts should be included in an intravenous hyperalimentation regimen. Antacids containing aluminum or magnesium which bind phosphates should be eliminated.

Table 31–1.   Some Available Phosphate Salts for Oral Use

Name	Content of Elemental Phosphorus (P)	Content of Other Electrolytes
K-Phos Neutral	250 mg P per tablet	approx. 45 mg potassium and 298 mg sodium per tablet
Neutra-Phos-K	250 mg P per capsule	approx. 15 mEq potassium per tablet. No sodium.
Phospho-Soda	645 mg P per 5 ml (a teaspoonful)	approx. 40 mEq sodium ions per 5 ml

Numerous preparations containing phosphate ions are available (Table 31–1). One should remember that one 8-ounce glass (250 ml) of skim or low fat milk contains approximately 250 mg elemental phosphorus and is useful if a patient can tolerate oral feedings and if calcium salts are not contraindicated.

An attempt should be made to raise the serum phosphate concentration to between 3 and 4 mg per dl. This may require 1000 mg or more elemental phosphorus a day.

Contraindications to the use of phosphate salts include hypercalcemia from any cause, hyperphosphatemia (usually due to renal failure or hypoparathyroidism), oliguria, or obvious tissue necrosis.

REFERENCES

Calcium
Agna, J.W., and Goldsmith, R.E.: Primary hyperparathyroidism associated with hypomagnesemia. N Engl J Med, *258*:222, 1958.
Akgün, S., and Ertel, N.H.: Chloride:phosphate ratio in hypercalcemia. Comments. Ann Intern Med, *81*:129, 1974.
AMA Drug Evaluations: *Blood Calcium Regulators,* 3rd ed. Acton (Mass.), Publishing Sciences Group, 1977.
Annesley, T.M., et al.: Artifactual hypercalcemia in multiple myeloma, Mayo Clin Proc, *57*:572, 1982.
Arnaud, C.D.: Familial benign hypercalcemia. Nature's solution to neonatal hyperparathyroidism, editorial, Mayo Clin Proc, *59*:864, 1984.
Aro, A., et al.: Hypercalcemia. Serum chloride and phosphate, letter. Ann Intern Med, *86*:664, 1977.
Aurbach, G.D., et al.: Hyperparathyroidism. Recent studies. NIH Conference. Ann Intern Med, *79*:566, 1973.
Barzel, U.S.: The differential diagnosis of hypercalcemia. Ann Intern Med, *76*:825, 1972.
Barzel, U.S.: Calcitonin therapy for bone disease and hypercalcemia. Editorial, Arch Intern Med, *142*:2076, 1982.
Bayat-Mokhtari, F., et al.: Parathyroid storm, Arch Intern Med, *140*:1092, 1980.
Bechtel, J.T., White, J.E., and Estes, E.H., Jr.: The electrocardiographic effects of hypocalcemia induced in normal subjects with ethamil disodium. Circulation, *13*:837, 1956.
Bilezikian, J.P.: The medical management of primary hyperparathyroidism, Ann Intern Med, *96*:198, 1982.
Bilezikian, J.P., et al.: Pseudogout after parathyroidectomy. Lancet, *1*:445, 1973.
Brown, J.E., and Palmisano, D.J.: Rapid identification of parathyroid adenoma by angiography. JAMA, *231*:177, 1975.

Burman, K.D., et al.: Ionized and total serum calcium and parathyroid hormone in hyperthyroidism. Ann Intern Med, *84*:666, 1976.

Caulfield, J.B., et al.: Blood calcium levels in the presence of arteriographic contrast material. Circulation, *52*:119, 1975.

Chakmakjian, Z.H., and Bethune, J.E.: Sodium sulfate treatment of hypercalcemia. N Engl J Med, *275*:862, 1966.

Chaplin, H., Clark, L.D., and Ropes, M.W.: Vitamin D intoxication. Am J Med Sci, *221*:369, 1951.

Christensson, T., et al.: Hypercalcemia and primary hyperparathyroidism. Prevalence in patients receiving thiazides as detected in a health screen. Arch Intern Med, *137*:1138, 1977.

Coe, F.D.: Magnitude of metabolic acidosis in primary hyperparathyroidism. Arch Intern Med, *134*:262, 1974.

Cunliffe, W.J., et al.: A calcitonin-secreting thyroid carcinoma. Lancet, *2*:63, 1968.

Cushard, W.G., Jr., et al.: Parathyroid function in sarcoidosis. N Engl J Med, *286*:395, 1972.

Davies, P.: Vitamin D poisoning. Ann Intern Med, *53*:1250, 1960.

deMorgan, N.P., and Waterhouse, C.: A case of tertiary hyperparathyroid crisis. Am J Med Sci, *256*:322, 1968.

Dent, D.E.: Emergency treatment of hypercalcemia. Lancet, *2*:613, 1967.

DeTorrente, A., et al.: Hypercalcemia of acute renal failure. Am J Med, *61*:119, 1976.

Duarte, C.G., et al.: Thiazide-induced hypercalcemia. N Engl J Med, *284*:828, 1971.

Dudley, F.J.: Extraskeletal calcification complicating oral neutral phosphate therapy. Lancet, *2*:628, 1970.

Editorial: Tertiary hyperparathyroidism after renal transplantation. JAMA, *209*:2048, 1969.

Edmonson, J.W.: Relationship of serum ionized and total calcium in primary hyperparathyroidism. J Lab Clin Med, *87*:624, 1976.

Elias, E.G., and Evans, J.T.: Hypercalcemic crisis in neoplastic diseases. Management with mithramycin. Surgery, *71*:631, 1972.

Esselstyn, C., Jr., et al.: Hyperparathyroidism after radioactive therapy for Graves' disease, Surgery, *92*:811, 1982.

Fialkow, P.J., et al.: Multicellular origin of parathyroid adenomas. N Engl J Med, *297*:696, 1977.

Frame, B., and Haubrich, W.S.: Peptic ulcer and hyperparathyroidism. Arch Intern Med, *105*:536, 1960.

Gabow, P.A., et al.: Furosemide-induced reduction in ionized calcium in hypoparathyroid patients. Ann Intern Med, *86*:579, 1977.

Gallagher, J.C., and Nordin, B.E.C.: Treatment with oestrogens of primary hyperparathyroidism in postmenopausal women. Lancet, *1*:503, 1972.

Gardner, R.J., and Koppel, D.M.: Hyperparathyroid crisis. Arch Surg, *98*:674, 1969.

Ginsberg, H., and Schwartz, K.V.: Hypercalcemia and complete heart block. Ann Intern Med, *79*:903, 1973.

Goldsmith, R.S., and Ingbar, S.H.: Inorganic phosphate treatment of hypercalcemia of diverse etiologies. N Engl J Med, *274*:1, 1966.

Halver, B.: Phosphates and hypercalcemia, letter. JAMA, *233*:551, 1975.

Heath, H., III: What is "normal" serum calcium? Ann Intern Med, *77*:329, 1972.

Heckman, B.A., and Walsh, J.H.: Hypernatremia complicating sodium sulfate therapy for hypercalcemic crisis. N Engl J Med, *276*:1082, 1967.

Heinemann, H.O.: Metabolic alkalosis in patients with hypercalcemia. Metabolism, *14*:1137, 1965.

Hodgkinson, A., Peacock, M., and Nordin, B.E.C.: Asymptomatic hyperparathyroidism. Lancet, *2*:49, 1971.

Hossain, M.: Vitamin D intoxication during treatment of hypoparathyroidism. Lancet, *1*:1119, 1970.

Johnson, R.D., and Conn, J.W.: Hyperparathyroidism with a prolonged period of normocalcemia. JAMA, *210*:2063, 1969.

Kahil, M., et al.: Hypercalcemia. Experience with phosphate and sulfate therapy. JAMA, *201*:721, 1967.

Kaplan, E.L., et al.: Acid-base balance and parathyroid function. Metabolic alkalosis and hyperparathyroidism. Surgery, *70*:198, 1970.

Keynes, W.M., and Caird, F.I.: Hypocalcemic primary hyperparathyroidism. Br Med J, 1:208, 1970.

Kutner, F.R.: Parathyroid crisis. Arch Surg, *91*:71, 1965.

Lentz, R.D., et al.: Treatment of severe hypophosphatemia. Ann Intern Med, *89*:941, 1978.

Leonard, A., and Helms, R.J., Jr.: Hypercalcemia in diuretic phase of acute renal failure. Ann Intern Med, *73*:137, 1970.

Lerner, R.: Tenderness above parathyroid adenoma. JAMA, *221*:716, 1972.

Livesay, J.J., and Mulder, D.C.: Recurrent hyperparathyroidism. Arch Surg, *111*:688, 1976.

Low, J.C., et al.: Ionic calcium determination in primary hyperparathyroidism. JAMA, *223*:152, 1973.

Mahadevia, P.S., et al.: Hypercalcemia in prostatic carcinoma, Arch Intern Med, *143*:1339, 1983.

Mallette, L.E., et al.: Neuromuscular disease in secondary hyperparathyroidism. Ann Intern Med, *82*:474, 1975.

Marx, S.J., et al.: Familial hypocalciuric hypercalcemia. The relation to primary hyperparathyroidism. N Engl J Med, *307*:416, 1982.

Massry, S.G., et al.: Inorganic phosphate treatment of hypercalcemia. Arch Intern Med, *121*:307, 1968.

Massry, S.G., et al.: Metabolic acidosis of hyperparathyroidism. Arch. Intern Med, *134*:385, 1974.

McMillan, D.E., and Freeman, R.B.: The milk-alkali syndrome. Medicine, *44*:485, 1965.

Moreau, J-F., et al.: Localization of parathyroid tumors by ultrasonography, letter. N Engl J Med, *302*:582, 1980.

Moses, A.M., and Notman, D.D.: Secondary hyperparathyroidism caused by oral contraceptives. Arch Intern Med, *142*:128, 1982.

Muggia, F.M., and Heinemann, H.O.: Hypercalcemia associated with neoplastic disease. Ann Intern Med, *73*:281, 1970.

Muggia, F.M., Chia, G.A., and Mickley, D.W.: Hyperphosphatemia and hypocalcemia in neoplastic disorders. N Engl J Med, *290*:857, 1974.

Mundy, C.R., et al.: The hypercalcemia of cancer. N Engl J Med, *310*:1718, 1984.

Orwoll, E.S.: The milk-alkali syndrome. Current concepts. Ann Intern Med, *97*:242, 1982.

Nathaniels, E.K., Nathaniels, A.M., and Wang, C-A.: Mediastinal parathyroid tumors. Ann Surg, *171*:165, 1970.

Newmark, S.R., and Himathongkam, T.: Hypercalcemic and hypocalcemic crises. JAMA, *230*:1438, 1974.

Paloyan, E., and Lawrence, A.M.: Primary hyperparathyroidism. Pathology and therapy, Editorial. JAMA, *246*:1344, 1981.

Pak, C.Y., et al.: A simple and reliable test for the diagnosis of hyperparathyroidism. Arch Intern Med, *129*:48, 1972.

Palmer, F.J., et al.: The chloride-phosphate ratio in hypercalcemia. Ann Intern Med, *80*:200, 1974.

Petersen, P.: Psychiatric disorders in primary hyperparathyroidism. J Clin Endocr, *28*:1491, 1968.

Purnell, D.C., et al.: Primary hyperparathyroidism. A prospective clinical study. Am J Med, *50*:670, 1971.

Rubens, R.D., et al.: Dissimilar adenomas in four parathyroids presenting as primary hyperparathyroidism. Lancet, *1*:596, 1969.

Rude, R.K., et al.: Treatment of thyrotoxic hypercalcemia with propranolol. N Engl J Med, *294*:431, 1976.

Samaan, N.A., et al.: Hyperparathyroidism and carcinoid tumor. Ann Intern Med, *82*:205, 1975.

Sataline, L.R., Powell, C., and Hamwi, G.J.: Suppression of the hypercalcemia of thyrotoxicosis by corticosteroids. N Engl J Med, *267*:646, 1962.

Segal, A.J., Miller, M., and Moses, A.M.: Hypercalcemia during the diuretic phase of acute renal failure. Ann Intern Med, *68*:1066, 1968.

Shackney, S., and Hasson, J.: Precipitous fall in serum calcium, hypotension, and acute renal failure after intravenous phosphate therapy for hypercalcemia. Ann Intern Med, 66:906, 1967.

Shen, F-H., and Sherrard, D.J.: Lithium-induced hyperparathyroidism. Ann Intern Med, 96:63, 1982.

Sherwood, L.M.: Hypernatremia during sodium sulfate therapy. N Engl J Med, 277:314, 1967.

Siddiqui, A.A., and Wilson, D.R.: Primary hyperparathyroidism and proximal renal tubular acidosis. Canad Med Assoc J, 100:654, 1972.

Silva, O.L., and Becker, K.L.: Salmon calcitonin in the treatment of hypercalcemia. Arch Intern Med, 132:337, 1973.

Singer, F.R., et al.: Mithramycin treatment of intractable hypercalcemia due to parathyroid carcinoma. N Engl J Med, 283:634, 1970.

Spiegel, A.M., et al.: Intrathyroidal parathyroid adenoma or hyperplasia. An occasionally overlooked cause of surgical failure in primary hyperparathyroidism. JAMA, 234:1029, 1975.

Spiegel, A.M., et al.: Persistent hyperparathyroidism caused by incomplete parathyroid resection and a hyperfunctioning parathyroid autograft, JAMA, 250:1896, 1983.

Stamp, T.C.B.: The hypocalcemic effect of intravenous phosphate administration. Clin. Sci. 40:55, 1971.

Suki, W.N., et al.: Acute treatment of hypercalcemia with furosemide. N Engl J Med, 283:836, 1970.

Torring, O., et al.: Urinary cyclic AMP corrected for glomerular filtration rate in the differential diagnosis of hypercalcemia. Acta Med Scand, 211:401, 1982.

Turchi, J.J., et al.: Hyperparathyroidism and pancreatitis. JAMA, 180:799, 1962.

Twycross, R.G., and Marks, V.: Symptomatic hypercalcemia in thyrotoxicosis. Br Med J, 2:701, 1970.

Walsh, F.B., and Howard, J.E.: Conjunctival and corneal lesions in hypercalcemia. J Clin Endocr, 7:644, 1947.

Weinberger, A., et al.: Chlorthalidone-induced hypercalcemia. JAMA, 231:134, 1975.

Wells, S.A., Jr., et al.: Repeated neck exploration in primary hyperparathyroidism. Localization of abnormal glands by selective thyroid arteriography, selective venous sampling, and radioimmunoassay. Surgery, 74:678, 1973.

Wills, M.R., and McGowan, G.K.: Plasma chloride levels in hyperparathyroidism and other hypercalcemic states. Br Med J, 1:1153, 1964.

Wills, M.R., et al.: Normocalcemic primary hyperparathyroidism. Am J Med, 47:384, 1969.

Yendt, E.R.: Disorders of calcium, phosphorus, and magnesium metabolism. In *Clinical Disorders of Fluid and Electrolyte Metabolism*, 2nd ed. (Maxwell, M.H., and Kleeman, C.R., Eds.). New York, McGraw-Hill Book Co., 1972.

Zweig, J.I.: Treatment of hypercalcemia with etidronate disodium, letter, JAMA, 244:437, 1980.

Phosphorus

Betro, M.G., and Pain, R.W.: Hypophosphatemia and hyperphosphatemia in hospital population. Br Med J, 1:273, 1972.

Darsee, J.R., and Nutter, D.O.: Reversible severe congestive cardiomyopathy in three cases of hypophosphatemia. Ann Intern Med, 89:867, 1978.

Fisher, J., et al.: Respiratory illness and hypophosphatemia, Chest, 83:504, 1983.

Jacobs, H.D., and Amsden, T.: Acute hemolytic anemia with rigid red cells in hypophosphatemia. N Engl J Med, 285:1446, 1971.

Knochel, J.P.: The pathophysiology and clinical characteristics of severe hypophosphatemia. Arch Intern Med, 137:203, 1977.

Lichtman, M.A., Miller, D.R., and Freeman, R.B.: "Mountain sickness" at low altitude due to hypophosphatemia. N Engl J Med, 281:567, 1969.

Lotz, M., Zisman, E., and Bartter, F.C.: Evidence for a phosphorus-depletion syndrome in man. N Engl J Med, 278:409, 1968.

Ludwig, G.D., et al.: Tertiary hyperparathyroidism induced by osteomalacia resulting from phosphorus depletion. Am J Med, 43:136, 1967.

Schonfeld, Y., et al.: Hypophosphatemia as diagnostic aid in sepsis. New York State J Med, *82*:163, 1982.

Territo, M.C., and Tanaka, K.R.: Hypophosphatemia in chronic alcoholism. Arch Intern Med, *134*:445, 1974.

Young, D.S.: "Phosphorus" or "Phosphate", Editorial, Ann Intern Med, *93*:631, 1980.

Zamkoff, K.W., and Kirshner, J.J.: Marked hypophosphatemia associated with myelo-monocytic leukemia. Arch Intern Med, *140*:1523, 1980.

CHAPTER 32

SYNDROMES ASSOCIATED WITH HYPOMAGNESEMIA AND HYPERMAGNESEMIA

The human body contains a large store of magnesium ions. Like potassium, magnesium is found primarily intracellularly. Magnesium has many functions. It acts as an activator for all the enzymes that require thiamine pyrophosphate as a cofactor, and plays a role in both carbohydrate and protein metabolism.

The intravenous injection of magnesium sulfate in the dog causes peripheral muscular paralysis. This is due to the curare-like effect of magnesium. This effect is due to a decreased liberation of acetylcholine at the neuromuscular junction and at sympathetic ganglia. It can be antagonized by an excess of calcium and by anticholinesterases such as physostigmine or neostigmine, or by the simultaneous administration of potassium.

In addition, the central nervous depression caused by magnesium ions is so great that magnesium can be used as a general anesthetic.

Magnesium produces a fall in blood pressure and can cause cardiac arrest in diastole. Toxic electrocardiographic signs include a prolongation of the P–R interval, widening of the QRS interval, and premature ventricular contractions.

Although there are similarities between the actions of magnesium and calcium, there are also curious differences between these two ions. Both a low serum magnesium and a low serum calcium concentration increase neuromuscular irritability, and a high concentration of these ions has a reverse effect. Magnesium narcosis, produced by injecting a magnesium preparation, can be promptly antagonized by the parenteral administration of calcium. However, the toxic effects of hypomagnesemia can be aggravated by calcium or phosphorus in the diet.

Most of the factors that control magnesium metabolism are not known. In animals, hypomagnesemia, like hypocalcemia, stimulates the secretion of parathyroid hormone, so that the serum calcium concentration rises. In humans, hypomagnesemia may prevent the action

341

of parathyroid hormone on bones, so that hypocalcemia may develop as a result of the hypomagnesemia. The renal excretion of magnesium ions is probably under the control of aldosterone. The normal serum magnesium concentration varies from approximately 1.5 to 2.5 mEq/L (1.8 to 3.0 mg/dl). A portion of the magnesium, approximately 35%, is bound to protein.

The normal diet supplies approximately 25 mEq (3.1 g) of magnesium ions daily. This is slightly more than the normal daily requirement. A large source of dietary magnesium is the chlorophyll in green vegetables. It is plentiful in nuts and legumes, fruits such as bananas, grapefruits, and oranges, and also in peanut butter and chocolate.

The kidneys are able to conserve magnesium ions, so that renal excretion may be less than 1 mEq a day, even when the patient is on a magnesium-free diet.

HYPOMAGNESEMIA

Hypomagnesemia is present when the magnesium serum concentration is less than 1.5 mEq/L (1.8 mg/dl). However, when symptomatic hypomagnesemia is present, the serum magnesium concentration is usually less than 1 mEq/L. (One should remember that there is no direct correlation between serum magnesium concentration and the body stores of magnesium ions.)

Etiology

Hypomagnesemia can occur in the following situations:

1. Impaired intake of magnesium salts, or impaired intestinal absorption of magnesium salts. It is difficult to produce magnesium deficiency or hypomagnesemia by means of dietary restriction. However, it can occur with prolonged malnutrition or starvation, or when a patient is given magnesium-free fluids intravenously, in association with no oral intake of food, and/or with nasogastric suction, for more than a week.

   Impaired intestinal absorption of magnesium ions occurs in steatorrhea and other intestinal malabsorption syndromes. In these conditions, the magnesium ions are excreted in the stool in the form of magnesium soaps. A high calcium intake or a low protein intake exacerbates the loss of magnesium ions this way. Magnesium ions are also lost with diarrhea, gastrointestinal fistulas, and so on.

2. Excessive urinary excretion of magnesium ions. The usual cause of this is diuretic therapy with the loop or thiazide diuretics, or ammonium chloride. Hypomagnesemia produced this way may be clinically significant because many of these patients are also taking digitalis, and there is evidence that digitalis toxicity can be precipitated or aggravated by hypomagnesemia.

   Hypomagnesemia due to excessive urinary losses also occurs for 24 hours after major surgery. It also occurs in primary aldosteronism, diabetic acidosis, primary hyperparathyroidism and other hypercalcemic states, acute intermittent porphyria with the syndrome of inappropriate secretion of ADH, acute pancreatitis, acute renal failure during the diuretic phase, renal tubular acidosis, chronic renal disease.

3. Other causes. Hypomagnesemia may occur in hypoparathyroidism in association with hypocalcemia, or postoperatively when all four parathyroid glands are removed, possibly due to some internal shift of magnesium ions from the extracellular water into bones ("hungry bones"). Excessive lactation may produce hypomagnesemia. Finally, hypomagnesemia may occur from drugs such as amphotericin B, gentamycin, carbenicillin, cisplatin, and for unknown reasons.

4. Chronic alcoholism with or without cirrhosis or delerium tremens. This is a common cause of hypomagnesemia. It is due to reduced caloric intake, including reduced intake of magnesium-containing foods, intestinal malabsorption, even a direct effect of alcohol. (Hypomagnesemia may exacerbate the increased neuroirritability of patients with delirium tremens.)

The cause of the decreased serum concentration of magnesium is not always clear. During the treatment of a patient with diabetic acidosis, for example, part of the magnesium passes from the extracellular water into the cells, but part is also excreted in the urine and lost. In patients with chronic lesions, malnutrition may be associated with a decreased intake of magnesium in the food. Patients with steatorrhea excrete a large amount of magnesium soaps in the stool. Another factor that may contribute to the loss of magnesium ions is a high intake of calcium salts when the diet is lacking in magnesium salts, because absorption of magnesium ions from the intestines varies inversely with the uptake of calcium salts. In hyperthyroidism, there is an increased protein-bound fraction of magnesium. Aldosteronism may cause increased fecal as well as urinary loss of magnesium ions. Alcoholic patients may develop hypomagnesemia because of chronic inadequate food intake.

Hypokalemia and a negative potassium balance may also occur because a diet that is lacking in magnesium salts is usually lacking in potassium salts also. Hypomagnesemia may also be associated with hypocalcemia or hypophosphatemia.

Pathology

In animals, experimental magnesium deficiency has resulted in pathological changes in the heart, vascular system, kidneys, liver and brain. Necrotic lesions without calcification have been found in the kidney glomeruli and tubules. In addition, tubular degeneration and fibrosis with calcium casts in the medullary loops and collecting tubules have been observed.

Symptoms and Signs

Investigators are not agreed on the clinical picture which magnesium deficiency produces in humans. The following psychiatric and neurological symptoms and signs have been described: personality changes with agitation, mental depression or confusion, hallucinations (usually auditory or visual), convulsions (grand mal or multifocal), increased reflexes, clonus, a positive Babinski sign, coarse tremor, athetoid and/or choreiform movements, ataxia, nystagmus, tetany with a positive Chvostek sign (usually with a negative Trousseau sign), muscle fasciculations, muscle cramps, paresthesias of the feet and legs, abnormal electroencephalographic signs such as diffuse slow waves.

Cardiovascular signs include tachycardia with atrial or ventricular premature contractions, hypotension, vasomotor changes such as painful cold hands and feet or increased perspiration, and nonspecific T-wave changes in the electrocardiogram.

Gastrointestinal symptoms such as dysphagia may develop.

Hypomagnesemia and hypocalcemia may coexist, especially in patients with an excessive loss of gastrointestinal fluids. The tetany of some of these patients responds to calcium rather than magnesium salts.

Hypomagnesemia and hypercalcemia may also coexist, not only in hyperparathyroid patients but also in neoplastic patients with osteolytic metastases.

Hypomagnesemia, rather than hypokalemia, may be a factor in some patients with digitalis toxicity.

Treatment

In the present state of our knowledge, it is questionable whether a patient, such as one with diabetic acidosis during the course of treatment, requires treatment for the hypomagnesemia. A parenteral solution such as Butler's solution contains about 2 mEq/L of magnesium.

Hypomagnesemia can be treated with magnesium salts intramuscularly, intravenously, or orally. Magnesium sulfate (hydrated), the most commonly used magnesium salt, contains 8.13 mEq magnesium ions per gram.

Magnesium sulfate can be given intramuscularly in a dose of 2 g (16.3 mEq) (4 ml of a 50% solution) every 8 hours, for 3 or more days, when significant hypomagnesemia is present. Serial serum magnesium concentrations can be used to regulate the dosage.

Magnesium balance can be maintained by giving as little as 25 mEq magnesium ions (6 ml of 50% magnesium sulfate) daily, if there are no abnormal losses.

Repeated intramuscular injections should be given at different sites because the injections may be painful. Procaine hydrochloride (1%) can be added to the injection if a large dose is used.

Magnesium sulfate can also be given intravenously when severe hypomagnesemia, associated with convulsions for example, is present. A dose of 4 ml of 50% magnesium sulfate solution (16.3 mEq), diluted to 100 ml should be given in 10 minutes (Parfitt and Kleerekoper).

Magnesium sulfate can also be given IV as a 1% solution (by adding 10 ml of a 50% magnesium sulfate solution (40.7 mEq) to 490 ml of 5% dextrose in water), in a period of 4 to 6 hours.

In patients with normal renal function, up to 50 mEq elemental magnesium can be given IV over 4 to 6 hours not to exceed 100 mEq every 12 hours.

When renal insufficiency is present, the dose should be reduced by 25 or 50%, depending on the severity of the renal impairment.

Magnesium salts can also be given orally to counteract continuous excessive losses, as in steatorrhea. For example, magnesium sulfate 2 g (16.3 mEq) can be given 3 times a day without producing a diarrhea. Magnesium citrate solution, N.F., can also be used in a dose of 15 ml 3 times a day, for example. (Each 100 ml contains 1.5 to 1.9 g of magnesium oxide with citric acid and sodium bicarbonate for effervescence.)

The principal dietary sources of magnesium ions are green vegetables, nuts and legumes, and fruits, as mentioned above.

One should remember that even if magnesium is given to a patient with magnesium deficiency, symptoms and signs may not be relieved for 60 to 80 hours.

HYPERMAGNESEMIA

An excess of magnesium can cause cardiac effects, such as a prolonged P–R interval, prolonged QRS interval, tall T waves, various degrees of a–v block, or ventricular premature contractions.

Hypermagnesemia is present when the serum magnesium concentration rises above 2.5 mEq/L (3.0 mg/dl).

Etiology

The most common cause of hypermagnesemia is renal failure. This can be aggravated when such a patient is given either magnesium sulfate to control convulsions or one of the many commercial antacids which contain magnesium salts—Aludrox, Camalox, Delcid, Gaviscon, Gelusil, Kolantyl, Maalox, Mylanta, and others.

It is possible that some of the clinical signs of uremia are due to hypermagnesemia.

Hypermagnesemia may also occur in diabetic acidosis when water loss is severe. It has also been reported as a result of frequent magnesium sulfate enemas, used in congenital magacolon.

Hypocalcemia may occur in association with hypermagnesemia. This may be due to the suppressive effects of hypermagnesemia on parathyroid hormone secretion. Or the hypermagnesemia may be associated with a shift of calcium ions either into the intracellular space or into bone.

Clinical Signs

When the serum magnesium concentration is between 3 and 5 mEq/L, there is a tendency to hypotension due to peripheral dilatation. In addition, the patient may experience a sense of heat and thirst. Nausea and vomiting may also occur.

When the concentration is 5 to 7 mEq/L, drowsiness appears. Deep tendon reflexes are lost at a serum magnesium concentration of 7 mEq/L. The respiratory center is depressed at a concentration of 10 mEq/L. Coma occurs at a concentration of 12 to 15 mEq/L, and cardiac arrest at a concentration of 15 to 20 mEq/L.

Prophylaxis

Magnesium salts should not be given to patients with acute or chronic renal disease.

Treatment

Magnesium toxicity can be treated by correcting water loss, if it is present, improving renal function, if possible, and the parenteral use of calcium gluconate (page 314). Artificial respiration may be necessary if respiratory failure occurs. Hypermagnesemia can also be corrected by dialysis.

REFERENCES

Aikawa, J.K.: *The Relationship of Magnesium to Disease in Domestic Animals and Humans.* Springfield, Charles C Thomas, 1971.

Bar, R.S., et al.: Hypomagnesemic hypocalcemia secondary to renal magnesium wasting. A possible consequence of high-dose gentamycin therapy. Ann Intern Med, *82*:646, 1975.

Barton, C., et al.: Renal magnesium wasting associated with amphotericin B therapy. Am J Med, *77*:471, 1984.

Beller, G.A., et al.: Correlation of serum magnesium levels and cardiac digitalis intoxication. Am J Cardiol, *33*:225, 1974.

Breidahl, H.D., and Nayler, W.G.: Plasma ionized calcium in hypomagnesemia. Br Med J, *1*:662, 1968.

Burch, G.E., and Giles, T.D.: The importance of magnesium deficiency in cardiovascular disease. Am Heart J *94*:649, 1977.

Cholst, I.N., et al.: The influence of hypermagnesemia on serum calcium and parathyroid hormone levels in human subjects. N Engl J Med, *310*:1221, 1984.

Dyckner, T., and Wester, P.O.: Clinical significance of diuretic-induced magnesium loss. Pract. Cardiol, *10*:124, 1984.

Fankushen, D., Raskin, D., Dimichi, A., and Wallach, S.: The significance of hypomagnesemia in alcoholic patients. Am J Med, *37*:802, 1964.

Ferdinandus, J., et al.: Hypermagnesemia as a cause of refractory hypertension, respiratory depression, and coma. Arch Intern Med, *141*:669, 1981.

Flink, E.B.: Role of magnesium depletion in Wernicke-Korsakoff syndrome, letter. N Engl J Med, *298*:743, 1978.

Flink, E.B., and Jones, J.E., Editors: The pathogenesis and clinical significance of magnesium deficiency. Ann New York Acad Sci, *162*:705, 1969.

Gerlach, K., et al.: Symptomatic hypomagnesemia complicating regional enteritis. Gastroenterology, *59*:567, 1970.

Gerst, P.H., Porter, M.R., and Fishman, R.A.: Symptomatic magnesium deficiency in surgical patients. Ann Surg, *159*:402, 1964.

Hall, R.C.W.: Hypomagnesemia. Physical and psychiatric symptoms. JAMA, *224*:1749, 1973.

Hamed, I.A., and Lindeman, R.D.: Dysphagia and vertical nystagmus in magnesium deficiency. Ann Intern Med, *89*:222, 1978.

Iseri, L.T., and French, J.H.: Magnesium. Nature's physiologic calcium blacker. Editorial, Am Heart J, *108*:188, 1984.

Juna, D.: Clinical review. The clinical importance of hypomagnesemia. Surgery, *91*:510, 1982.

Lim, P.: Magnesium deficiency in patients on long term diuretic therapy for heart failure. Br Med J, *3*:626, 1972.

Lyman, N.W., et al.: Cisplatin-induced hypocalcemia and hypomagnesemia. Arch Intern Med, *140*:1513, 1980.

Massry, S.G., Coburn, J.W., and Kleeman, C.R.: Evidence for suppression of parathyroid gland activity by hypermagnesemia. J Clin Invest, *49*:1619, 1970.

McDonald, S.J., et al.: Magnesium metabolism in chronic renal failure. Clin Sci, *28*:107, 1965.

Monif, G.R.G., and Savory, J.: Iatrogenic maternal hypocalcemia following magnesium sulfate therapy. JAMA, *219*:1469, 1972.

Mordes, J.P., et al.: Extreme hypermagnesemia as a cause of refractory hypotension. Ann Intern Med, *83*:657, 1975.

Parfitt, A.M., and Kleerekoper, M.: Clinical disorders of calcium, phosphorus, and magnesium metabolism. In *Clinical Disorders of Fluid and Electrolyte Metabolism,* 3rd ed. Edited by M.H. Maxwell and C.R. Kleeman, New York, McGraw-Hill Book Co., 1980.

Potts, J.T., Jr., and Roberts, B.: Clinical significance of magnesium deficiency and its relation to parathyroid disease. Am J Med Sci., *235*:206, 1958.

Randall, R.E., Jr., et al.: Hypermagnesemia in renal failure. Ann Intern Med, *61*:73, 1967.

Rosler, A., and Rabinowitz, D.: Magnesium-induced reversal of vitamin D resistance in hypoparathyroidism. Lancet, *1*:803, 1973.

Sawyer, R.B., et al.: Postoperative magnesium metabolism. Arch Surg, *100*:343, 1970.

Seelig, M.S., and Berger, A.R.: Range of normal serum magnesium values. N Engl J Med, *290*:974, 1974.

Shils, M.E.: Experimental human magnesium depletion. Medicine, *48*:61, 1969.

Smith, W.O., and Hammarsten, J.F.: Intracellular magnesium in delirium tremens and uremia. Am J Med Sci, *237*:413, 1959.

Specter, M.J., et al.: Studies on magnesium's mechanism of action in digitalis-induced arrhythmias. Circulation, *52*:1001, 1975.

Triger, D.R., and Jockes, A.M.: Severe muscle cramps due to acute hypomagnesemia in hemodialysis. Br Med J, *2*:804, 1969.

Vallee, B.L., Wacker, W.E.C., and Ulmer, D.D.: The magnesium-deficiency tetany syndrome in man. N Engl J Med, *262*:155, 1960.

Wacker, W.E.C., Moore, F.D., Ulmer, D.D., and Vallee, B.L.: Normocalcemic magnesium deficiency tetany. JAMA, *180*:161, 1962.

Wacker, W.E.C., and Parisi, A.F.: Magnesium metabolism. N Engl J Med, *278*:658, 712, 772, 1968.

Wan-chun, C., et al.: ECG changes in early stage of magnesium deficiency, letter. Am Heart J, *104*:1115, 1982.

Wong, E.T., et al.: A high prevalence of hypomagnesemia and hypermagnesemia in hospitalized patients. Am J Clin Path, *79*:348, 1983.

Wiegmann, T., and Kaye, M.: Hypomagnesemic hypocalcemia. Arch Intern Med, *137*:953, 1977.

Wilson, T.A., et al.: Hypermagnesemia, serum calcium, and parathyroid hormone levels, letter. N Engl J Med, *311*:601, 1984.

Zimmet, P.: Role of magnesium in tetany. N Engl J Med, *279*:109, 1968.

PART 5

THE PRINCIPLES OF FLUID THERAPY

CHAPTER 33

GENERAL PRINCIPLES OF WATER AND ELECTROLYTE THERAPY

In the preceding pages of this book, it has been emphasized that the *patient* must be treated, not an electrolyte or chemical disturbance. In this way, the physician will avoid many errors in therapy, which would otherwise result.

The aims of water and electrolyte therapy are:

1. To treat shock.
2. To replace electrolyte and water deficits.
3. To provide water, electrolytes, and nutriments for maintaining the daily needs of the patient.
4. To avoid creating new disturbances as a result of the therapy.

In the previous chapters, the daily requirements of water and the various electrolytes have been described. This information can now be summarized.

ROUTE OF ADMINISTRATION

Food and fluids should be given by the oral route (either by mouth or by nasogastric tube). If this is not possible, intravenous therapy, rather than subcutaneous therapy (hypodermoclysis), should be used.

Hypodermoclysis

Hypodermoclysis is the administration of a solution subcutaneously. The most commonly used solution for this purpose is isotonic sodium chloride solution, with or without 5% dextrose. Stronger strengths of dextrose should not be used. Half-isotonic (0.45%) sodium chloride solution, with or without 5% dextrose can also be used. Other solutions that can be given subcutaneously are Darrow's solution, Ringer's solution, lactated Ringer's solution, and 1/6 molar sodium lactate. However, dextrose in water, or any solution without sodium chloride or other extracellular electrolyte in at least half-isotonic concentration, should never be given subcutaneously. If this is done, extracellular water and electrolytes will diffuse into the hypodermoclysis area. When this happens, the circulating blood volume will decrease and shock may occur or become aggravated.

The lateral chest, lateral abdomen, or lateral thigh areas can be used for the hypodermoclysis.

When one needle is used for the hypodermoclysis, 250 to 500 ml of the solution can be administered in 1 hour. This volume can be doubled by injecting the solution in two separate areas.

The rate of absorption of the solution can be greatly increased by injecting the enzyme hyaluronidase into the injection area. One hundred fifty turbidity reducing units (1 ml) can be used for each liter of solution injected. Hypodermoclysis is valuable when it is impossible to find a patient's vein. However, the procedure may allow a staphylococcus skin infection to develop.

RATE OF ADMINISTRATION

The rate of administration depends on the need for fluids and the nature of the fluid. It is important for the physician to prescribe exactly how fast the fluid should be given intravenously. Infusion sets from various manufacturers deliver different-sized drops. Therefore, it is necessary to know how many drops are required to deliver 1 ml of fluid.

The rate of administration of fluids intravenously can be determined from the following rule:

drops per minute × drop factor = ml per hour.

The *drop factor* is obtained by dividing 60 by the number of drops that are needed to deliver 1 ml. For example, if 15 drops from an infusion set deliver 1 ml, the drop factor is 60/15 = 4. Therefore, if the infusion drips at a rate of 25 drops per minute, 25 × 4 = 100 ml of fluid will be infused in 1 hour. If a different infusion set is used with a smaller aperture, so that 20 drops are required to deliver 1 ml (drop factor 60/20 = 3) and the infusion drips at a rate of 25 drops per minute, only 75 ml (25 × 3) will be infused in 1 hour.

If the number of drops that deliver 1 ml is not known, one can assume that the drop factor is 4. However, the volume of fluid infused in 1 hour should be checked with the number of drops flowing per minute.

Microdrip bulbs are also available. They deliver 60 drops per minute. Such microdrip bulbs are helpful when a "KVO" ("Keep vein open") order is written and one does not want an excessive amount of fluid infused. (When a microdrip bulb is used, the 24-hour intravenous fluid volume can be maintained at approximately 350 ml. If a regular drip bulb had been used, the patient would receive a liter or more in this time.)

DAILY WATER AND ELECTROLYTE REQUIREMENTS

Daily Water Requirements

Approximately 30 ml per kg body weight (15 ml per pound). Thus, a 70-kg adult would require 2000 ml water daily.

Fever will increase the water needs by approximately 15% for each 1° C rise in the patient's temperature.

Daily Electrolyte Requirements

Sodium, 100 mEq (5.9 g NaCl) (also see below). If fever and sweating are present, sodium chloride will be needed in addition to water. It is difficult to determine volume losses of sweat (which may vary from 0 to 1000 ml per hour). A significant volume of sweat will be lost if the patient's temperature is above 38.3° C (101° F), or if the room temperature is 32° C (90° F) or higher.

One can replace the lost sweat by infusing 1 part isotonic saline solution and 2 parts dextrose in water (or a solution of one-third strength saline) which has the approximate composition of sweat. The daily volume needed may vary from 500 to 2000 ml.

Potassium, 60 mEq daily (4.5 g KCl). If fever or sweating is present, 4 mEq more potassium ions will be needed.

Magnesium, 8 to 20 mEq daily (1 to 3 g $MgSO_4$).

The use of multiple electrolyte solutions is described below.

Calorie Requirements

During fasting, an average 70-kg male loses approximately 80 g of body protein daily. If 100 g or more of dextrose are given, the protein loss decreases by one-half. Therefore, 100 to 150 g of dextrose should be infused daily when the patient is not able to eat. This supplies 340 to 510 kilocalories (kcal). (One gram of *hydrous* dextrose supplies 3.4 kcal.) This is equivalent to 1000 to 1500 ml of a 10% solution of dextrose in water, or 2000 to 3000 ml of a 5% solution.

(One gram of carbohydrates provides 4 kcal, 1 g of ethyl alcohol provides 7 kcal; 1 g of fat provides 9 kcal; and 1 g of protein provides 4 kcal.)

When a patient is unable to eat or drink for a period of 4 to 8 days, a high calorie solution can be infused, with or without electrolytes, as needed. For example, a solution of 20% dextrose in water provides 200 g of dextrose—680 kcal per liter. Two liters will therefore provide 1360 kcal. This is adequate to prevent ketosis and the breakdown of protein temporarily. However, such a concentrated dextrose solution is irritating and will frequently cause a local thrombophlebitis or thrombosis when it is used for more than several days. Therefore, it should be infused, if possible, into a large vein, such as the subclavian vein or superior vena cava.

Regular crystalline insulin can be added to such a concentrated dextrose solution to increase the metabolism of the infused dextrose and to decrease hyperglycemia and/or glycosuria. Usually, 1 unit of regular insulin to every 4 g of dextrose is used. When a concentrated dextrose solution infusion is stopped, it should be followed by an infusion of 5 to 10% dextrose solution, to prevent a reactive hypoglycemia.

(Insulin is stable in a solution of 5 or 10% dextrose in water, with or without electrolytes. However, up to 30% of the added insulin can adhere to the glass infusion flask or to the intravenous tubing. This insulin never reaches the patient. However, this can be overcome (see page 236). The insulin, of course, can be given intramuscularly or subcutaneously.)

A liter of 5% amino acids in 5% dextrose in water can also be infused daily when the patient has not been able to eat for several days.

Commercial solutions containing ethyl alcohol can be used for short-term intravenous infusions, because each 1 g ethyl alcohol provides 7 kcal.

When a patient is unable to eat for 8 or more days, nasogastric tube feeding with ordinary liquefied food and added vitamin supplements, or with an elemental diet, can be used. An alternative is peripheral parenteral nutrition (see below), or total parenteral nutrition (intravenous hyperalimentation). Tube feedings or total parenteral nutrition can be continued for months.

Protein Requirements

40 g a day. This can be supplied by 1000 ml of 5% amino acids in 5% dextrose.

Vitamins

A daily dose of 2 ml parenteral vitamin B complex and 500 mg vitamin C can be added to the infusion.

Summary

Therefore, the following solutions can be given daily for the first 2 or 3 days:

1. 1500 ml 10% dextrose in water.
2. 500 ml isotonic sodium chloride (or lactated Ringer's) solution in 5% dextrose.
3. 3 g potassium chloride (added to a liter of the dextrose solution, or to the sodium chloride solution).
4. Vitamin B complex, 2 ml; vitamin C, 500 mg, added to one of the infusion bottles.
5. If there is fever, add 500 ml 10% dextrose in water, plus 500 ml isotonic sodium chloride solution.

If the patient is receiving parenteral therapy for 3 or more days and is not taking food orally, 1000 ml 5% amino acids in 5% dextrose in water can be added.

One should remember that errors may occur in calculating fluid intake and output: a liter bottle of an intravenous fluid may actually contain 1100 ml, a pint bottle of blood or plasma may contain 600 ml and a sip of water or mouth rinsing, if repeated often, may add up to 1000 ml per day.

CHARTING WATER AND ELECTROLYTE BALANCES

It is important to keep accurate and adequate records of the patient's water and electrolyte intake and output. If this is done, the physician will frequently be able to prevent many of the water and electrolyte syndromes from developing.

In the research laboratory, complicated measurements can be done. In the hospital, simple methods must be used. The following simple procedures are of great value:

1. Daily weight, if possible.
2. Daily intake of both water and electrolytes.
3. Daily urine volume, including the specific gravity (or osmolality) of the urine.
4. Serum sodium, potassium, bicarbonate (CO_2 content), chloride, and osmolality determinations, on admission and as often as necessary.

REFERENCES

Abbott, W.E., Levey, S., Foreman, R.C., Krieger, H., and Holden, W.D.: Danger of administering parenteral fluids by hypodermoclysis. Surgery, *32*:305, 1952.

Bridenbaugh, P.O., et al.: Limitations of lactated Ringer's solution in massive fluid replacement. JAMA, *206*:2313, 1968.

Brooke, C.E., and Anast, C.S.: Oral fluid and electrolytes. JAMA, *179*:792, 1962.

Gamble, J.L.: *Chemical Anatomy, Physiology and Pathology of Extracellular Fluid,* 6th ed. Cambridge, Harvard University Press, 1954.

Glick, S.M.: Insulin. Not recommended in infusions. JAMA, *230*:468, 1974.

Rigor, B., Bosomworth, P., and Rush, B.F., Jr.: Replacement of operative blood loss of more than 1 liter with Hartmann's solution. JAMA, *203*:399, 1968.

Tarail, R.: Practice of fluid therapy. JAMA, *171*:131, 1959.
Trudnowski, R.J.: Hydration with Ringer's lactate solution. JAMA, *195*:545, 1966.
Weisberg, H.F.: *Electrolyte and Acid-Base Balance,* 2nd ed. Baltimore, Williams & Wilkins, 1962.
Wilson, M.G., and Tovey, G.H.: Graphic fluid-balance chart. Lancet, *1*:1207, 1961.

CHAPTER 34

PARENTERAL THERAPY IN SURGICAL PATIENTS

PATHOPHYSIOLOGY

A major surgical operation, trauma, or other acute stress can produce numerous physiological changes, including the following:

Even before an operation, there is increased sympathetic stimulation and increased secretion, of catecholamines (epinephrine and norepinephrine), which last at least 2 to 3 days and are associated with tachycardia, vasoconstriction, and an increased blood sugar, even to diabetic levels.

Stimulation of the anterior pituitary gland causes numerous effects. Increased secretion of anterior pituitary growth hormone also raises the blood sugar level. More important, an increased secretion of ACTH (corticotropin) occurs. This stimulates the adrenal glands to secrete large amounts of hydrocortisone and other corticosteroids to combat the stress. This hypersecretion lasts for approximately 1 to 2 days or more.

In addition, the stress stimulates the posterior pituitary gland to secrete ADH. As a result, water retention occurs and the urinary output the first day postoperatively may become as low as 500 ml or less. The serum sodium concentration also becomes low due to the dilution of the plasma with water. The hypersecretion of ADH usually lasts approximately 2 to 4 days.

Increased secretion of aldosterone by the adrenal glands also occurs. This is partly due to stimulation of the adrenals by ACTH. Aldosterone secretion also occurs as a result of the decreased circulating blood volume and/or loss of extracellular fluids which are often present after a major operation. The aldosterone secretion causes an increased diuresis of potassium ions, and a retention of sodium ions. However, the serum sodium concentration remains low. The increased aldosterone secretion usually also lasts 2 to 4 days.

There may also be a marked increase in oxygen consumption and a

357

rise in body temperature, so that the caloric needs after a major surgical operation may rise to more than 3000 kcal a day, for the first 4 to 5 days. These calories are usually supplied by the metabolism of body fat. For example, 250 to 500 g of fat can be oxidized daily after major surgery. Since each gram of fat produces 9 kcal, 250 g of fat would produce 2250 kcal. The oxidation of lean muscle also occurs. (Each gram of protein provides 4 kcal.) As a result, a patient usually loses 0.5 kg daily in the first 5 days after surgery.

Disturbances in water and electrolyte balance also occur postoperatively. The antidiuresis due to ADH has already been mentioned. The metabolism of body fat and protein produces approximately 460 ml water of oxidation daily (Chap. 3). In addition, there is a moderate retention of sodium and chloride ions and a loss of potassium ions (due to aldosterone). These electrolyte changes usually disappear within three to six days.

WATER AND ELECTROLYTE SYNDROMES IN SURGICAL PATIENTS

Preoperative Water and Electrolyte Management

It is not unusual for preoperative patients to have severe water and/or electrolyte losses due to inadequate intake of water or food, vomiting, nasogastric suction, diarrhea, diuretics, and so on. These losses should be replaced prior to surgery, to prevent hypotension or acute renal failure during or immediately after the operation.

Intraoperative Fluid Therapy

Many different routines are used for giving IV fluids intraoperatively. These range from no fluids at all in minor operations to various combinations of saline, other electrolytes, blood, and colloid expanders. The apparent success of these various regimens indicates that patients can adapt to various fluid and electrolyte treatment.

The following regimen (adapted from Giesecke) applies to adult patients with no preexisting fluid or electrolyte imbalance. It may require changes depending on the clinical situation.

Stage 1. At the start of a general anesthesia, a 70-kg patient can receive 500 ml of 5% dextrose in water in the first 30 to 45 minutes of anesthesia.

A patient who has been without oral intake for 6 or more hours ("NPO after midnight" order) will show an insensible water loss of 2 ml/kg/hr. This can be replaced with the above hypotonic maintenance solution.

Stage 2. The IV replacement treatment depends on the type of surgery.

A. *Hypotonic Maintenance* fluid therapy, using 5% dextrose in water, or 0.45% sodium chloride solution in 5% dextrose in water, given at a rate of 2 ml/kg/hr, is continued in patients when there is minimal loss of blood or fluids.

Such operations include most ophthalmic surgery, cystoscopy, and so on.

B. Minimal *replacement* fluid therapy using lactated Ringer's solution with or without 5% dextrose, 0.9% sodium chloride (full strength saline), or similar solutions, given at a rate of 6 ml/kg/hr.

Such operations include those with minimal surgical traumas, such as tonsillectomy, plastic operations, and so on.

C. Moderate *replacement* fluid therapy, using lactated Ringer's solution with or without 5% dextrose, 0.9% sodium chloride, or similar solutions given at a rate of 8 ml/kg/hr.

Such operations include herniorrhaphy, appendectomy (without peritonitis), thoracotomy, and so on.

D. Severe *replacement* fluid therapy using lactated Ringer's solution with or without 5% dextrose, 0.9% sodium chloride, or similar solutions, given at a rate of 10 ml/kg/hr.

Such operations include bowel resection for intestinal obstruction, total hip replacement, radical mastectomy, and so on.

Regardless of the type of surgery, the patient's vital signs and circulation should be continuously monitored. A urine output of 1 ml/kg/hr should be maintained.

Special operations require changes in this regimen. For example 5% dextrose in water should be omitted in a transurethral prostatectomy because such patients will absorb a large amount of hypotonic irrigating solution during the resection. Such patients should receive initially lactated Ringer's solution with or without 5% dextrose, 0.9% sodium chloride or similar solutions.

Similarly, additional fluids must be given IV for third space fluid losses.

Third-Space Fluid Losses

In addition, so-called "third-space" fluid losses, due to sequestration of fluids in the body, may be present. This can occur in the following conditions: acute intestinal obstruction (as much as 5 liters or more can accumulate within the lumen of the obstructed intestines); acute gastric dilatation; acute peritonitis, or acute pancreatitis; burns, crush injuries, acute spreading cellulitis; following abdominal surgery, particularly pelvic surgery (the fluid accumulates in the peritoneum, bowel wall and other traumatized tissues); and following surgery on the abdominal aorta after the aortic clamp has been released *(declamping phenomenon)* (the fluid accumulates in the ischemic lower extremities).

The sequestration of fluids in these patients will decrease the circulating blood volume and produce signs of hypotension or shock, since, when plasma exudes out of the bloodstream into a sequestered third space, the red blood cells are now suspended in a smaller volume of plasma. Therefore, the hematocrit rises. This rise in hematocrit can be used to determine the extent of the plasma loss, *vis:*

Plasma deficit (ml) = Normal blood volume −

$$\frac{\text{Normal bl vol.} \times \text{Normal (or initial) HCT.}}{\text{Measured HCT.}}$$

It is assumed that the normal blood volume equals approximately 7% of body weight, and that the normal hematocrit is 45%.

Example: Patient with acute intestinal obstruction, weight 70 kg. Measured HCT, 55%. The normal blood volume in this patient is 70,000 × 0.07 = 4900 ml

$$\text{Plasma deficit} = 4900 - \frac{4900 \times 0.45}{0.55}$$

$$= 4900 - 4000$$

$$= 900 \text{ ml}$$

Theoretically, a third-space fluid loss should be treated with plasma or another colloid solution. However, as was pointed out in the treatment of burns (Chap. 9), this may not be necessary. A multiple electrolyte solution, such as lactated Ringer's solution, can be infused instead. The volume of solution needed can be calculated in a general way by infusing 2½ times the estimated plasma volume deficit.

Thompson and his associates have used the following regimen for their patients undergoing major aortoiliac reconstructive surgery: At the start of the operation, a liter of 5% dextrose in lactated Ringer's solution is infused rapidly as the abdomen is opened and the initial dissection is started. Then the solution is given throughout the operation at a rate of 500 ml for every hour of surgery. Blood loss is replaced volume for volume simultaneously with the infusion. The patient also receives approximately 250 ml of 5% dextrose in water during surgery.

The principal criterion for the rate of infusion of the lactated Ringer's solution during the operation is to maintain a satisfactory blood pressure without using vasoconstrictors, and a urinary output between 30 and 50 ml per hour.

Similar third-space fluid losses occur in medical patients with marked ascites or pleural effusion. However, the decreased circulating blood volume and hypotension occur after the sequestered fluid has been rapidly removed, because the fluid reaccumulates quickly. It is better to treat these patients medically, using water restriction if necessary, digitalis if indicated, increasing the sodium content of the diet, and so on.

Blood Losses

During the operation, blood loss can be calculated in the following ways:

If 500 ml or more of blood is lost, it should be replaced immediately. (If whole blood cannot be given because of a patient's religious convictions, for example, lactated Ringer's solution can be infused, equal to 2½ times the volume of blood lost. However, if more than 1000 or 1200 ml of blood has been lost, the patient should also receive supplemental plasma or another colloid solution, to maintain the circulation. No specific rules can be given for the volume of colloid solution needed. Empirically, one can give 500 ml colloid solution for each 1500 ml lactated Ringer's solution infused.)

A simple way to estimate blood loss during a surgical operation is to weigh the sponges before and after use. The difference in grams is equivalent to the volume in ml of blood they have absorbed. Add to this the volume of blood in the operating-room suction bottle. Then increase the total by one-half, to approximate the actual blood loss.

Postoperative Water and Electrolyte Management

There is also controversy about the volume and type of intravenous fluids needed postoperatively. The immediate goal of postoperative fluid therapy is to maintain a blood pressure of approximately 90/60, a pulse rate of less than 120 per minute, and an hourly urine flow between 30 and 50 ml in association with an adequate level of consciousness, pupillary size, patent airway and breathing pattern, warm skin and skin color, and normal body temperature (Shires).

If an uncomplicated operation has been performed, and if there have been no third-space fluid losses and if acute renal failure is not anticipated, it is necessary only to supply an adequate amount of water. If the patient is able to take 500 ml water by mouth and retain it the first day, there is no need for parenteral water. However, if an abdominal or anastomotic operation has been performed and oral intake is forbidden, from 500 to 1000 ml of water is adequate.

Water needs will be greater if fever, dyspnea, or other causes of water loss are present. Similarly, electrolytes will be needed if abnormal electrolyte losses are present. For example, nasogastric suction drainage can be replaced volume for volume with half-strength saline solution. (Each liter contains 77 mEq sodium and 77 mEq chloride ions.) Potassium chloride should not be added the first postoperative day. From the second postoperative day, 20 mEq potassium ions (1.5 g of potassium chloride) per liter can be added to the half-strength saline solution.

When pyloric obstruction or postoperative malfunction of a gastrointestinal stoma is present, massive volumes of gastric juice can be withdrawn by nasogastric suction. Attempts to replace this loss with a large volume of intravenous fluids, particularly sodium- and potassium-free fluids such as dextrose in water, can cause a self-perpetuating, abnormal, high-output, high-intake cycle that is similar to the situation that may develop during the diuretic phase of acute renal failure when too many fluids are given intravenously. Electrolyte balance does not occur in these patients with a large volume of gastric aspirate. Instead, water excess with hyponatremia, hypochloremia, and hypokalemia may develop, and renal blood flow may decrease, so that the BUN concentration may rise and urine output may decrease.

Berry suggests that when the gastric aspirate reaches 2500 ml or more in a 24-hour period, the nasogastric suction should be stopped temporarily, the volume of intravenous fluids should be decreased one-half, and the patient's clinical condition and electrolyte concentrations should be carefully observed. If severe water excess has developed, hypertonic sodium chloride intravenously may be necessary. If mechanical gastrointestinal obstruction is present, it must be corrected surgically.

Some surgeons give isotonic sodium chloride solution postoperatively or lactated Ringer's solution, even on the first postoperative day. I prefer to use a solution of quarter-strength sodium chloride solution in dextrose. Each liter supplies water and, in addition, 38.5 mEq sodium and 38.5 chloride ions. Most postoperative patients are able to tolerate this amount of sodium chloride without developing pulmonary edema or edema of the lower extremities. (This volume should be considered as part of the total water intake.)

By the second or third postoperative day, the routine maintenance requirements, described on page 353, can be supplied.

If a complicated operation has been performed with third-space losses or if there is a possibility of acute renal failure, a large amount of fluids and electrolytes may be required to prevent hypotension and renal failure.

Thompson uses the following regimen *postoperatively* for his patients who have undergone abdominal aortic surgery:

1. The intravenous fluids are continued at a rate of approximately 125 ml per hour. The rate of infusion is varied, depending on the blood pressure, urinary output, and any unusual extrarenal losses.
2. In the first 24 hours postoperatively, the patient receives approximately 1 liter of lactated Ringer's solution and 2½ liters of 5% dextrose in water.
3. In the second 24 hours postoperatively, the patient receives approxi-

mately 500 ml of 5% dextrose in *isotonic sodium chloride,* and 2000 ml of 5% dextrose in water.

4. On the third postoperative day, the nasogastric tube is removed and fluids are given orally, but 1 to 2 liters of 5% dextrose in water are infused. Thereafter the infusions are stopped.

Many other water, electrolyte, and acid-base syndromes may occur in surgical patients. Acute respiratory acidosis may occur during operation; metabolic acidosis is common after any general surgical operation; operations on the upper gastrointestinal tract may induce an acute hypokalemic alkalosis; respiratory alkalosis is common, particularly if the patient is receiving assisted respiration; the liberal administration of fluids intravenously to postoperative patients frequently produces hyponatremia due to water excess and occasionally water intoxication. These have been discussed in the various chapters of the book.

REFERENCES

Berry, R.E.L.: The "third kidney" phenomenon of the gastrointestinal tract. A complication of parenteral fluid therapy and intestinal trauma. Arch Surg, *81*:193, 1960.

Duncalf, D., and Underwood, P.S.: Transfusion during and after surgical operations. In H. Laufman and R.B. Erichson (Eds) *Hematologic Problems in Surgery,* Philadelphia, W.B. Saunders Co., 1970.

Gaensler, E.A.: Respiratory acidosis as seen following surgery. Am J Surg, *103*:289, 1962.

Giesecke, A.H.: Perioperative fluid therapy-crystalloids. In R.D. Miller (Ed.) *Anesthesia,* New York, Churchill Livingstone, vol 2, 1981.

Goggin, M.J., and Joekes, A.M.: Gas exchange in renal failure. 1. Dangers of hyperkalemia during anaesthesia. Br Med J, *2*:244, 1971.

Gollub, S., et al.: Electrolyte solution in surgical patients refusing transfusion. JAMA, *215*:2077, 1971.

Hogbin, B.M., et al.: An evaluation of peripheral essential amino acid infusion following major surgery. J Parenteral and Enteral Nutrition, *8*:511, 1984.

Irvin, T.T., et al.: Plasma volume deficits and salt and water excretion after surgery. Lancet, *2*:1159, 1972.

Lauria, J.I.: Intraoperative management of fluid deficits. New York State J Med, *72*:691, 1972.

Mason, E.E.: *Fluid Electrolyte and Nutrient Therapy in Surgery.* Philadelphia, Lea & Febiger, 1974.

Moore, F.D.: *Metabolic Care of the Surgical Patient.* Philadelphia, W.B. Saunders Co., 1959.

Moran, W.H., Jr., Miltenberger, F.W., Shuaby, W.A., and Zimmerman, B.: The relationship of antidiuretic hormone secretion to surgical stress. Surgery, *56*:99, 1964.

Orloff, M.J., and Hutchin, P.: Fluid and electrolyte response to trauma and surgery. In *Clinical Disorders of Fluid and Electrolyte Metabolism.* 2nd ed. (Maxwell, M.H., and Kleeman, C.R., Eds.). New York, McGraw-Hill Book Co., 1972.

Passi, R.B., et al.: Pathophysiologic mechanisms of shock in acute gastric dilatation. Surgery, *65*:298, 1969.

Powers, S.R., Jr., et al.: Prevention of postoperative acute renal failure with mannitol in 100 cases. Surgery, *55*:15, 1964.

Rigor, B., Bosomworth, P., and Rush, B.F., Jr.: Replacement of operative blood loss of more than 1 liter with Hartmann's solution. JAMA, *203*:111, 1968.

Shires, G.T.: Fluid and electrolyte therapy. In *American College of Surgeons Committee on Manual of Preoperative and Postoperative Care,* 2nd ed. Philadelphia, W.B. Saunders Co., 1971.

Shires, T.C., and Canizaro, P.C.: Fluid, electrolyte and nutritional management of the surgical patient. In *Principles of Surgery,* 3rd ed., Editor in Chief S.I. Schwartz, New York, McGraw-Hill Book Co., 1979.

Tasker, P.R.W., et al.: Prophylactic use of intravenous saline in patients with chronic renal failure undergoing major surgery. Lancet *2*:911, 1974.

Thompson, J.E., et al.: Prevention of hypotensive and renal complications of aortic surgery using balanced salt solution. Ann Surg, *167*:767, 1968.

Underwood, P.S.: Fluid management in the recovery room. In Frost, E.A.M., and Andrews, I.C. (Eds). *Recovery Room Care,* International Anesthesiology Clinics, *21*: Spring, 1983.

CHAPTER 35

SOLUTIONS AVAILABLE FOR FLUID THERAPY

The term *tonicity* is usually used to describe the osmolality of a parenterally given solution in relation to the normal osmolality of the blood and extracellular water. A solution is described as *isotonic* or *isosmotic* when it has the same osmolality of the blood and extracellular water. Therefore, when such a solution is infused, it will not cause the red blood cells to swell or to shrink. A *hypotonic* solution has an osmolality less than that of blood and extracellular water. A *hypertonic* solution has a greater osmolality. Usually, isotonic solutions are infused. However, hypotonic or hypertonic solutions can be used under special conditions.

CARBOHYDRATE IN WATER SOLUTIONS

Physiological Properties

Carbohydrate in water solutions can be used in the following ways:

1. They supply water. Pure water cannot be given parenterally because it is markedly hypotonic and would cause the red blood cells to swell and hemolyze. It therefore must be given with carbohydrates or electrolytes, or other substances, in an isotonic solution.

   A 5% dextrose (glucose) solution in water is approximately isotonic. However, a 10% dextrose, a 10% fructose, or a 10% invert sugar (which is half dextrose, half fructose) solution, or even 20, 25, or 50% dextrose solutions can be given intravenously if given slowly. When this is done, adequate mixing and dilution of the sugar solution with blood occur. This prevents local phlebitis.

   Carbohydrates supply water in the following way: The oxidation of each gram of dextrose or fructose supplies 0.6 ml of water of oxidation per gram (Chap. 3). Therefore, the oxidation of 100 g of dextrose, which is present in an infusion of 1 liter of 10% dextrose in water, would supply 60 ml of water in addition to the 1000 ml of water in the solution.

2. In addition, the dextrose or fructose provides calories for part of the daily metabolic needs of the patient. An average adult at rest requires approximately 1500 calories a day. Since each gram of dextrose provides 4.1 calories, a total of approximately 375 g of dextrose would be needed if

the dextrose were the only source of calories. This would be equivalent to 3750 ml of a solution of 10% dextrose in water. However, such a large amount of dextrose in water daily is dangerous, and therefore dextrose should not be used primarily for caloric purposes.

3. The ingestion of 100 to 150 g of dextrose decreases the catabolism of endogenous protein. In this way, it decreases the amount of water needed by the kidneys for the excretion of waste products (Chap. 3). The dextrose also prevents depletion of liver glycogen and therefore prevents the production of an excessive amount of ketone acids.

4. Fructose theoretically has the following advantages over dextrose:
   a. Fructose can be metabolized in the absence of insulin. Therefore, it can be utilized more rapidly than dextrose in a patient with diabetic acidosis or with disturbed liver function, as postoperatively, during fevers, and in liver disease.
   b. A 10% fructose solution can be given at the same rate as a 5% dextrose solution, without any of the sugar spilling into the urine.

      However, recent studies in children indicate that fructose may cause a transient increase in the lactic acid content of the blood, and a decrease in the CO_2 content. A fructose infusion can also cause hypophosphatemia.

Dextrose in water solutions may have a pH as low as 4 to 5 to minimize degradation and the resulting caramelization of the dextrose during sterilization. This may be one of the reasons for the development of postinfusion thrombophlebitis. The danger of this can be decreased by using small scalp-vein needles, and by changing the infusion site every 3 days.

Solutions Available

Dextrose in water is available in the following strengths: 2.5, 5, 10, 20, 25, and 50%; fructose in water is available in a 10% solution; *invert sugar* (half dextrose-half fructose) is available in a 5 or 10% solution.

Volume of Solution Needed

This is discussed on pages 353 and 355. In addition, the administration of an excessive amount of dextrose in water may actually cause a loss of water from the body, rather than water excess. This will occur if the circulating blood volume is increased to such an extent that aldosterone secretion stops. As a result, the kidneys may begin to excrete a large amount of sodium ions and water.

Route of Administration

Dextrose or fructose in water should be given intravenously, and should never be given subcutaneously.

Rate of Administration

Dextrose in water can be given intravenously at a rate of 0.5 g per kg body weight, per hour, without causing glycosuria. Therefore, it requires about 3 hours for the infusion of 1000 ml of a solution of 10% dextrose in water. This is equivalent to 333 ml per hour (see page 352). A 5% dextrose solution, or a 10% fructose or invert sugar solution, can be given at twice this rate, namely, 666 ml per hour (see page 352).

Some patients may be able to tolerate 0.85 g dextrose per kg body weight (1000 ml of a 10% dextrose solution in 2 hours, or 1000 ml of a 5% dextrose solution in 1 hour). It is useful to test the urine for sugar at regular intervals when dextrose is being infused. A moderate glycosuria of 3 plus or less may develop. This will not cause a urinary loss of water or electrolytes because not enough dextrose is being lost in the urine to act as an osmotic diuretic.

If dextrose is infused too rapidly, it may cause a transient reactive hyperinsulinism and the patient may experience weakness, apprehension, sweating, decreased blood pressure, and even disorientation or a convulsive seizure. These symptoms disappear if the infusion is continued (also seen Chap. 36).

A solution of 20% dextrose in water can be used when carbohydrates are needed, but the intake must be kept low. One liter of 20% dextrose in water can be given in a period of 6 hours. It should be infused into a large vein, such as the superior vena cava, to prevent thrombosis.

ISOTONIC AND HYPOTONIC SODIUM CHLORIDE SOLUTIONS

Physiological Properties

Isotonic sodium chloride solution, or saline, is often called "physiologic" or "normal" saline, or salt solution. However, these terms are not correct, because 1 liter of blood contains approximately 142 mEq sodium and approximately 103 mEq chloride, but isotonic saline solution contains approximately 150 mEq sodium and 150 mEq chloride per liter. Therefore, only the sodium concentration of isotonic sodium chloride solution is similar to that of blood. Its chloride concentration is much higher than the chloride concentration of blood. Therefore, if a large amount of isotonic sodium chloride solution is given to a patient who has lost more sodium than chloride (as in diarrhea, for example) and if the kidneys are not able to excrete the excess chloride ions, a severe hyperchloremic metabolic acidosis can occur (Chap. 17). However, it is isosmotic, and will not cause hemolysis of the red blood cells when infused, either alone, or with 2.5, 5, or 10% glucose, 5% fructose or 5 or 10% invert sugar, or with potassium, alcohol, plasma expanders such as dextran, vitamins, or other electrolytes.

Composition	% Sol.	Grams per liter	Concentration mEq/L	
Composition	% Sol.	Grams per liter	Na^+	Cl^-
NaCl	0.9	9.	154	154
NaCl	0.45	4.5	77	77
NaCl	0.33	3.3	56	56
NaCl	0.3	3.	51	51
NaCl	0.225	2.25	38.5	38.5
NaCl	0.2	2.	34	34

Isotonic sodium chloride solution contains sodium and chloride ions, and has been used principally in syndromes associated with sodium loss, such as diabetic acidosis, loss of gastrointestinal fluids, adrenocortical insufficiency, and burns. It should not be used to replace water loss.

Solutions Available

The following types of isotonic and hypotonic sodium chloride solutions are available:

Sodium chloride, 0.9% solution: plain or with 5 or 10% dextrose.
Sodium chloride, 0.45% (Half-strength): plain or with 2.5, 5, or 10% dextrose.
Sodium chloride, 0.33% (slightly more than third-strength): with 5% dextrose.
Sodium chloride, 0.3% (third-strength): with 5% dextrose.
Sodium chloride, 0.2% (slightly less than quarter-strength): with 5% dextrose.

Volume of Solution Needed

This is discussed on page 355, and in various chapters throughout the book.

Route of Administration

Isotonic 0.9% sodium chloride, or hypotonic 0.45% saline solution can be given intravenously or subcutaneously, either alone or with 5%

Table 35–1. Equivalent Values of Some of the Salts Used for Replacement Therapy

1 g NaCl = 17 mEq Na (approx.)	1 mEq Na = 59 mg NaCl (approx.)
1 g NaHCO₃ = 12 mEq Na	1 mEq Na = 84 mg NaHCO₃
1 g Na lactate = 9 mEq Na	1 mEq Na = 112 mg Na lactate
1 g KCl = 13.9 mEq K	1 mEq K = 74.5 mg KCl
1 g K acetate = 10 mEq K	1 mEq K = 100 mg K acetate
1 g K citrate = 8.3 mEq K	1 mEq K = 120 mg K citrate
0.92 g K₂HPO₄ plus	1 mEq Ca = 55 mg CaCl₂
0.2 mg KH₂PO₄ = 12.5 mEq P	1 mEq Ca = 224 mg Ca gluconate
1 g CaCl₂ = 20 mEq Ca	1 mEq Cl = 53.5 mg NH₄Cl
1 g Ca gluconate = 5 mEq Ca	1 mEq P = 74 mg K₂HPO₄
1 g MgSO₄ = 8.3 mEq Mg	plus 16 mg KH₂PO₄
	1 mEq Mg = 120 mg MgSO₄

dextrose. A 10% dextrose, fructose, or invert sugar in sodium chloride solution should not be used subcutaneously, because it is hypertonic and will cause water to leave the bloodstream and accumulate in the injection area. This may precipitate or worsen shock. Dextrose in 0.33, 0.3, 0.225 or 0.2% sodium chloride solution should only be given intravenously.

Rate of Administration

Isotonic sodium chloride solution is usually given at a rate up to 400 ml per hour (see page 352). However, if shock due to sodium loss is present, it can be given at a rate of 2000 ml per hour (see page 84).

HYPERTONIC SODIUM CHLORIDE SOLUTIONS

Physiological Properties

Hypertonic sodium chloride solution is indicated when there is a severe sodium loss in association with a relative water excess, or when there is primary water excess (water intoxication). In these cases, it raises the osmotic pressure of the extracellular water.

Solutions Available

Hypertonic sodium chloride solution is available in 3 and 5% concentrations.

			Concentration mEq/L	
		Gram		
Composition	*% Sol.*	*per liter*	*Na+*	*Cl−*
NaCl	3	30	513	513
NaCl	5	50	855	855

Volume of Solution Needed

This is discussed on page 62.

Route of Administration

Hypertonic sodium chloride solution can only be given intravenously.

Rate of Administration

Hypertonic sodium chloride solution must be given slowly, because it can precipitate pulmonary edema. The rate of infusion is described on page 62.

ACIDIFYING SOLUTIONS

Ammonium chloride is the solution commonly used.

Physiological Properties

When ammonium chloride is administered, the ammonium ion is converted to urea by the liver. The chloride ion reacts with hydrogen ions in the extracellular water, forming hydrochloric acid which is able to correct a metabolic alkalosis, particularly if the alkalosis is associated with a loss of chloride ions.

Ammonium chloride has been used in the treatment of patients with metabolic alkalosis, due to vomiting and loss of hydrochloric acid. However, in these patients, a solution containing isotonic or hypotonic sodium chloride solution with potassium chloride (see page 82) is usually more effective.

Ammonium chloride is contraindicated in patients with disturbed liver function and a high blood ammonia content, as in right-sided heart failure, cirrhosis of the liver, or azotemia. If an excessive amount of ammonium chloride is given, a metabolic acidosis may develop with drowsiness, mental confusion, disorientation, hyperpnea, and coma. In patients with liver disease, the ammonium chloride can precipitate hepatic coma.

Solutions Available

Ammonium chloride is available as a hypertonic, 2.14% solution in water.

| Composition | % Sol. | Gram per liter | Concentration mEq/L | |
			NH_4^+	Cl^-
NH_4Cl	2.14	21.4	400	400

Ammonium chloride concentration can also be added to isotonic sodium chloride solution. It is available in 20 ml vials. Each ml contains 5 mEq ammonium ions and 5 mEq chloride ions. (To prepare a solution containing approximately 400 mEq/L (2.14%) for example, 80 ml of ammonium chloride concentrate is added to 920 ml isotonic sodium chloride solution.)

Volume of Solution Needed

This is discussed on page 272.

Route of Administration

Ammonium chloride solutions should only be given intravenously. If an excessive amount of ammonium chloride is infused, signs of ammonia intoxication (page 172) can develop.

Rate of Administration

The 2.14% ammonium chloride solution can be given at a rate up to 120 ml per hour (see page 352).

ALKALINIZING SOLUTIONS

These solutions contain sodium bicarbonate, or sodium racemic lactate, or acetate, which is oxidized in the body to bicarbonate. THAM (tromethamine) is also an alkalinizing salt.

Physiological Properties

Alkalinizing solutions can be used in the treatment of metabolic acidosis. It is important not to raise the CO_2 content above 18 mEq/L, because of the danger of producing a metabolic alkalosis and tetany. In addition, calcium salts should also be given when alkalinizing solutions are used, to prevent tetany (page 201).

Sodium bicarbonate is the drug of choice in the treatment of metabolic acidosis. If the acidosis is not severe it can be given orally (page 190), or it can be given intravenously as a 1.5% solution in 5% dextrose in water, or in lesser concentrations (see page 180).

When a severe metabolic acidosis is present, hypertonic 7.5% sodium bicarbonate solution can be given intravenously. It is usually diluted with at least a similar volume of dextrose in water. However, in an emergency, as in cardiac arrest, it can be given intravenously undiluted. Hypertonic sodium bicarbonate solution can also be given to a patient with renal failure and metabolic acidosis who develops sodium loss and hyponatremia.

| Composition | % Sol. | Gram per liter | Concentration mEq/L | |
			Na^+	HCO_3
Sodium bicarbonate, isotonic	1.5*	15.	178	178
Sodium bicarbonate, hypertonic $NaHCO_3$	7.5	†	†	†
Sodium r-lactate 1/6 molar isotonic) $NaC_3H_5O_3$	1.72	17.2	167	167

*A 1.5% solution of sodium bicarbonate can be prepared by adding 4 ampuls of the hypertonic 7.5% solution to 800 ml 5% dextrose in water. Less concentrated solutions, using 1, 2, or 3 ampuls in 1000 ml dextrose in water, can also be prepared. (Two ampuls in a liter will supply approximately 88 mEq sodium and bicarbonate ions; 3 ampuls in a liter will supply approximately 133 mEq sodium and bicarbonate ions.)

†Hypertonic sodium bicarbonate is commercially available in 50 ml ampuls, containing 3.75 g of sodium bicarbonate (45 mEq sodium, and 45 mEq bicarbonate.) It should be diluted with at least an equal volume of dextrose in water solution before use.

One-sixth molar (isotonic) sodium racemic lactate, which consists of equal parts of d- and l-lactate, can be used if there is no need for fluid restriction. The lactate ions in sodium lactate are metabolized by the liver into bicarbonate ions, so that the effect of using a lactate salt is the same as using sodium bicarbonate.

One-sixth molar lactate should not be used if liver disease, shock, or right-sided heart failure is present, because the metabolism of lactic acid is impaired. Lactate and bicarbonate solutions are also contraindicated in respiratory alkalosis, where the low CO_2 content may simulate a metabolic acidosis (Chap. 25).

Volume of Solution Needed

To raise the CO_2 content 1 mEq/L, give 1.2 ml of the 1/6 molar sodium lactate per kg body weight.

This rule is derived in the following way: An adult has an extracellular water content of 20% of the body weight. Therefore, there is 0.2 liter extracellular water for every 1 kg body weight. If an ion, such as lactate, has a concentration in the extracellular water of 1 mEq/L, there would be 0.2 mEq of the ion per kg body weight.

If one uses a solution of 1/6 molar sodium lactate, which contains 167 mEq/L of solution, 1 ml of the solution contains 0.167 mEq of the lactate ion. Therefore, 1.2 ml of the 1/6 molar solution will contain 0.2 mEq/L.

If 1.2 ml of the 1/6 molar sodium lactate solution per kg body weight is now given, this would raise the lactate concentration 0.2 mEq per kg of body weight, or 1 mEq/L of extracellular water. The bicarbonate concentration would be raised similarly, because 1 mEq sodium lactate is converted into 1 mEq sodium bicarbonate.

When the patient's water intake must be restricted, as in acute renal failure, hypertonic sodium bicarbonate can be used instead of the 1/6 molar sodium lactate.

The negative base excess concentration has also been used to determine the amount of sodium bicarbonate which is needed to correct a metabolic acidosis (see page 182).

Route of Administration

The 1/6 molar sodium lactate or the isotonic (1.5% sodium bicarbonate is given intravenously.

Rate of Administration

Either of these solutions can be given at a rate up to 300 ml per hour (see page 352).

Molar lactate of hypertonic bicarbonate should be given at the same rate as hypertonic sodium chloride solution (page 62).

TROMETHAMINE

Tromethamine (tris buffer) is an amino alcohol. Its formula is $(CH_2OH)_3C-NH_2$. When given intravenously, it acts as a hydrogen ion (proton) acceptor and prevents or corrects acidosis by actively binding H^+ (hydrogen) ions. It can bind the H^+ ions of lactic, pyruvic and other metabolic acids, as well as carbonic acid. In this way it increases the concentration of HCO_3^- ions. Tromethamine also acts as an osmotic diuretic, increasing urine flow, urinary pH, and the urinary excretion of fixed acids, such as phosphoric and sulfuric acids, carbonic acid, and electrolytes.

Approximately 30% of tromethamine is not ionized and is therefore capable of diffusing into the cells. In this way it can correct intracellular as well as extracellular acidosis.

Tromethamine is rapidly eliminated by the kidneys (unless renal insufficiency is present). Seventy-five per cent or more appears in the urine after 8 hours. Urinary excretion continues over a period of 3 days.

Tromethamine is marketed in the form of THAM or as THAM-E, as a 0.3 molar solution, which contains sodium chloride and potassium chloride which have been added to the lyophilized tromethamine, to anticipate the loss of these electrolytes when the osmotic diuresis occurs.

Tromethamine has been used in:
1. Metabolic acidosis associated with cardiac bypass surgery. It is primarily indicated in such cases.
2. Correction of the acidity of ACD (acid-citrate-dextrose) blood in cardiac bypass surgery. Such blood has a low pH and becomes more acid on storage.

Overdosage of THAM or THAM-E can produce severe hypoglycemia which may last for 24 hours. In addition, hyperkalemia or apnea may occur. Therefore, it is contraindicated in patients with chronic respiratory acidosis. Other contraindications include anuria and azotemia.

The manufacturer's literature should be consulted for dosage.

SPECIAL SOLUTIONS

Ringer's Solution

Ringer's solution (triple chloride solution) is essentially an isotonic saline with potassium and calcium in concentrations approximately equal to their concentrations in the blood and extracellular water. However, if potassium of calcium loss is present, a much larger amount of these ions will be needed than is present in the Ringer's solution.

Ringer's solution can be given intravenously in the same way as isotonic saline.

Composition	% Sol.	Gram per liter	Na^+	K^+	Ca^+	Cl^-
				Concentration mEq/L		
NaCl	0.86	8.6	147.5			147.5
KCl	0.03	0.3		4		4
CaCl$_2$	0.033	0.33			4.5	4.5
Total			147.5	4 (156)	4.5	156

Saline-Lactate Solutions

Hartmann devised the first practical saline-lactate solution to avoid the excessive chloride content of isotonic saline solution and to supply bicarbonate ions. It consisted of 6 g of sodium chloride (103 mEq sodium and 103 mEq chloride ions) and 5.6 g of sodium lactate (51 mEq sodium and 51 mEq lactate ions) per liter. Bicarbonate ions were formed from the metabolism of the lactate ions. This solution, however, has been superseded by a modified form, which is commercially available. It is called lactated Ringer's solution (Hartmann's modified solution).

Composition	% Sol.	Gram per liter	Na^+	K^+	Ca^{++}	HCO_3^-	Cl^-
					Concentration mEq/L		
NaCl	0.6	6.	102				102
KCl	0.03	0.3		4			4
CaCl$_2$	0.02	0.2			3		3
Sodium lactate	0.3	3.	28			28	
Total			130	4 (137)	3	28 (137)	109

An acetated Ringer's solution is also available. It is similar to Ringer's lactate solution except that the sodium lactate is replaced by sodium acetate.

Theoretically, sodium acetate is preferable to sodium lactate because a significant part of the administered sodium lactate is converted into liver glycogen. This reduces the amount of bicarbonate ions formed. Acetate ions are not metabolized by the liver, but by muscles and other peripheral tissues. In addition, the acetate ions are metabolized in a different way from the lactate ions and require less oxygen for their metabolism to carbon dioxide and bicarbonate ions. This may be important if shock is present.

Several of the pharmaceutical firms are now using sodium acetate instead of sodium lactate in various electrolyte replacement solutions.

Lactated Ringer's solution is superior to isotonic sodium chloride solution because its electrolyte concentration is similar to that of blood. For example, the sodium concentration is higher than the chloride concentration; and the lactate supplies bicarbonate in a concentration which is similar to that present in normal plasma.

Lactated Ringer's solution can be used in place of isotonic sodium chloride solution. It is particularly valuable in metabolic acidosis syndromes.

MULTIPLE ELECTROLYTE SOLUTIONS

Physiological Properties

Talbot and Butler devised multiple electrolyte solutions which are based on the concept that the amount of water and electrolytes which the patient retains is not related to the amount of water and electrolytes received, but instead is dependent on the regulatory mechanisms of the body. In other words, they believe that the apparent success of many different types of fluid therapy has been due, not to the types of solutions used, but to the regulatory or homeostatic mechanism of the body, especially of the kidneys. In this way, needed amounts of water and electrolytes are utilized, and what is not needed is excreted. These "multiple electrolyte solutions" are available with modifications under numerous trade names, such as Ionosol solutions (Abbott), Isolyte solutions (American McGraw), Polysal solutions (Cutter). They are hypotonic and therefore contain free water in addition to electrolytes. They contain sodium, chloride, and lactate ions, which are extracellular electrolytes, as well as potassium and phosphate ions, which are intracellular ions. Some of the solutions also contain magnesium ions.

Originally it had been hoped that a "multiple electrolyte solution" could be used as an "all-purpose" solution, regardless of the water and electrolyte deficit. Multiple electrolyte solutions have been used successfully in the following situations:

1. For water and electrolyte maintenance in patients who are not taking fluids orally.

2. When gastrointestinal fluids are lost, as by vomiting, gastric suction, diarrhea, or fistulas.
3. In moderate sodium loss syndromes.
4. In moderate potassium loss syndromes.
5. In metabolic acidosis syndromes, as in diabetic acidosis, due to excessive administration of chloride ions, and severe infections.
6. In metabolic alkalosis syndromes, due to excessive administration of alkali, or loss of hydrochloric acid and potassium ions from vomiting or gastric suction.

However, multiple electrolyte solutions are contraindicated in the following situations:

1. When severe sodium loss is present, especially if the serum sodium concentration is below 125 mEq/L. These patients may require a hypertonic sodium chloride solution.
2. When a severe burn is present. The serum potassium concentration may be abnormally high due to tissue destruction and acidosis. In addition, these patients require large amounts of a solution such as lactated Ringer's solution rather than a hypotonic solution.
3. In adrenocortical insufficiency. These patients have an abnormally high serum potassium concentration and should not receive fluids with potassium.
4. With severe water loss, or diabetes insipidus. These patients primarily require water without electrolytes.
5. When water excess (water intoxication) is present. These patients require cessation of water therapy, and may require hypertonic sodium chloride solution.
6. When a severe metabolic acidosis or metabolic alkalosis is present.
7. When renal insufficiency is present.
8. When a severe calcium loss is present with tetany. Such patients should receive 10% calcium gluconate intravenously.
9. When hypoparathyroidism is present. These patients have an abnormally high phosphate concentration and should not receive a phosphate salt, which is present in the multiple electrolyte solutions.

Solutions Available

In general, two types of multiple electrolyte solutions are available:
Maintenance Therapy Solutions. This type of *hypotonic* multiple electrolyte solution has been used as a substitute for dextrose and water when the patient cannot take fluids orally, as after surgery. Table 35–2 shows the composition of available maintenance solutions.

A similar maintenance solution can be prepared as follows:

830 ml 5% dextrose in water.
20 ml molar potassium chloride solution. (This supplies 20 mEq potassium ions and 20 mEq chloride ions.)
150 ml 1/6 molar sodium lactate, *or* 150 ml isotonic (1.5%) sodium bicarbonate solution. (This supplies 26 mEq sodium ions and 26 mEq lactate *or* bicarbonate ions.)

Volume of Solution Needed. The maintenance therapy solutions contain a large amount of potassium. Therefore, they can be used only when the patient

Table 35–2. Maintenance Therapy (Hypotonic Multiple Electrolyte) Solutions

Solution	Manufacturer	Na⁺	K⁺	mEq/L Ca⁺⁺	Mg⁺⁺	Cl⁻	HCO₃⁻	HPO₄⁻	Carbohydrate
Isolyte R	American McGraw	40	16	5	3	40	24 (acetate)		5% dextrose
Normosol M	Abbott	40	13	—	3	40	16 (acetate)	—	plain or 5% dextrose
Maintenance solution	Self-prepared	25	20			20	25 (bicarbonate, or lactate)		5% dextrose

Table 35–3.   Relations Between Body Weight and Approximate Surface Area (After Crawford et al)

Weight kg	lb	Approximate surface area* (square meters)
50	110	1.50
60	132	1.65
70	154	1.75
80	176	1.85
90	198	1.95
100	220	2.05

*For adults of average height.

is passing an adequate amount of urine. If kidney function is not adequate, the patient should receive ½ isotonic or ¼ isotonic saline solution, or dextrose in water, depending on the disturbance present, until the circulation improves and adequate urine output returns.

The required volumes of maintenance therapy solution can be calculated on the basis of the surface area of the body.

A *maintenance* 24-hour volume is approximately 1500 ml per square meter of body surface. (See Table 35–3.)

When a *moderate* fluid deficit is present (weight loss up to 5%), a 24-hour volume of approximately 2400 ml per square meter of body surface will provide the maintenance volume needs and correct the fluid deficit.

When a *severe* fluid deficit is present (weight loss more than 5%), a 24-hour volume of approximately 3000 ml per square meter of body surface will provide the maintenance volume needs and correct the fluid deficit.

Table 35–3 shows the approximate relations between body weight and surface area.

Route of Administration. Maintenance therapy solutions should be given only intravenously.

Rate of Administration. One method of calculating the rate of administration is to divide the total daily volume of the solution by 24 (hours).

In adults, up to 400 ml per hour can be given.

Replacement Therapy Solutions. This type of *isotonic* multiple electrolyte solution has been used as a substitute for isotonic saline solution, when there is a marked loss of water and electrolytes, as in severe vomiting or diarrhea, or after surgery, burns, trauma. Table 35–4 shows the composition of available replacement solutions.

The "1-2" solution is a similar replacement solution. It can be prepared by mixing 1 part of 1/6 molar sodium lactate with 2 parts of isotonic saline. (This supplies 150 mEq sodium ions, 100 mEq chloride ions, and 50 mEq bicarbonate ions [as lactate].)

Volume of Solution Needed. This depends on the clinical condition and the serum electrolyte concentrations. The general rules (page 355) will have to be modified for each patient.

Route of Administration. Replacement therapy solutions should be given only intravenously.

Rate of Administration. Up to 400 ml per hour can be given. One method of calculating the rate of administration is to divide the total daily volume of the solution by 24 (hours).

Table 35–4. Replacement Therapy (isotonic Multiple Electrolyte) Solutions

Solution	Manufacturer	Na⁺	K⁺	Ca⁺⁺ mEq/L	Mg⁺⁺	Cl⁻	HCO₃⁻	Carbohydrate
Hartmann's	Several	130	4	3	—	109	28 (as lactate, or acetate)	None, or 5% dextrose
Normosol-R	Abbott	140	5	—	3	98	50 (acetate 27, gluconate 23)	None, or 5% dextrose
Plasmalyte	Travenol	140	10	5	3	103	47 (acetate 47)	None, or 5% dextrose
Isolyte E	American McGraw	140	10	5	3	103	57 (acetate 49) citrate 8)	None, or 5% dextrose
"1–2"	Self-prepared	150	—	—	—	100	50 (lactate)	None

POTASSIUM-CONTAINING SOLUTIONS

Physiological Properties

Potassium-containing solutions supply potassium ions which are necessary for cellular metabolism. Potassium chloride is generally used. However, potassium acetate or potassium phosphate can also be used.

Theoretically, it would seem that potassium phosphate should be more valuable than the potassium chloride because there is usually phosphate loss in association with the potassium loss. However, potassium chloride is satisfactory for most patients. In addition, it is extremely important to use potassium *chloride* and not any of the other potassium salts in patients who have been receiving the thiazide diuretics, furosemide, or ethacrynic acid.

Potassium acetate can be used in patients with potassium loss associated with metabolic acidosis, as in renal tubular acidosis, and potassium-losing nephritis. The acetate is metabolized to bicarbonate which helps restore the pH to normal.

Solutions Available

Potassium chloride ampuls are available, and the required amount of the potassium ion can be added to dextrose in water, or to isotonic saline solution. However, one should remember that if a severe potassium loss is present the administration of sodium ions aggravates the potassium loss.

Numerous solutions are available for IV use containing 10, 20, 30, or 40 mEq K/L with varying concentrations of sodium chloride and 5% dextrose in water.

Volume of Solution to Be Given

The amount of potassium salt to be used is discussed on page 286.

Route of Administration

Potassium-containing solutions should be given intravenously or orally.

Rate of Administration

Potassium salts should not be prepared in a concentration greater than 80 mEq/L, and should not be given at a rate greater than 20 mEq/hr (rarely 40 mEq/hr). In addition, no potassium-containing solution should be used until there is an adequate urine output.

COLLOIDAL SOLUTIONS

Physiological Properties

Whole blood, plasma, packed red blood cells, pooled plasma, concentrated salt-poor albumin, or colloidal plasma expanders such as dextran are valuable for increasing the circulating blood volume when shock is present, because most of these solutions are retained within the vascular system, where they increase the osmotic pressure of the blood above that of the extracellular fluid spaces. As a result, water passes from the extracellular fluid space into the blood, increasing the circulating blood volume.

Solutions Available

Whole Blood. This is the solution of choice when shock is due to hemorrhage or severe anemias.

One unit of blood will raise the hemoglobin from 1 to 1.5 g/dl. Common dangers of whole blood transfusion are serum hepatitis, transient fever due to bacterial contamination, incompatible transfusion reactions, allergic reactions, sensitization to Rh or other blood factors, or acute pulmonary edema due to overtransfusion. This latter can occur either during the transfusion or one hour afterward. In addition, a large transfusion of citrated blood can also cause hypocalcemia (page 316).

		Concentration		
	Volume	*(mEq per stated volume)*		
Composition	*ml.*	*Na+*	*K+*	*Cl−*
Whole blood	1000	142	5	103
Packed red blood cells	250	5	20	13
Plasma	250	38	1	25
Concentrated salt-poor albumin	100	16	—	2
Dextran in isotonic saline	250	36		36

It is advisable not to give whole blood and 5% dextrose in water simultaneously, because of the danger of hemolysis.

Packed Red Blood Cells. Blood can be centrifuged and the plasma drawn off. The packed red cells can then be transfused, either with the small amount of plasma remaining, or they can be resuspended in a small volume of isotonic saline solution or 5% dextrose in saline solution. Packed red blood cells are valuable when patients who show congestive heart failure or sodium excess require blood.

Pooled Plasma. A good physiological plasma expander, it is better than blood because it is not necessary to type and cross-match the patient. However, viral hepatitis can be transmitted through plasma also unless it has been stored at 34° C for 6 months. It is preferable to use Plasmanate (Cutter), which contains human plasma protein fractions because this has been treated with heat to destroy hepatitis viruses.

Concentrated Salt-Poor Albumin. This is valuable in cirrhotic and nephrotic patients whose edema or ascites is due partly to a low serum albumin concentration.

Dextran

Dextran is available in two forms- with a molecular weight of 70,000 (dextran 70) or 75,000 (Dextran 75), or with a molecular weight of 40,000 (low molecular weight dextran, dextran 40).

Dextran 70 or 75

This is used to expand the plasma volume as an adjunct treatment of shock or impending shock when the circulating blood volume is low, as in burns, hemorrhage, surgery, etc., and when blood or blood products are not available. However, dextran is not a substitute for whole blood because it has no oxygen-carrying properties. It is also not a substitute for plasma proteins because its effects are limited.

Adverse effects include hypersensitivity reactions, such as nasal congestion, urticaria, tightness in the chest and wheezing, and hypotension. Severe anaphylactoid reactions with shock and even death have also occurred. Anaplylactoid reactions can be treated with the administration of 1:1000 epinephrine, 0.5 ml subcutaneously, followed, if necessary, by IV injection of 0.25 to 0.5 ml of a 1:10,000 solution.

Because death from an anaphylactic reaction can occur after as little as 10 ml dextran 75 has been given, blood pressure should be monitored and the patient observed closely during at least the first 30 minutes of infusion of any dextran preparation.

Dextran can interfere with platelet function and can increase the bleeding time, especially if the dose exceeds 1 to 1.5 L. This reaction may not appear for 6 to 9 hours after the infusion and bleeding may occur. The hematocrit should be checked after a dextran infusion and care should be taken not to depress the hematocrit below 30%.

Dextran is contraindicated with patients who are hypersensitive to it, and in patients with severe bleeding disorders or severe cardiac or renal failure. It can cause circulatory overload, particularly if dextran in 0.9% sodium chloride solution is used.

Dextran 70 or 75 is given IV as a 6% solution. The total dose should not exceed 1.2 gm/kg (20 ml/kg) in the first 24 hours. If dextran is needed after this, the dosage should not exceed 0.6 g/kg (10 ml/kg). In adults, the usual dose is 30 g (500 ml). In an emergency, dextran can be given to adults at a rate of 1.2 to 2.4 g (20 to 40 ml) per minute. If the patient has normal or near normal blood volume, the rate of infusion should not exceed 0.24 g (4 ml) per minute.

Dextran 70 and dextran 75 are available in 5% dextrose in water, or in a 0.9% sodium chloride solution. The containers have no preservatives and any unused solution should be discarded.

(The numerical designation: 70, 75, 40, is simply the weight-average molecular weight divided by 1000.)

Dextran 40

Dextran 40 has a molecular weight of approximately 40,000. Its uses are similar to those of dextran 70 or 75. In addition, it can be used as a priming fluid, alone, or with additives, for pump oxygenators during extracorporeal circulation.

It can cause the same kind of anaphylactoid reactions as dextran 70 or 75.

When dextran 40 is given by rapid IV infusion, it may cause the central venous pressure (CVP) to rise precipitously and may provoke congestive heart failure, especially if it is given in a 0.9% sodium chloride solution.

It must be given cautiously to patients with active bleeding because it improves the micro-circulation and may increase the bleeding. It is contraindicated in patients with thrombocytopenia or hypofibrinogenemia, and in patients with severe dehydration.

The dosage depends on the patient's needs. A total dose of 10% solution should not exceed 2 g/kg (20 ml/kg) in the first 24 hours. If it is continued beyond this time the dose should not exceed 1 g/kg (10 ml/kg). Therapy should not be continued longer than 5 days.

The first 500 ml of dextran 40 can be infused rapidly while the CVP is monitored. The remaining dose should be infused slowly.

Dextran 40 is available as a 10% solution in 5% dextrose in water, or in 0.9% sodium chloride solution. The containers have no preservative and any unused solution should be discarded.

Mannitol

Mannitol is a low-molecular hexahydric alcohol. It has marked hydroscopic activity, and acts as an osmotic diuretic by raising the osmotic pressure of the glomerular filtrate to such an extent that there is a decrease in the tubular reabsorption of water and ions such as sodium potassium chloride, calcium, magnesium, which are excreted in the urine. Also, if the patient is taking lithium, an increased urinary excretion of this also occurs. When given intravenously, it is associated with a rapid rise in serum osmolality. As a result, water moves from the cells into the extracellular water and the blood, and the serum sodium concentration falls. Mannitol is also able to increase renal blood flow and urine volume even when an antidiuretic state is present, as postoperatively, and after trauma to the kidneys.

Mannitol has been used under the following conditions:

1. In acute renal failure treatment should be started as soon as possible after oliguria is noted. A test dose is necessary, approximately 0.2 g/kg, or 12.5 g—62.5 ml.—as a 20% solution, infused in 3 to 5 minutes to produce an adequate urine flow-at least 30 to 50 ml/hr. If the urine flow does not increase within 2 to 3 hours a second test dose may be given. If there is an inadequate response, no further mannitol should be given until the patient is reevaluated.

    If there is an adequate response to mannitol, a regular dose of 100 g can be given as a 15 or 20% solution in a period of 90 minutes to several hours.
2. To prevent oluguria or acute renal failure, 50 to 100 g of mannitol may be given. Generally a concentrated solution is given initially, followed by a 5 or 10% solution. When used prophylactically in surgical operations, the mannitol may be started before or immediately after surgery and may be continued postoperatively.
3. A dose of 100 g of mannitol, given in a period of 2 to 6 hours, has been used in nephrotic, cardiac or cirrhotic patients who show refractory edema and ascites. Either the 10 or 20% solution can be used. However, the physician should observe these patients carefully for signs of increasing edema or the development of pulmonary edema.
4. A 5 to 10% solution of mannitol can be used as an adjuvant treatment of exogenous poisoning, as long as indicated clinically, and as long as the urinary output remains at a high level, or until a maximum of 200 g is given.
5. Mannitol has also been used in ophthalmology and in neurological surgery to reduce elevated intraocular pressure, cerebrospinal pressure, and cerebral edema, as a 20% solution.

Mannitol in water is available in concentrations of 5, 10, 15, 20, and 25%. It is chemically stable. However, the 20 and 25% solutions have a tendency to crystallize when exposed to a low temperature. If this occurs, the bottle should be warmed to 60° C in a water bath and then cooled to body temperature (38° C) before administering. As the bottle cools enough to be handled, it should be shaken vigorously several times. An alternate solution, if a 20 or 25% solution is used, is to administer it with a filter to prevent mannitol crystals from entering the circulation. This problem will not occur if solutions of 15% or less concentration are used.

The usual adult dose of mannitol is 100 g in 24 hours. Doses as high as 200 g/24 hours and even higher have been given. However, when large doses are used, a water excess syndrome (Chap. 6) may develop. The mannitol can be stopped when the patient is able to maintain a urine flow of 100 ml/hour. If he or she cannot produce more than 100 ml/hour in response to mannitol, he or she should not receive more than 100 g in any 24-hour period. The physicians should also give the patient water and other electrolytes that may be needed.

Side reactions may occur. Thirst is common. Headache, chills, an anaphylactoid reaction, a sensation of constriction or pain in the chest may occur if a large amount of mannitol is given rapidly; convulsions due to water excess may occur, or the patient may develop pulmonary edema due to the sudden increase in circulating blood volume. If repeated doses of mannitol are given, they may produce such an extensive osmotic diuresis that a water loss syndrome (Chap. 4) develops. Although urine which is formed as a result of mannitol infusion shows a low sodium concentration, significant hyponatremia may occasionally develop. Renal changes consisting of swelling of the epithelium of the proximal convoluted tubules may occur in patients who receive more than 100 g of mannitol. Extravasation of the solution may cause local edema or thrombophlebitis.

Mannitol should not be combined with whole for transfusing blood.

Mannitol intoxication is treated with hemodialysis.

Mannitol infusions are contraindicated if the patient does not respond to a test dose, or if a small dose precipitates or increases pulmonary edema. They should also not be used in metabolic edema associated with abnormal capillary fragility or membrane permeability, where the heart, liver, and kidneys are normal.

Hetastarch

Hetastarch is a synthetic polymer derived from a waxy starch composed mostly of amylopectin. It closely resembles glycogen and has a range of molecular weights ranging from 10,000 to 1,000,000. The smaller molecules are excreted in the urine. The larger molecules require enzymatic degredation before they are excreted.

It expands the circulating plasma volume like serum albumin and like dextran. It has a calculated osmolality of approximately 310 mOsm/liter, and the expansion of plasma volume is slightly in excess of the volume infused. Maximal plasma volume expansion occurs a few minutes after the infusion. The expanded plasma volume may last for 24 hours or longer. However, small amounts of the hetastarch may persist for weeks in the body.

Hetastarch increases the sedimentation rate when added to whole blood. It also raises the blood sugar concentration as it is metabolized. It also raises the blood amylase concentration because it binds amylase and prevents its normal excretion in the urine. This increased amylase concentration may persist for 3 to 5 days after the hetastarch is stopped. Therefore blood amylase concentration cannot be used to diagnose acute pancreatitis during this time.

Hetastarch is not antigenic. However, allergic or sensitivity reactions can occur, for example, vomiting, slight rise in temperature with flu-like symptoms, enlargement of submaxillary and parotid glands, urti-caria, wheezing. The blood platelet count and hematocrit can decrease as a result of the volume-expanding effects of hetastarch. One should avoid having the hematocrit fall below 30% after an infusion.

Hetastarch is contraindicated in patients with bleeding disorders, cogestive heart failure, or impaired renal function.

The dose of hetastarch depends on the patient's needs. The usual adult dose of the hetastarch 6% solution is 30 to 60 g (500 ml to 1 L). The total daily dose should not exceed 1.2 g/kg (20 ml/kg), or 90 g (1500 ml). In patients in hemorrhagic shock, it can be given at a rate ap-proaching 1.2 g/kg/hr (20 ml/kg/hr). Slower rates are generally used in patients with burns or septic shock.

In patients with severe renal impairment or a creatinine clearance less than 10 ml/min the usual initial dose can be given, but subsequent doses should be reduced to about ¼ or ½ of the usual dose.

Hetastarch is available as Hespan (American Critical Care) as a 6% solution in 0.9% sodium chloride solution. It has no preservatives and any unused solution should be discarded.

Urea

Urea, like mannitol, is an osmotic diuretic. It is not metabolized and it diffuses rapidly through the glomeruli. Therefore, when it is given orally or intravenously, it is associated with the passage of a large amount of water from the extracellular spaces into the bloodstream, and, when it is excreted by the kidneys, it carries along a large amount of water and sodium ions.

Urea can be given IV or orally. IV urea has been used to lower intra-cranial and intraocular pressure, and also to treat the syndrome of inappropriate secretion of antidiuretic hormone (SIADH).

Oral urea has also been used to treat SIADH and also as a diuretic in refractory heart failure. It can be used in conjunction with furosem-ide.

In treating SIADH, it can be given IV as a 30% solution, in a dose of 80 g infused over 6 hours. Or it can be given orally as two or three 30-g doses in 24 hours.

When used as an oral diuretic, large doses, 45 to 90 g a day can be used. It has a bitter taste which can be masked by putting the urea in grape juice. Or, 30 g of urea crystals and 10 ml of an aluminum and magnesium hydroxide antacid, such as Maalox, can be dissolved in 100 ml of water.

For IV use, urea is available in vials of 40 g of lyophilized urea (Ureaphil-Abbott). 105 ml of a 5 or 10% dextrose in water solution, or

10% invert sugar solution is added to the 40 g of lyophilized urea. The resultant solution contains 300 mg urea per ml (30% solution).

The solution is irritating and may result in thrombosis, thrombophlebitis, or sloughing of the tissues. Therefore, it should not be given in the veins of the lower limbs of elderly patients. It should not be given faster than 4 ml of the 30% solution per minute to prevent side effects, such as nausea, vomiting, nervousness, tachycardia, hypotension, syncope, mental confusion, or hyperthermia. The infusion should not be stopped abruptly. No more than 1.5 g/kg or 120 g should be given IV in a 24-hour period. Headache may also occur as a result of excessive diuresis, and intraocular hemorrhage may occur in patients with absolute glaucoma, if the urea is infused too rapidly. Abnormal ECG changes may also occur.

Urea is contraindicated in patients showing a severe decrease in renal or hepatic function, or if marked sodium or water loss or active intracranial hemorrhage is present.

PARENTERAL SOLUTIONS WHICH PROVIDE NOURISHMENT

Carbohydrate Solutions

These have already been described in the beginning of this chapter.

Alcohol Solutions

Physiologic Properties. Intravenous alcohol can be used to supply calories because it is rapidly and completely metabolized. It therefore prevents carbohydrate, protein and fat breakdown. It has also been used as a sedative and analgesic agent, and can inhibit the secretion of ADH, the antidiuretic hormone.

Volume of Solution to Be Used. A total daily dose of 1000 to 2000 ml can be given.

Route of Administration. Alcohol solutions should be given only intravenously.

Rate of Administration. An adult can metabolize approximately 10 ml of pure alcohol per hour. This is equivalent to 200 ml of a 5% alcohol solution. Therefore, 200 to 300 ml of a 5% alcohol solution per hour can be given without causing symptoms of intoxication.

Solutions Available. Alcohol is available in a 5% solution with 5% dextrose in water.

One gram of ethyl alcohol provides 7.1 kcalories. Therefore, 1 liter of a 5% alcohol, 5% dextrose solution will provide 525 kcalories (50 g alcohol-355 kcal; 50 g dextrose-170 kcal) in contrast to 170 kcal which 1 liter of 5% dextrose would provide.

Alcohol solutions are contraindicated if shock is present, in epilepsy, or if severe liver or renal disease is present. There is potentiation of ethyl alcohol by sodium pentothal, and these two should not be given together.

Amino Acid Solutions

When a patient is receiving parenteral fluids for a day or a short time, it is not necessary to provide proteins. However, if parenteral fluid therapy is maintained more than three or four days, the patient should receive protein parenterally in the form of amino acids. One liter of a solution of 3.5% amino acid contains 5.5 g of nitrogen. This is the equivalent of 35 g of protein, or 140 kcal.

Side Effects. Patients with hepatic insufficiency may develop metabolic alkalosis, prerenal azotemia, hyperammonia, stupor and coma. Patients with impaired renal function may develop a marked rise in BUN. However, a modest rise in BUN occurs normally. Metabolic or respiratory alkalosis may be exacerbated because of the acetate ions in the amino acid solution. Also, amino acid preparations should be used in burn patients only during the convalescent phase.

Amino acid solutions may cause the following reactions especially if given at an excessive rate; nausea, vomiting, headache, flushing, chills or fever. Local venous thrombosis may also occur.

Solutions Available. Numerous amino acid preparations are available. The 3.5% solution (without additives) is essentially isotonic. The 5% solution (without additives) is slightly hypertonic.

Amino acid solutions can be given in conjunction with 5 or 10% dextrose solutions or with intravenous fat emulsion.

Volume of Solution to be Used. For peripheral IV infusion, 1 to 1.5 g/kg/day of total amino acids will achieve optimum sparing of protein catabolism. If one uses a 3.5% solution, 1 L will contain 35 g of the amino acids. Therefore, if one decides to infuse 1 g/kg/day, a 70-kg (154 pound) patient will need 70 g of the amino acids, or 2 L of the 3.5% solution daily.

Route of Administration. All amino acid preparations should be given IV.

Rate of Administration. One should calculate the amino acid and fluid needs per 24 hours and give the amino acid solution over a 24-hour period.

Fat Emulsions

Several fat emulsions are available for IV use, containing soybean or safflower oil stabilized with egg phosphotides and made isotonic with glycerol. The 10% emulsion supplies 1.1 kcal per ml of the emulsion. The 20% emulsion supplies 2 kcal per ml.

Indications. Fat emulsion can be used as a source of calories and essential fatty acids when a patient needs parenteral nutrition for an extended period (usually for more than 5 days).

Contraindications. Fat emulsion is contraindicated if a patient has a disturbance of normal fat metabolism, such as pathological hyperlipemia, lipoid nephrosis, or if the patient has acute pancreatitis accompanied by hyperlipemia. It must also be used cautiously if a patient has severe liver damage, pulmonary disease, anemia, a disorder of blood coagulation, or when there is danger of fat embolism.

Side Effects. These may be immediate (acute) or long-term (chronic).

Immediate side effects may include allergic reactions, hyperlipemia, dyspnea, cyanosis, flushing, dizziness, headache, sleepiness, nausea, vomiting, increased temperature, sweating, chest and back pain, thrombocytopenia, hypercoagulability, and transient increases in liver enzyme values.

Long-term side effects include hepatomegaly, jaundice due to central lobular cholestasis, splenomegaly, thrombocytopenia, leukopenia, transient increases in liver enzyme values, *overloading syndrome* (which consists of focal convulsive seizures, fever, leukocytosis, splenomegaly, and shock), and the deposition of a brown "fat" pigment in the reticuloendothelial cells of the liver (the significance of which is unknown).

Other side effects include irritation at the site of the infusion, or thrombophlebitis. This can be avoided if the infusion site is changed every 12 hours.

Dosage and Administration. The fat emulsion can be given intravenously either through a peripheral vein or through a central venous catheter. The initial rate of infusion in adults for the first 15 minutes should be 1.0 ml per minute for the 10% solution, or 0.5 ml per minute for the 20% solution. If no adverse reactions occur (see Side Effects above) the infusion rate can be increased to allow no more than 500 ml of the 10% solution or 250 ml of the 20% solution to be given over a period of four to six hours.

The daily dosage of the fat emulsion should not exceed 2.5 g/kg body weight. In addition, it should provide no more than 60% of the total caloric intake of the patient. (The remaining 40% of the calories should be supplied by carbohydrates and amino acids.)

The fat emulsion should be infused separately from any other intravenously administered solution, to avoid disturbing the stability of the emulsion. However, it can be infused into the same peripheral vein as a carbohydrate or amino acid solution, by means of a Y-connector located near the infusion site. The flow rate of each solution should be controlled separately by infusion pumps. A filter should *not* be used with the fat emulsion.

Periodic liver function tests should be done when fat emulsions are used for a long term.

Peripheral Parenteral Nutrition. Total parenteral nutrition, using an amino acid solution with a concentrated dextrose solution, intravenously through a central venous catheter, is available. However, a 10 or 20% lipid emulsion in combination with a 10% dextrose solution and amino acid solution, can be infused through a peripheral vein, if a patient is only moderately debilitated or cachectic. This procedure is known as *peripheral parenteral nutrition.*

The following is an example of solutions that can be used:

Solution	*kcalories*
750 ml 10% fat emulsion (1.1 kcal/ml)	825
500 ml 10% dextrose (50 g) 3.5% in water (3.4 kcal/ml)	170
1000 ml 3.5% amino acid solution in 5% dextrose solution (50 g)	
35 g protein-eqivalent (4 kcal/g)	140
50 g dextrose (3.4 kcal/g)	160
total kcalories	1290

REFERENCES

AMA Drug Evaluations, 5th ed., American Medical Association, Chicago, Ill., 1983.

American Hospital Formulary Service, Drug Information 84.

Borges, H.F., et al.: Mannitol intoxication in patients with renal failure. Arch Intern Med, *142*:63, 1982.

Blackburn, G.L., et al.: Peripheral intravenous feeding with isotonic amino acid solutions. Am J Surg, *125*:447, 1973.

Decaus, G., et al.: Treatment of syndrome of inappropriate secretion of antidiuretic hormone by urea. Am J Med, *69*:99, 1980.

Diehl, J.T., et al.: Clinical comparison of hetastarch and albumin in postoperative cardiac patients. Surg Forum, *32*:260, 1981.

Clemetson, C.A.B., and Moshefghi, M.M.: Strange effects of "dextrose 5% in water." N Engl J Med, *280*:332, 1969.

Cooke, R.E., and Crowley, L.G.: Replacement of gastric and intestinal fluid losses in surgery. N Engl J Med, *246*:637, 1952.

Crossley, K., and Matsen, J.M.: The scalp-vein needle. JAMA, *220*:985, 1972.

Darrow, D.C., et al.: Disturbances of water and electrolytes in infantile diarrhea. Pediatrics, *3*:129, 1949.

Davidsohn, I.: Dextrose and transfused blood. JAMA, *174*:332, 1960.

Downs, J.W.: The problem of overtransfusion in massive hemorrhage. Ann Surg, *148*:73, 1958.

Editorial: Postinfusion hypoglycemia. JAMA, *160*:876, 1956.

FDA Drug Bulletin: Users reminded about adverse reactions to dextran. *13*:no 3, Nov. 1983.

Felig, P.: Intravenous nutrition. Fact and fancy. N Engl J Med, *294*:1455, 1976.

Flatau, E., and Resnitzky, P.: Fatal anaphylactoid reaction after dextran 40 administration, letter. JAMA, *243*:1035, 1980.

Fonkalsrud, E.W., et al.: Reduction of infusion thrombophlebitis with buffered glucose solutions. Surgery, *63*:280, 1968. Also N Engl J Med, *280*:1480, 1969.

Frazer, I.H., et al.: Is infusion phlebitis preventable? Br Med J, *2*:232, 1977.

Freeman, J.B., et al.: The current status of protein sparing. Surg Gynecol Obstet, *144*:843, 1977.

Fye, W.B.: Sydney Ringer, calcium, and cardiac function. Circulation, *69*:849, 1984.

Grady, G.F.: Transfusions and hepatitis. Update in '78, N Engl J Med, *298*:1413, 1978.

Grindon, A.J.: The use of packed red blood cells. JAMA, *235*:389, 1976.

Hanson, S.M.: Ringer, Hartmann, and their solutions. JAMA, *204*:272, 1968.

Hartmann, A.F., et al.: Further observations on metabolism and clinical uses of sodium lactate. J Pediat, *13*:692, 1938.

Hartmann, A.F., and Senn, M.J.E.: Studies on the metabolism of sodium-r-lactate. J Clin Invest, *11*:327, 337, 345, 1932.

Heller, W.M.: Ringer, JAMA, *207*:2103, 1969.

Kohen, M., Mattikow, M., and Middleton, E., Jr.: Study of three untoward reactions to dextran. J Allerg, *46*:109, 1970.

Letters to the Editor: pH of intravenous solution. N Engl J Med, *280*:900, 1969.

Mailloux, L., et al.: Acute renal failure after administration of low molecular weight dextran. N Engl J Med, *277*:1113, 1967.

Makim, D.G., Goldmann, D.A., and Rhame, F.S.: Infection control in intravenous therapy. Ann Intern Med, *79*:867, 1973.

Mannsmann, H.C., Jr.: Tris buffer vs. sodium bicarbonate, letter. N Engl J Med, *275*:1203, 1966.

Mead, W.B.: Particles in intravenous fluids. N Engl J Med, *287*:1152, 1972.

Nahas, G.G.: Tris buffer vs sodium bicarbonate. N Engl J Med, *275*:1024, 1966.

Oliver, T.K., Jr.: Tris buffer vs sodium bicarbonate. N Engl J Med, *275*:1203, 1966.

Oliver, W.J., Graham, B.D., and Wilson, J.L.: Lack of scientific validity of body surface as basis for parenteral fluid dosage. JAMA, *167*:1211, 1958.

Questions and Answers: Parenteral fluids by hypodermoclysis to elderly patients may be hazardous. JAMA, *226*:1127, 1973.

Sarma, D.P.: Use of blood in elective surgery, JAMA, *243*:1536, 1980.

Siberman, H., et al.: Parenteral nutrition with lipids. JAMA *238*:1380, 1977.

Talbot, N.B., Crawford, J.D., and Butler, A.M.: Medical progress; homeostatic limits to safe parenteral fluid therapy. N Engl J Med, *248*:1100, 1953.

Talbot, N.B., et al.: Medical progress; application of homeostatic principles to the practice of parenteral fluid therapy. N Engl J Med, *252*:856, 1955.

The Medical Letter: Parenteral water and electrolyte solutions. *7*:17, 1965.

The Medical Letter: Parenteral water and electrolyte solutions. *12*:19, 1970.

The Medical Letter: Plastic containers for intravenous solutions. *17*, no. 10, May 9, 1975.

Tse, R.L., and Lee, M.W.: pH of infusion fluids. A predisposing factor in thrombophlebitis. JAMA, *215*:642, 1971.

Tullis, J.L.: Albumin, 1. Background and use. 2. Guidelines for clinical use. JAMA, *237*:355, and 460, 1977.

Turco, S., and Davis, N.M.: Glass particles in intravenous injections. E Engl J Med, *287*:1204, 1972.

Vidt, D.G.: Use and abuse of intravenous solutions. JAMA *232*:533, 1975.

Wakim, K.G.: "Normal" 0.9% salt solution is neither "normal" nor physiological. JAMA, *214*:1710, 1970.

Weisberg, H.F.: Osmolarity of parenteral fluids. JAMA, *194*:471, 1965.

Wolf, A.V.: The dehydrating effect of continuously administered water. Am J Physiol, *143*:567, 1945.

Zintel, H.A., Rhoads, J.E., and Ravdin, I.S.: Use of intravenous ammonium chloride in treatment of alkalosis. Surgery, *14*:728, 1943.

Appendix I

METHOD OF CALCULATING
OSMOTIC SHIFTS OF WATER

The osmotic shift of water in Figure 1 can be calculated from the osmotic formula, namely:

Osmotic concentration × volume = total osmolatity

In the NaCl compartment, 14 liters of sodium chloride are present with an osmolal concentration of 290 mOsm/L, and a total osmolality of $14 \times 290 = 4060$ milliosmoles.

In the K_2HPO_4 compartment, 28 liters of potassium phosphate are present, with an osmolal concentration of 310 mOsm/L, and a total osmolality of $28 \times 310 = 8680$ milliosmoles.

The total volume of solution is therefore $14 + 28 = 42$ liters, with a total osmolality of $4060 + 8680 = 12,740$ milliosmoles.

When osmotic equilibrium occurs, the 12,740 milliosmoles will be equally divided among the 42 liters, giving an average osmolal concentration of $12740/42 = 303$ mOsm/L.

The 4060 milliosmoles will remain in the NaCl compartment but will be now contained in $4060/303 = 13.4$ liters.

The 8680 milliosmoles will remain in the K_2HPO_4 compartment, but will now be contained in $8680/303 = 28.6$ liters.

In other words, the NaCl solution has a lower osmotic pressure than the K_2HPO_4 solution. Therefore 0.6 liter of water will flow from the NaCl solution to the K_2HPO_4 solution to equalize the osmotic pressure in this example.

before osmotic equilibrium

14 liters 290 mOsm/L 4060 mOsm NaCl	28 liters 310 mOsm/L 8680 mOsm K₂HPO₄	A.

after osmotic equilibrium

13.4 liters 303 mOsm/L 4060 mOsm NaCl	28.6 liters 303 mOsm/L 8680 mOsm K₂HPO₄	B.

Fig. 1.   Diagram showing the effect of osmotic pressure. See text.

Appendix II

CALCULATION OF THE OSMOTIC SHIFT OF WATER WHICH OCCURS AS A RESULT OF WATER LOSS

Figure 2A shows the normal volumes of extracellular and cellular water in a 70-kg male. (The total body water volume is 60% of the body weight: $0.6 \times 70 = 42$ liters. The extracellular water is 20% of the body weight: $0.2 \times 70 = 14$ L:42 $- 14 = 28$ L, the volume of the cellular water.)

Notice that the osmolality of both the extracellular and cellular water is the same, namely, 310 milliosmoles per liter, and the serum sodium concentration is 142 mEq/L. The total osmolality of the extracellular water equals the osmolal concentration per liter times the volume of the extracellular water: $310 \times 14 = 4340$ milliosmoles. The total osmolality of the cellular water also equals the osmolal concentration per liter times the cellular water volume: $310 \times 28 = 8680$ milliosmoles. The body water equals $4340 + 8680 = 13020$ milliosmoles.

In Figure 2B, 3 liters of extracellular water have been lost. Osmotic equilibrium has not yet occurred. Notice that the volume of the extracellular water has decreased to 11 liters, and its osmolal concentration has increased to 394 milliosmoles per liter. (The reason for this is that only water [but no electrolytes] has been lost.) Therefore, 4340 milliosmoles are now contained in 11 liters. This gives a concentration of $4340/11 = 394$ milliosmoles per liter. Notice also that the serum sodium concentration has also risen proportionately to 180 mEq/L:

$$142:X = 310:394$$

$$X = \frac{142 \times 394}{310} = 180$$

normal

14 liters 310 mOsm/L 4340 mOsm ECW serum Na 142 mEq/L	28 liters 310 mOsm/L 8680 mOsm cellular water	A

Water Loss—3 Liters
before osmotic equilibrium

11 liters 394 mOsm/L 4340 mOsm serum Na 180 mEq/L	no change	B

Water Loss
after osmotic equilibrium

13 Liters 334 mOsm/L 4340 mOsm serum Na 152 mEq/L	26 liters 334 mOsm/L 8680 mOsm	C

Fig. 2. Diagrams showing the effect of water loss on osmotic equilibrium. See text.

Notice also that the osmotic pressure of the extracellular water (394 mOsm/L) is now greater than that of the cells, which is still 310 mOsm/L.

Figure 2C shows the volume and osmolal changes after water has flowed from the cells to the extracellular water. The new osmolal concentration in the extracellular water and in the cells can be calculated from the following osmotic formula:

osmolal concentration × volume = total osmolality.

Because 3 liters of water have been lost, the total volume of body water is now 42 − 3 = 39 liters. The total osmolality of the extracellular and cellular water remains the same as before the water loss, namely, 13010 milliosmoles.

The formula can now be rewritten:

$$\text{osmolal concentration X volume} = \text{total osmolality}$$

$$X \times 39 \quad = 13010$$

$$X = \frac{13010}{39} = 334 \text{ mOsm/L}$$

Just as the osmolality falls from 394 to 334 mOsm/L, the serum sodium concentration also falls proportionately from 180 to 152 mEq/L (180:X = 394:334).

The osmotic formula can now be used to calculate the volumes of extracellular and cellular water which are present after osmotic equilibrium occurs:

$$\text{osmotic concentration} \times \text{volume V} = \text{total osmolality}$$

$$334 \times V = 4340$$

$$V = \frac{4340}{334} = 13 \text{ liters (extracellular water).}$$

$$334 \times V = 8680$$

$$V = 26 \text{ liters (cellular water).}$$

Appendix III

THE AMOUNT OF SODIUM CHLORIDE NEEDED TO RAISE THE SERUM SODIUM CONCENTRATION BY 10 mEq/L

To raise the serum sodium concentration by 10 mEq/L, a volume of 5% sodium chloride solution should be given which is equal (in ml) to 6 times the patient's weight in kilograms.

This rule is derived in the following way: Even though the sodium chloride is confined to the extracellular water, it causes a shift of water between the cells and the extracellular water when it is either added to, or removed from, the extracellular water. Therefore, its osmotic effect is distributed throughout the entire volume of body water.

Example: Man, weighing 70 kg. Total body water is 60% of the body weight, or 42 liters. The extracellular water volume is 20% of the body weight, or 14 liters; the cellular water is 40% of the body weight, or 28 liters.

If the serum sodium concentration is 132 mEq/L, this represents a deficiency of 10 mEq/L (142, normal—132). This is equivalent to a deficit of 20 mOsm/L (because sodium chloride ionizes into sodium and chloride ions—see page 20). Since the normal osmolal concentration is 310 mOsm/L, the present osmolal concentration must be 290 mOsm/L. Furthermore, since the extracellular water volume is 14 liters, there is a deficit of 20 × 14 = 280 milliosmoles per liter in the extracellular water.

When sodium chloride is added, it will increase the osmolality of the extracellular water above that of the cells. As a result, pure water will flow from the cells into the extracellular water. Therefore, as Welt has pointed out, enough sodium chloride must also be added to raise the osmolality of this water to 310 mOsm/L. Since the initial volume of the cell water in this patient is 28 liters, and its osmotic concentration is 290 mOsm/L, the cells have a total of 28 × 290 = 8120 milliosmoles. When water flows from the cells to the extracellular water, the osmotic concentration of the cells will be raised to 310 mOsm/L.

Using the osmotic formula (on page 393), we know that:

$$\text{Osmotic concentration} \times \text{volume V} = \text{total osmolality}$$

$$310 \times V = 8120$$

$$V = \frac{8120}{310} = 26.194 \text{ liters of cell water.}$$

Therefore, the volume of water that flows out of the cells is 28 − 26.194 = 1.806 liters.

Since the osmolality of these 1.806 liters must be raised from 0 to 310 mOsm/L, it will require 310 × 1.806 = 560 milliosmoles of sodium chloride.

The total sodium chloride requirement is therefore:

> 280 milliosmoles to raise the extracellular water osmolality from 290 to 310 mOsm/L.
> plus
> 560 milliosmoles of sodium chloride to raise the osmolality of the pure water that flows from the cells to the extracellular water from 0 to 310 mOsm/L.
> 280 + 560 = 840 milliosmoles of sodium chloride needed. This is equivalent to 840/2 = 420 millimoles or milliequivalents of sodium chloride.

Notice that the value 420 mEq is identical with that obtained by multiplying the patient's weight by the factor 6.

Since 420 mEq of sodium chloride are contained in 420 ml of 5.85% sodium chloride, 420 ml of 5.85% sodium chloride solution will raise the serum sodium concentration by 10 mEq/L. However, as was pointed out on page 62, 420 ml of 5% sodium chloride solution can be used instead.

(A 5.85% solution of NaCl contains 58.5 g per liter. Since the molecular weight of NaCl is 58.5 [Na, 23; Cl, 35.5], each ml of 5.85% NaCl contains 1 mEq Na.)

It should also be pointed out that all these calculations are merely approximations and do not represent absolute amounts or volumes of sodium chloride which must be used. In addition, the above calculations assume that 420 mEq of solid sodium chloride have been added. However, the sodium chloride is dissolved in 420 ml of water. This will also dilute the body water and cause the serum sodium concentration to rise less than 10 mEq/L.

As has been pointed out earlier, the body is not a closed system. As soon as the hypertonic sodium chloride solution is infused, the blood volume rises, aldosterone secretion stops, and the kidneys begin to excrete this excess sodium. However, the sodium is infused in a hypertonic solution, but is excreted in a hypotonic solution. As a result, a large amount of water is excreted along with the sodium. This also causes the serum sodium concentration to rise.

REFERENCES

Welt, L.G.: *Clinical Disorders of Hydration and Acid-Base Balance.* Boston, Little Brown & Co., 1955.
Wynn, V.: The osmotic behavior of the body cells in man. Lancet, *2*:1212, 1957.

Appendix IV

THE EFFECT OF HYPERGLYCEMIA ON THE SERUM SODIUM CONCENTRATION

Since glucose does not penetrate cell membranes passively, it has an osmotic pressure. However, its normal concentration in the blood (100 mg/dl) is relatively low. Therefore, it does not normally exert a significant osmotic pressure. However, in a patient with severe diabetes mellitus, for example, where the blood glucose concentration may be very high, the glucose will exert a significant osmotic pressure. This will cause the osmotic pressure of the extracellular water to rise above that of the cells, and the serum osmolality will rise.

As a result, water will flow from the cells to the extracellular water, which will become diluted. This will lower the concentration, not only of glucose, but of all the electrolytes. As a result, the serum sodium concentration may appear to be low. This really represents a dilutional effect and not a true decrease or loss of sodium.

The following rule can be used to determine the effect of hyperglycemia on the serum sodium concentration:

The serum sodium concentration will decrease 1.6 mEq/L for each 100 mg/dl increase of serum glucose concentration (above the normal level of 100 mg/dl).

Proof of this is as follows (Katz): When the serum glucose concentration rises, it increases the osmolality of the blood and extracellular water above that of the cells. Therefore, water flows from the cells into the extracellular water to equalize this difference. As the water flows from the cells, the osmolality of the extracellular water will decrease and the osmolality of the cells will increase, until a point is reached when the extra- and intracellular osmolalities will be equal. This point can be calculated from the osmotic formula (page 393): osmotic concentration × volume = total osmolality.

Example:

Patient's weight, 70 kg; serum sodium concentration, 140 mEq/L; blood glucose concentration, 100 mg/dl. (5.5 mOsm/L:* plasma (and cell) osmolality, 285 mOsm/L.

If 1000 mOsm glucose are now added to the blood and extracellular water (assuming that the water in which the glucose is dissolved has negligible volume), the osmolality of the blood and extracellular water will rise as follows:

Since the extracellular water is 20% of body weight, a 70-kg person has 70 × 0.2 = 14 liters of extracellular water (and a total of 285 × 14 = 3990 mOsm).

Since the cell water is 40% of body weight, this person has 70 × 0.4 = 28 liters of cell water (and a total of 285 × 28 = 7980 mOsm).

The total body water is therefore 14 + 28 = 42 liters (and a total of 3990 + 7980 = 11,970 mOsm).

When the 1000 mOsm glucose are added, the total body water osmolality increases to 12,970 mOsm. However, this is still contained in 42 liters of body water. Therefore, each liter of body water now contains 12,970/42 = 308.8 mOsm/L.

The cell water that originally contained 7980 mOsm in 28 liters now has 7980/308.8 = 25.8 liters—a loss of 2.2 liters, which have moved to the extracellular water. The extracellular water volume now is therefore 14 + 2.2 = 16.2 liters.

The final serum glucose concentration is therefore

$$\frac{1000 + (5.5 \times 14)}{16.2} = 66.48 \text{ mOsm/L, or 1197 mg/dl.}$$

The final serum sodium concentration is $\dfrac{140 \times 14}{16.2} = 121 \text{ mEq/L}$

*The molecular weight of glucose is 180. Therefore, 1 mOsm equals 180 mg, and a concentration of 5.5 mOsm/L is equivalent to a concentration of 100 mg per dl.

When these results are repeated for different amounts of added glucose, the results indicate that the serum sodium concentration decreases 1.6 mEq/L for each 100 mg/dl rise in serum glucose concentration (above a normal level of 100 mg/dl).

In early editions of the book the classic rule was stated, namely, that each 100 mg/dl excess of serum glucose concentration (above the normal level of 100 mg/dl) is associated with a decreased serum sodium concentration of 2.8 mEq/L. However, this rule disregards the fact that, as glucose enters the extracellular water and raises its osmolality, it immediately causes a shift of water from the cells to equalize this increased osmotic pressure.

REFERENCES

Crandall, E.D.: Serum sodium response to hyperglycemia. N Engl J Med, *290*:465, 1974.

Jenkins, P.G., and Larmore, C.: Hyperglycemia-induced hyponatremia. N Engl J Med, *290*:573, 1974.

Katz, M.A.: Hyperglycemia-induced hyponatremia. Calculation of expected serum sodium depression. N Engl J Med, *289*:843, 1973.

Robin, A.P., Ing, T.S., et al.: Hyperglycemia-induced hyponatremia. A fresh look. Clin Chem, *125*:496, 1979.

Index